Lippincott's Primary Care

Orthopaedics

Lippincott's Primary Care

Orthopaedics

EDITORS

Paul A. Lotke, MD

Professor of Orthopaedic Surgery
University of Pennsylvania
Philadelphia, Pennsylvania
Llanerch Medical Center
Havertown, Pennsylvania

Joseph A. Abboud, MD

Clinical Assistant Professor of Orthopaedic Surgery
University of Pennsylvania Health System
Shoulder and Elbow Reconstructive Surgeon
Pennsylvania Hospital
Philadelphia, Pennsylvania

Jack Ende, MD

Professor of Medicine
University of Pennsylvania School of Medicine
Chief, Department of Medicine
Penn Presbyterian Medical Center
Philadelphia, Pennsylvania

 Wolters Kluwer | **Lippincott Williams & Wilkins**
Health

Philadelphia • Baltimore • New York • London
Buenos Aires • Hong Kong • Sydney • Tokyo

Acquisitions Editor: Sonya Seigafuse
Managing Editor: Ryan Shaw
Project Manager: Alicia Jackson
Senior Manufacturing Manager: Benjamin Rivera
Marketing Manager: Kimberly Schonberger
Creative Director: Doug Smock
Cover Designer: Larry Didona
Production Service: Aptara, Inc.

© 2008 by LIPPINCOTT WILLIAMS & WILKINS, a WOLTERS KLUWER business
530 Walnut Street
Philadelphia, PA 19106 USA
LWW.com

Printed in China

Library of Congress Cataloging-in-Publication Data

Lippincott's primary care orthopaedics / editors, Paul A. Lotke, Joseph A. Abboud, Jack Ende.
     p. ; cm.
   Includes bibliographical references and index.
   ISBN-13: 978-0-7817-7182-5 (case : alk. paper)
   ISBN-10: 0-7817-7182-X (case : alk. paper) 1. Orthopedics. 2. Primary care (Medicine) I. Lotke, Paul A. II. Abboud, Joseph A. III. Ende, Jack. IV. Title: Primary care orthopaedics.
   [DNLM: 1. Musculoskeletal Diseases—Handbooks. 2. Primary Health Care—Handbooks. WE 39 L765 2008]
   RD732.L58 2008
   617.4'7—dc22

                                                                              2008009612

Care has been taken to confirm the accuracy of the information presented and to describe generally accepted practices. However, the authors, editors, and publisher are not responsible for errors or omissions or for any consequences from application of the information in this book and make no warranty, expressed or implied, with respect to the currency, completeness, or accuracy of the contents of the publication. Application of the information in a particular situation remains the professional responsibility of the practitioner.

The authors, editors, and publisher have exerted every effort to ensure that drug selection and dosage set forth in this text are in accordance with current recommendations and practice at the time of publication. However, in view of ongoing research, changes in government regulations, and the constant flow of information relating to drug therapy and drug reactions, the reader is urged to check the package insert for each drug for any change in indications and dosage and for added warnings and precautions. This is particularly important when the recommended agent is a new or infrequently employed drug.

Some drugs and medical devices presented in the publication have Food and Drug Administration (FDA) clearance for limited use in restricted research settings. It is the responsibility of the health care provider to ascertain the FDA status of each drug or device planned for use in their clinical practice.

To purchase additional copies of this book, call our customer service department at (800) 638-3030 or fax orders to (301) 223-2320. International customers should call (301) 223-2300.

Visit Lippincott Williams & Wilkins on the Internet: at LWW.com. Lippincott Williams & Wilkins customer service representatives are available from 8:30 am to 6 pm, EST.

10 9 8 7 6 5 4 3 2 1

Contents

Introduction to Lippincott's Primary Care Series

Welcome to Lippincott's Primary Care Series. The intended goal of this series is to help assist you in all of the use-case scenarios that you might encounter each day.

In this product, <u>Primary Care Orthopaedics</u>, you will find:

1. **Book:** The book contains both bulleted points for quick look-up access when you need an answer right away, as well as longer text for the occasions when you need a little more information.

   Additionally we have included pedagogy to highlight certain aspects of the text. These elements include:

 Patient Assessment—Quick reference for the physical examination

 Not to Be Missed—Things to watch out for or possible diagnoses to keep in mind during the examination

 When to Refer—When to suggest further options to your patient

 Patient Education Information Available in Print and Online

 Physical Therapy Available in Print and Online

2. **Website** that includes:
   - Fully searchable text of the book
   - Image bank that can be downloadable into PowerPoint for presentations
   - Video clips of some "how to" procedures
   - PDF downloadable Patient Information Sheets and Rehabilitation and Home Physical Therapy

3. **Anatomical Chart for Your Office**

We certainly hope this product is useful and meets your needs.

Please look for other titles in the Lippincott's Primary Care Series.

Preface

The text is designed as a contemporary primer and treatment guide for the most common musculoskeletal problems seen by primary care physicians.

Problems related to the musculoskeletal system can be complex and confusing to manage. Some have long term implications and require chronic supervision, while others are self limited and resolve in short periods of time. The variety and complexity of these problems can be intimidating to the primary care physician. Therefore, this text has selected the 71 most common problems presenting in the outpatient setting. The text is organized basically by anatomic divisions, except for a few chapters on common systemic problems or universal treatment modalities. Each chapter includes strategies and clinical suggestions for how to establish the diagnosis and suggests treatment alternatives. Other diagnoses to consider are highlighted and suggestions as to when to refer for subspecialty care are noted. Each chapter is designed to deliver the most useful information in an efficient and defined format. This text is not a complete reference text for each disease process, but a quick synopsis of the problem, followed by treatment recommendations and clinical pearls. It is for the busy practitioner who needs an up-to-date efficient guide as to how to manage common musculoskeletal problems.

Acknowledgments

We would like to recognize the efforts expended by the publisher in helping to create this textbook. Especially important has been the organizational and creative efforts of Ryan Shaw and the foresight and zeal of Sonya Seigafuse. In addition, and most importantly, this text could not have been possible without the efforts of the physician authors who have contributed so generously with their time and expertise. Without their dedication to teaching and patient care, this book could not be possible.

Contributors

Joseph A. Abboud, MD
Clinical Assistant Professor of Orthopaedic
    Surgery
University of Pennsylvania Health System
Shoulder and Elbow Reconstructive Surgeon
Pennsylvania Hospital
Philadelphia, Pennsylvania

Rocco Bassora, MD
Orthopaedic Resident
Department of Orthopaedics
University of Pennsylvania
Orthopaedic Resident
Department of Orthopaedics
Hospital of the University of Pennsylvania
Philadelphia, Pennsylvania

Timothy J. Bayruns, PT, DPT, OCS
Musculoskeletal Team Leader
Department of Physical Medicine and
    Rehabilitation
University of Pennsylvania Health System
Philadelphia, Pennsylvania

Andrea L. Bowers, MD
Clinical Instructor
Department of Orthopaedic Surgery
Hospital of the University of Pennsylvania
Philadelphia, Pennsylvania

David Bozentka, MD
Associate Professor
Department of Orthopaedic Surgery
University of Pennsylvania
Chief
Department of Orthopaedic Surgery
Penn Presbyterian Medical Center
Philadelphia, Pennsylvania

Lan X. Chen, MD
Division of Rheumatology
Hospital of the University of Pennsylvania
Philadelphia, Pennsylvania

Kingsley R. Chin, MD
Assistant Professor
Department of Orthopaedics
University of Pennsylvania
Chief of Spine Surgery
Department of Orthopaedics
Hospital of the University of Pennsylvania
Philadelphia, Pennsylvania

Marc L. Cohen, MD
Instructor
Department of Medicine
Harvard Medical School
Attending Physician
Division of General Medicine and Primary Care
Department of Medicine
Beth Israel Deaconess Medical Center
Boston, Massachusetts

Jonathan Dunham, MD
Division of Rheumatology
Hospital of the University of Pennsylvania
Philadelphia, Pennsylvania

Brian J. Eckenrode, PT, MSPT, OCS
Associate Faculty Member
Physical Therapy Department
Arcadia University
Glenside, Pennsylvania
Senior III Physical Therapist
Sports Medicine and Performance Center
The Children's Hospital of Philadelphia
Philadelphia, Pennsylvania

Jack Ende, MD
Professor
Department of Medicine
University of Pennsylvania School of Medicine
Chief
Department of Medicine
Penn Presbyterian Medical Center
Philadelphia, Pennsylvania

Mitchell Fagelman, MD
Metocrest Orthopaedics and Sports Medicine
Carrollton, Texas

Monica Ferguson, MD
Assistant Professor of Clinical Medicine
Department of General Internal Medicine
University of Pennsylvania School of Medicine
Assistant Professor of Clinical Medicine
Department of General Internal Medicine
Hospital of the University of Pennsylvania
Philadelphia, Pennsylvania

Christian Fras, MD, FACS
Director of Orthopaedic Surgery
Lankenau Spine Center
Lankenau Hospital
Wynnewood, Pennsylvania

Matthew Garberina, MD
Summit Medical Group
Berkeley Heights, New Jersey

Charles L. Getz, MD
Assistant Professor of Orthopaedics Surgery
Rothman Institute
Thomas Jefferson University
Philadelphia, Pennsylvania

Joseph Gianoni, DPT, MS, PT, OCS, ATC
Facility Director
Phoenix Rehabilitation and Health Services
Sellersville, Pennsylvania

B. David Horn, MD
Department of Pediatric Orthopaedic Surgery
The Children's Hospital of Philadelphia
Philadelphia, Pennsylvania

Kristofer J. Jones, MD
Resident
Department of Orthopaedic Surgery
Weill-Cornell Medical College
Resident
Department of Orthopaedic Surgery
Hospital for Special Surgery
New York, New York

Ankur A. Karnik, MD
Resident
Hospital of the University of Pennsylvania
Philadelphia, Pennsylvania

Christopher J. Kauffman, MSPT
Associate Faculty Member
Physical Therapy Department
Arcadia University
Glenside, Pennsylvania
Lead Physical Therapist
Department of Occupational and Physical
    Therapy
Hospital of the University of Pennsylvania
Philadelphia, Pennsylvania

Jaehon M. Kim, MD
Resident
Department of Orthopaedic Surgery
Harvard Combined Orthopaedic Residency
    Program
Boston, Massachusetts

Sharat Kusuma, MD, MBA
Fellow and Clinical Instructor
Adult Reconstruction and Arthroplasty
Department of Orthopaedic Surgery
Rush University Medical Center/Midwest
    Orthopaedics at Rush
Chicago, Illinois

Jennifer Kwan-Morley, MD
Department of Rheumatology
Paoli Hospital
Paoli, Pennsylvania

Brian G. Leggin, PT, DPT, OCS
Team Leader
Department of Rehabilitation Medicine,
    Occupational and Physical Therapy
Penn Presbyterian Medical Center
Philadelphia, Pennsylvania

David S. Logerstedt, PT, MPT, MA, SCS
Sport Team Leader
Department of Occupational and Physical
    Therapy
University of Pennsylvania Health System
Philadelphia, Pennsylvania

Jess H. Lonner, MD
Director of Knee Replacement Surgery
Department of Orthopaedic Surgery
Pennsylvania Hospital
Philadelphia, Pennsylvania

Paul A. Lotke, MD
Professor of Orthopaedic Surgery
University of Pennsylvania
Philadelphia, Pennsylvania
Llanerch Medical Center
Havertown, Pennsylvania

Jonas L. Matzon
Resident
Department of Orthopaedic Surgery
Hospital of the University of Pennsylvania
Philadelphia, Pennsylvania

Charles L. Nelson, MD
Associate Professor
Department of Orthopaedic Surgery
University of Pennsylvania
Attending Surgeon
Department of Orthopaedic Surgery
Penn Presbyterian Medical Center
Philadelphia, Pennsylvania

Enyi Okereke, PharmD, MD
Associate Professor
Department of Orthopaedics
University of Pennsylvania School of Medicine
Chief
Foot and Ankle Services
University of Pennsylvania Health System
Philadelphia, Pennsylvania

David Pedowitz, MS, MD
Orthopaedic Surgeon
Crystal Run Healthcare LLC
Middletown, New York

Stephan G. Pill
Resident
Department of Orthopaedic Surgery
Hospital of the University of Pennsylvania
Philadelphia, Pennsylvania

Sudheer Reddy, MD
Resident Instructor
Department of Orthopaedic Surgery
Hospital of the University of Pennsylvania
Philadelphia, Pennsylvania

Eric T. Ricchetti, MD
Instructor
Department of Orthopaedic Surgery
University of Pennsylvania School of Medicine
Resident
Department of Orthopaedic Surgery
Hospital of the University of Pennsylvania
Philadelphia, Pennsylvania

Gayle K. Severance MS, OTR/L, CHT
Occupational Therapist, Senior II
Occupational and Physical Therapy Department
University of Pennsylvania Health System
Philadelphia, Pennsylvania

Heather L. Smith, PT, MHS, OCS
CEQI Specialist
Clinical Effectiveness and Quality Improvement
    Department
University of Pennsylvania Health System
Philadelphia, Pennsylvania

David A. Spiegel, MD
Assistant Professor of Orthopaedic Surgery
Department of Orthopaedic Surgery
University of Pennsylvania School of Medicine
Division of Orthopaedic Surgery
Children's Hospital of Philadelphia
Philadelphia, Pennsylvania

David R. Steinberg, MD
Associate Professor and Director of Hand
    Fellowship
Department of Orthopaedic Surgery
University of Pennsylvania
Philadelphia, Pennsylvania

Won Sung, PT, DPT
Adjunct
Department of Physical Therapy
Arcadia University
Glenside, Pennsylvania
Physical Therapist
Penn Therapy and Fitness
University of Pennsylvania Health System
Philadelphia, Pennsylvania

Fotios P. Tjoumakaris, MD
Resident
Department of Orthopaedic Surgery
Hospital of the University of Pennsylvania
Philadelphia, Pennsylvania

Joan M. Von Feldt, MD, MSEd
Associate Professor
DM—Division of Rheumatology
University of Pennsylvania
Division of Rheumatology
Hospital of the University of Pennsylvania
Philadelphia, Pennsylvania

Laura Walsh, MS, OTR/L, CHT
Hand Therapy Team Leader
Upper Extremity Center
Penn Presbyterian Medical Center
Philadelphia, Pennsylvania

Keith Wapner, MD
Clinical Professor
Department of Orthopedic Surgery
University of Pennsylvania
Foot and Ankle Fellowship Director
Department of Orthopedic Surgery
Pennsylvania Hospital
Philadelphia, Pennsylvania

Gautam P. Yagnik, MD
Chief Resident
Department of Orthopaedic Surgery
University of Pennsylvania
Chief Resident
Department of Orthopaedic Surgery
Hospital of the University of Pennsylvania
Philadelphia, Pennsylvania

Lippincott's Primary Care

Orthopaedics

Lumbosacral Spine

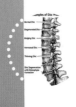

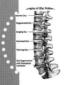

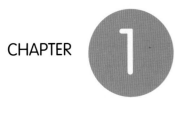 Degenerative Disc Disease

Christian I. Fras

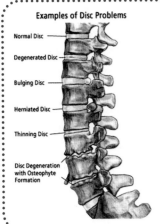

Examples of Disc Problems

- Normal Disc
- Degenerated Disc
- Bulging Disc
- Herniated Disc
- Thinning Disc
- Disc Degeneration with Osteophyte Formation

A 57-year-old man presents with back pain aggravated with activity, particularly with standing and walking. It is relieved with sitting down and especially by lying down. The patient complains of no persisting symptoms of weakness.

CLINICAL POINTS

- Disc degeneration occurs as part of the aging process.
- Chronic low back pain that increases in frequency is typical.
- Many patients also complain of leg pain.
- Pain is worse with activity.

Clinical Presentation

Degenerative disc disease of the lumbar spine is defined as premature aging of one or more of the lumbar intervertebral discs with subsequent pain, most commonly low back pain. The typical patient with degenerative disc disease will be in the third to sixth decade of life with chronic low back pain that had been intermittent in nature and is becoming increasingly frequent and painful.

In virtually all people, the discs of the spine, and in particular the discs of the lumbar spine, will undergo degeneration as part of the aging process. In the young, healthy disc, the internal aspect of the disc, the nucleus pulposus, is composed primarily of water with the addition of proteoglycans. As the disc degenerates, the nucleus pulposus loses much of its water content and tends to collapse; as this collapse progresses, other degenerative changes may be noted, including arthritic changes in the facet joints in the posterior aspect of the spine. Ultimately, this process occurs to some degree in virtually all discs of the spine in virtually all people. Degenerative disc disease, however, is defined as the condition whereby one or a few discs in the lower back have become degenerated in a premature fashion, while the remainder of the discs remain healthy in appearance; this is accompanied by painful symptoms, most commonly back pain but also with occasional leg pain as well. The existence of this clinical condition (degenerated discs causing back pain) is controversial because many individuals with no back pain or leg pain symptoms have been noted on MRI studies to have evidence of disc degeneration. Furthermore, there are a great number of individuals who have severe back pain but have no evidence of any disc degeneration. Thus, it can be difficult to identify those individuals whose complaints of back pain are specifically referable to a prematurely degenerated disc.

The clinical presentation of the patient with degenerative disc disease is typically of an individual complaining of low back pain. Many of these individuals will also complain of a component of radicular leg pain. Often, this leg pain will involve only the posterior aspect of the thighs but may occasionally involve the entire leg. Very rarely, the patient may complain primarily of radicular-type leg pain and very little low back pain. In some cases, the patient may complain of feelings of instability in the spine and a sense that the vertebrae in the lower back are moving back and forth excessively. This can be explained by the fact that the disc functions biomechanically, not just as a shock-absorbing cushion but also to impart stability to the spine. As the disc degenerates, it may allow excessive motion to take place; initially, this excessive motion is resisted by other elements within the spine such as the ligaments, muscles, and the facet joints. However, if these other elements ultimately become degenerated as well, instability may result. If the patient has symptoms from the disc degeneration, these symptoms are typically chronic in nature. When questioning the patient, a typical history that emerges is one of back pain that began many years ago and was intermittent, with the episodes of severe back pain becoming more and more frequent, lasting for longer periods of time, and becoming progressively more intense. A subset of patients will remain asymptomatic for many years and then become acutely, and thereafter chronically, symptomatic after a trauma. Frequently, this trauma may be related to a motor vehicle accident or a work-related injury. Unfortunately, this population of patients has a more guarded prognosis with regard to improvement of symptoms with conservative or surgical management.

Most patients suffering from back pain secondary to degenerative disc disease find that their pain is aggravated with activity, particularly with standing and walking. It is relieved with sitting down and in particular is relieved by lying down. Patients may complain of subjective numbness, pins and needles, or tingling in their legs and feelings of intermittent weakness in their legs with intermittent giving way but no persisting symptoms of weakness.

Physical Findings

The physical examination of patients with degenerative disc disease is relatively unremarkable. Most patients do not exhibit any clear focal neurologic deficits. Care must be taken when examining the patients to distinguish between weakness related to pain or psychologic difficulties and weakness secondary to true neurologic dysfunction and nerve root compression; the former is suggested by global weakness in multiple muscle groups in the lower extremity as well as "cogwheeling" and "giving way" when attempting to test strength; the latter is suggested by weakness in muscles referable to one or perhaps two nerve roots and a smooth inability to offer resistance on manual strength testing. Reflexes are typically intact in these patients, and sensation in the lower extremities is typically unaltered. There may be some tenderness to palpation over the lower back, particularly in the area of the paraspinous muscles, but this is not

PATIENT ASSESSMENT

1. Low back pain that is worse with activity
2. No focal neurologic deficits
3. X-rays, MRI, and possibly discography helpful in making diagnosis

always present. Evaluation of range of motion of the lumbar spine is relatively unhelpful, as many patients will have diminished range of motion in that area because of pain and muscle spasms. Significant tenderness to palpation over the lumbar spine is suggestive of a potential nonorganic cause for a patient's back pain in the setting of degenerative disc disease. Straight-leg-raise testing in these patients will often cause back pain but will not typically reproduce radicular leg pain.

Studies (Labs, X-rays)

Radiographic evaluation of the patient with suspected degenerative disc disease begins with plain x-ray studies. At the very least, these should include AP, lateral, and L5-S1 spot lateral x-rays of the lumbar spine and oblique x-rays of the lumbar spine. Flexion and extension x-rays of the lumbar spine may prove useful as well. X-rays can be useful to rule out such pathology as fractures or tumors; they can also rule out spinal deformity such as scoliosis or spondylolisthesis. Finally, suggestion of disc degeneration is often evident by loss of space between vertebra and associated osteophyte formation, particularly in the anterior aspect of the vertebral bodies. More accurate suggestion of degenerative disc disease is by way of MRI studies; sagittal T2-weighted images are particularly useful to evaluate disc height and hydration (Fig. 1.1). On these images, a disc that is degenerated will appear internally "black," while a healthy disc will internally appear "white" (i.e., the same density and appearance as cerebrospinal fluid, which is also primarily composed of water). Disc collapse

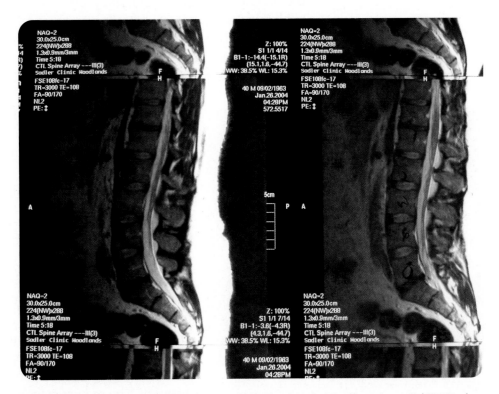

Figure 1.1 A 40-year-old man with chronic, intractable back pain and minimal leg pain; sagittal T2 MRIs show significant loss of disc height and hydration at L5-S1.

can also be seen on these images. Disc bulging commonly occurs in association with disc degeneration; this disc bulging may contact the neural elements and may potentially be a source for irritation of the nerves and thereby provide a source for a patient's radicular leg symptoms. Occasionally, a frank disc herniation can also be identified. The typical patient with degenerative disc disease will have one or perhaps two discs that are obviously degenerated on MRI study, with significant loss of disc height and hydration evident; by far, the most commonly affected discs are L4-5 and L5-S1. Typically, the remainder of the discs in the lumbar spine appear healthy and well hydrated. The patients in whom all of the discs appear to be lacking hydration and to have lost height (degeneration of all the discs in the lumbar spine) are often the patients with a nonorganic source for back discomfort. When disc degeneration is severe, changes within the endplates of the vertebral bodies may be seen, with edema noted in the area of the endplates of the vertebral body (Modic changes).

Discography is an interventional radiographic test that some practitioners employ to verify the existence of the degenerated disc as the "pain generator." Discograms are controversial studies that do not enjoy universal acceptance within the spine surgery community; however, in recent years, they have become increasingly recognized as useful in identifying and confirming that a disc is actually the source of a patient's back pain. Briefly stated, a discogram is an interventional maneuver whereby a needle is introduced into a disc and fluid is injected (most commonly contrast dye) (Fig. 1.2). In theory, if a disc is degenerated and contributing to the patient's pain, injection of this fluid will stimulate the pain fibers within the annulus of the disc and will provoke the patient's typical pain; if, however, the disc is not contributing to the patient's pain, such an injection may be moderately uncomfortable for the patient but will not provoke a typical, "concordant" pain response.

Other studies have a relatively limited role in evaluating degenerative disc disease. EMG studies are of little benefit in this entity, and laboratory workup is of minimal benefit except in cases where other pathology is potentially suspected (such as infection or neoplasm).

Treatment and Clinical Course

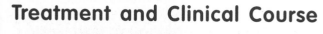

1. NSAIDs
2. Physical therapy
3. Consideration of epidural steroid injections
4. Surgical treatment controversial

Treatment of degenerative disc disease is controversial. The vast majority of patients with degenerative disc disease realize significant benefit from conservative management. The mainstay of conservative treatment is physical therapy, with the possible combined use of NSAIDs.

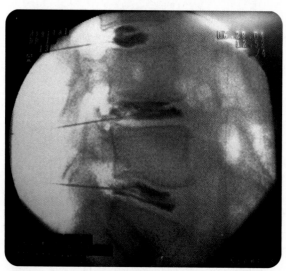

Figure 1.2 Fluoroscopic image of discography performed at L3-4, L4-5, L5-S1, with normal nucleogram at L3-4 and abnormal (degenerated) nucleograms at L4-5 and L5-S1.

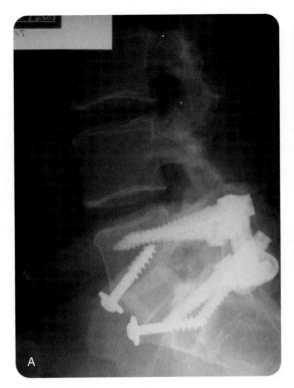
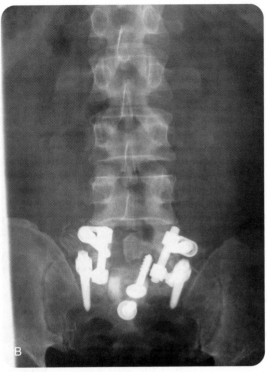

Figure 1.3 A: Lateral postoperative x-ray of fusion at L5-S1 for degenerative disc disease (see MRI in Fig. 1.1); the patient underwent anterior lumbar interbody fusion with femoral ring allograft and placement of "buttress" screws followed by posterior spinal fusion with instrumentation (pedicle screws). **B:** AP x-ray of the same patient.

Other treatments may involve various injections into the spine, such as epidural steroid injections, nerve root blocks, or facet joint injections. The success rate of these injections for isolated degenerative disc disease is debated and appears to be relatively modest but can be of benefit in a small subset of patients. Other experimental treatments involve intradiscal electrothermal coagulation (IDET). Results of IDET are unclear, with several studies showing conflicting outcomes. Thus far, IDET appears not to have gained widespread acceptance, although further studies on its efficacy need to be performed.

The natural history of degenerative disc disease of the lumbar spine is relatively poorly understood. There are some suggestions in the literature that if a patient simply waits long enough (5–10 years), the back pain will substantially dissipate. However, no long-term outcome studies following large numbers of patients over many years have been performed to evaluate this in greater detail.

Surgical treatment for degenerative disc disease remains controversial. Surgical management involves either fusion procedures or artificial disc replacement. A wide variety of fusion operations can potentially be performed (Fig. 1.3A,B). In theory, a spinal fusion operation prevents motion at the particular level involved and thereby prevents stimulation of the pain fibers at that level, thus reducing a patient's pain. The optimal surgery proposed for a patient may vary from surgeon to surgeon based on individual bias regarding the risks versus benefits of the various procedures.

Recently, artificial disc replacements have become commercially available in the United States and have been offered as alternatives to spinal fusion

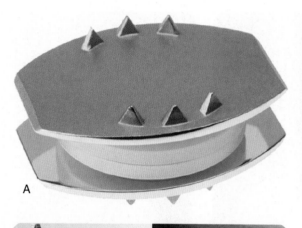

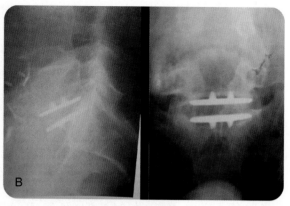

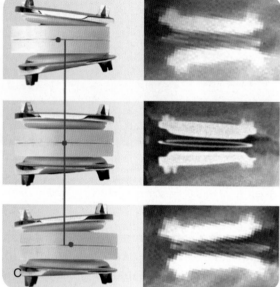

Figure 1.4 **A:** Charité total disc replacement (TDR). Mobile center core is made of plastic (same plastic as used in hip and knee replacements), sandwiched between two metal plates that attach to the vertebral body. (Courtesy of DePuy Spine.) **B:** The motion of the plastic central core is designed to mimic that of the natural activity of the disc during normal body movement (Courtesy of DePuy Spine.) **C:** Lateral and AP postoperative x-rays of TDR at L5-S1. (From Bridwell KH, Dewald RL, eds. *The Textbook of Spinal Surgery*. Philadelphia: JB Lippincott; 1991.)

operations for the treatment of degenerative disc disease in the lumbar spine (Fig. 1.4A–C). Long-term outcome studies regarding these implants are not available from the United States; some European studies with 10 years or more of follow-up suggest no long-term problems regarding these implants.

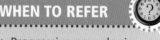

WHEN TO REFER

- Progressive neurologic deficit
- Patient not responding to conservative treatment after 4 to 6 months

 Refer to Physical Therapy

ICD9

722.4 Degeneration of cervical intervertebral disc
722.51 Degeneration of thoracic or thoracolumbar intervertebral disc
722.52 Degeneration of lumbar or lumbosacral intervertebral disc
722.6 Degeneration of intervertebral disc, site unspecified

References

1. Carragee E. Surgical treatment of lumbar disk disorders. JAMA 2006;296(20):2485–2487.
2. Hanley EN. The surgical treatment of lumbar degenerative disease. In: Garfin SR, Vaccaro AR, eds. *Orthopaedic Knowledge Update: Spine*. Rosemont, IL: American Academy of Orthopaedic Surgeons; 1997:121–140.
3. Turner JA, Ersek M, Herron L, et al. Patient outcomes after lumbar spinal fusions. JAMA 1992;268:907–911.
4. Zdeblick TA. A prospective, randomized study of lumbar fusion: preliminary results. Spine 1993;18:983–991.

② Herniated Disc

Christian I. Fras

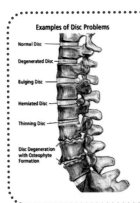

Examples of Disc Problems

Normal Disc
Degenerated Disc
Bulging Disc
Herniated Disc
Thinning Disc
Disc Degeneration with Osteophyte Formation

A 46-year-old man presents with back pain that tends to dissipate, and the patient begins to experience increasing buttock and, thereafter, increasing radicular leg pain. Patient notes that sitting is the most uncomfortable position and that standing and lying down is more comfortable.

CLINICAL POINTS

- Pain in the lower back may not be severe and often is not associated with trauma.

- The most common disc in the lumbar spine to herniate is L4-5.

- Besides pain, common symptoms include numbness, pins and needles, and tingling.

Clinical Presentation

A lumbar disc herniation is defined as a prolapse of the annulus fibrosis of the lumbar disc into the spinal canal causing compression of the neural elements or frank rupture of the annulus fibrosis with extrusion of nucleus pulposus material into the spinal canal causing compression of the neural elements (Fig. 2.1). The typical patient with a lumbar disc herniation presents in the third to sixth decade of life. The classic description of pain given by the patient is that of an early period of low back pain, which is often described as being comparatively modest in severity. This pain tends to last 7 to 14 days and often is not precipitated by any kind of specific trauma. Over the course of several days, the back pain tends to dissipate and the patient begins to experience increasing buttock and, thereafter, increasing radicular leg pain, more commonly in one leg than the other. The distribution of leg pain follows a dermatomal pattern consistent with the nerve root compressed.

The most common disc to herniate in the lumbar spine is L4, L5, followed by L5-S1. Nerves compressed at these levels would involve L4, L5 or S1 nerve roots; this would typically cause pain that starts in the buttock and goes down the posterior aspect of the thigh into the calf and into the foot. Many patients will note that sitting is their most uncomfortable position and that standing and lying down are more comfortable for them. Numbness, pins and needles, and tingling accompanying the pain are common. Weakness in a particular muscle group may occur, but it is rare for multiple muscle groups to be affected. Very rarely, a massive disc herniation can compress all of the nerves in the spinal canal at that level, including the lower sacral nerve roots; such a situation, known as *cauda equina syndrome*, will produce severe pain down both legs, significant derangement in bowel and bladder function (incontinence or retention), and "saddle anesthesia" (numbness in the buttocks around the anus and

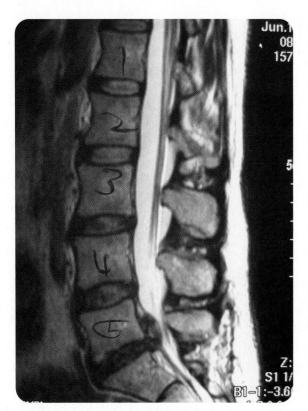

Figure 2.1 Sagittal T2 MRI of L5-S1 herniated nucleus pulposus, with cephalad migration of extruded fragment.

genitals and in the inner aspects of the thighs). Severe weakness may also accompany this syndrome. Fortunately, the development of cauda equina syndrome is an exceedingly rare phenomenon.

Very rarely, a lumbar disc herniation will cause only back pain; however, by far, the more common clinical presentation that of buttock and radicular leg pain (excepting the initial prodrome of mild low back pain).

Physical Findings

Physical examination of the patient with a lumbar disc herniation will typically reveal minimal, if any, low back tenderness. Range of motion of the lower back will usually be restricted secondary to pain. Some patients have pain with deep palpation in their buttock (in the area of the "sciatic notch"). Root tension signs will typically exist. These signs include positive straight-leg-raise testing; positive contralateral straight-leg-raise testing; and occasionally, positive femoral stretch testing. The straight-leg-raise test was originally described with the patient lying supine and elevating the painful leg; in the patient with a lumbar disc herniation, such a maneuver will exacerbate and reproduce a typical radicular leg pain, sometimes as early as at 45 degrees of elevation. It should be noted that back pain produced by straight-leg-raise testing is nondiagnostic; for a straight-leg-raise test to be truly considered positive, it must reproduce the patient's typical buttock and radicular leg pain. A contralateral straight-leg-raise test involves elevating the uninvolved (i.e., nonpainful) leg and finding that this reproduces a patient's typical radicular leg pain in the opposite limb. A positive contralateral straight-leg-raise test is considered to be pathognomonic for a lumbar disc herniation. Many patients are aware that a straight-leg-raise test "should" cause pain and will, therefore, report significant back and sometimes even leg pain with straight-leg-raise testing even when ultimately no intraspinal pathology is found to exist. To exclude this confounding factor, many clinicians will perform the straight-leg-raise test with the patient seated. A positive straight-leg-raise test typically indicates a lumbar disc herniation at the L5-S1 or L4-5 levels and sometimes at the L3-4 levels. A femoral stretch test is performed by having the patient lie prone and extending the involved leg back off the table; such a maneuver will be considered positive if it reproduces the typical leg pain. The femoral stretch test can be useful in identifying patients with disc herniations at L1-2 or L2-3 and rarely also at L3-4.

A thorough neurologic examination should be performed as well. This involves evaluating the reflexes, especially the patellar tendon and Achilles tendon reflexes, as well as strength testing of all muscle groups in the lower extremity. An excellent way to assess the strength of the muscles innervated by the L4, L5, or S1 nerve roots is to ask the patient to walk on the heels and toes. Assessing the strength of the muscles innervated by the

PATIENT ASSESSMENT

1. Typically, there will be minimal, if any, back tenderness.
2. Straight-leg-raise testing will produce radicular pain.
3. Thorough neurologic evaluation is needed.
4. X-rays are useful in ruling out a structural abnormality.

L2, L3, and to some degree L4 nerve roots can be performed by asking the patient to rise, unassisted, from a seated or squatting position. Sensation to light touch can also be evaluated but is often unchanged. The patient with an L4-5 disc herniation can have compression of the L4, L5, or both, nerve roots. The patient with a lumbar disc herniation at L5-S1 can have compression of the L5, S1, or both nerve roots. The patient with L4 nerve root compression can be found to have weakness of ankle dorsiflexion, some difficulty walking on the heels, and a diminished patella tendon reflex on that side. The patient with L5 nerve root compression may be found to have weakness of dorsiflexion of the great toe (extensor hallucis longus function) and will have difficulty walking on the heels. There is no reflex to assess L5 nerve function. The patient with compression of the S1 nerve root will have weakness of the gastroc-soleus muscle group with difficulty walking on the toes or doing repeated toe raises; there may be a diminished Achilles tendon reflex. It is important for the clinician to take note of such neurologic deficits, although most patients with lumbar disc herniations will not have such frank neurologic deficits, and indeed most patients with a lumbar disc herniation will have no neurologic deficits.

NOT TO BE MISSED

- Lumbar spinal stenosis
- Neoplasm
- Infection
- Sacroiliac disease
- Hip arthritis
- Knee arthritis
- Vascular claudication
- Diabetic neuropathy
- Visceral disorder

Studies (Labs, X-rays)

Diagnostic imaging studies for a suspected lumbar disc herniation include plain x-rays and most commonly an MRI scan. A plain x-ray is useful to rule out a structural abnormality of the spine such as scoliosis, spondylolisthesis, or a fracture; it will not, however, show anything but the osseous structures and will therefore not show a lumbar disc herniation. A lumbar disc herniation is best and most easily shown with MRI of the lumbar spine. Contrast administration is of no benefit, unless the patient has had previous lumbar spine surgery. MRI studies have been shown to have a very high sensitivity and specificity for detecting lumbar disc herniations. In patients who have a contraindication for MRI (such as a pacemaker or morbid obesity), CT scanning can be performed and in many cases may accurately show the lumbar disc herniation; accuracy of the CT scan is increased if it is preceded by a myelogram.

If the diagnosis of a symptomatic lumbar disc herniation is uncertain, an EMG-NCS study can be performed to help clarify the situation. However, this type of study should be approached with caution, as its results often lack sufficient sensitivity and specificity to be of great value in routine clinical practice.

Treatment and Clinical Course

1. NSAIDs
2. Physical therapy
3. Medrol Dosepak
4. Epidural steroid injections
5. Surgical treatment for distinct indications

SECTION 1 Lumbosacral Spine

The vast majority of lumbar disc herniations do not require surgical intervention. Indeed, many patients find that spontaneous resolution of their symptoms occurs without any treatment whatsoever within 4 to 6 weeks of the onset of symptoms. Conservative management includes a short period of bed rest (3–5 days); NSAIDs, if not medically contraindicated; short courses of oral steroids (such as Medrol Dosepak); physiotherapy; and epidural steroid injections. The influence of these interventions on the natural history of a lumbar disc herniation is controversial, and their utility in changing the ultimate outcome of the patient's symptoms is the subject of great debate in the spine surgery community. However, it does appear that these interventions can shorten the duration of the patient's symptoms. Some studies have suggested that these conservative measures are unlikely to provide any significant relief if the patient's pain has persisted for more than 3 to 6 months, but this is a subject of debate as well. Natural history studies have suggested that up to 80% of patients with a lumbar disc herniation will ultimately have resolution of symptoms without surgical intervention and possibly without any intervention whatsoever.

Strict indications for surgical intervention of lumbar disc herniation involve a progressive neurologic deficit or the presence of cauda equina syndrome. A nonprogressive (static) neurologic deficit is not in and of itself an absolute indication for surgery, as several studies have shown that the chance for recovery of a neurologic deficit is the same with surgical or nonsurgical intervention. Other relative indications for surgical intervention involve persisting radicular pain despite appropriate conservative treatment that would ideally last at least 4 to 6 weeks. However, some patients find themselves to be so incapacitated by their pain that they are unable to tolerate waiting this length of time for conservative measures to take effect. Several studies have shown surgery for lumbar disc herniations that produce radicular leg pain to be highly effective in relieving the patient of leg pain; furthermore, some studies have indicated that the success rate of surgical intervention is higher than that of nonsurgical intervention and relieves the patient of disability more rapidly. However, this information must be balanced against the natural history of lumbar disc herniations, which is shown to be generally (although not universally) positive.

The standard operation for a lumbar disc herniation is a laminectomy-discectomy. This typically involves an incision approximately 1.5 to 3.0 inches in length and takes approximately 1 hour. Success rates for surgery vary in different studies in the literature, but many studies have shown satisfaction rates in excess of 90%. Those patients contemplating surgery should be advised that the laminectomy-discectomy procedure has a relatively small role in improving back pain but can assist in improving radicular leg pain. A traditional axiom is, "the back pain you have before surgery will be the same back pain you have after surgery." While this is not universally true, the patient should nonetheless be cautioned against unreasonable expectations regarding improvement of back pain following surgery.

WHEN TO REFER

- Patient not responding to conservative treatment
- Progressive neurologic deficit
- Cauda equina syndrome

 Refer to Patient Education

 Refer to Physical Therapy

ICD9

722.0 Displacement of cervical intervertebral disc without myelopathy
722.10 Displacement of lumbar intervertebral disc without myelopathy
722.11 Displacement of thoracic intervertebral disc without myelopathy
722.2 Displacement of intervertebral disc, site unspecified, without myelopathy

References

1. Carragee E. Surgical treatment of lumbar disk disorders. *JAMA* 2006;296(20):2485–2487.
2. Hanley EN. The surgical treatment of lumbar degenerative disease. In: Garfin SR, Vaccaro AR, eds. *Orthopaedic Knowledge Update: Spine.* Rosemont, IL: American Academy of Orthopaedic Surgeons; 1997: 121–140.
3. Weinstein JN, Lurie JD, Tosteson TD, et al. Surgical vs nonoperative treatment for lumbar disk herniation. the Spine Patient Outcomes Research Trial (SPORT) observational cohort. *JAMA* 2006;296(20):2451–2459.
4. Weinstein JN, Tosteson TD, Lurie JD, et al. Surgical vs nonoperative treatment for lumbar disk herniation. the Spine Patient Outcomes Research Trial (SPORT): a randomized trial. *JAMA* 2006;296(20):2441–2450.

A 42-year-old woman presents with low back pain and no associated leg pain. Patient complains of decreased back range of motion. (Figure from LifeART image, © 2007 Lippincott Williams & Wilkins. All rights reserved.)

CLINICAL POINTS

- Low back pain is one of the most common causes of disability.

- Almost all cases result from low back sprain.

- The majority of patients recall the event that triggered the pain.

Clinical Presentation

The lifetime prevalence of low back pain is estimated at 50% to 80%, with up to 5% of the population affected yearly. It is the most common cause of disability in patients younger than 45 years of age and second only to arthritis as the most common cause in those age 45 to 60 years. The vast majority of cases of low back pain (97%) are due to low back sprains.

Most patients with an acute low back sprain are young (20–45 years old). Back pain in the very young (adolescent or younger) is distinctly unusual and classically considered to be a worrisome sign of significant pathology until proven otherwise. Most patients will recall an inciting event, although the forces involved may be relatively modest. Patients will typically deny any true radicular leg pain, although some may show pseudoradicular symptoms, with pain in the proximal aspect of the posterior thigh. Weakness and numbness are typically absent.

While there are no risk factors that have been strongly linked to the development of back sprains, weak associations have been found to exist between back pain/back sprains and obesity, smoking, heavy lifting, vibrational stresses, prolonged sitting, and job dissatisfaction.

Care should be taken to ensure that constitutional symptoms are not reported, such as fever, chills, pain that wakes the patient from sleep, weight loss, malaise, and the like; these warning signs can signify more ominous conditions such as infection or malignancy.

Physical Findings

Physical examination may reveal spasm of the paraspinous muscles with tenderness about them; midline back tenderness is typically absent. Range of motion of the lower back is typically diminished secondary to pain.

Neurologic evaluation is unremarkable, with full strength in all muscle groups of the lower extremities, normal/symmetric reflexes, and normal sensation in the legs. Care must be taken to distinguish between giving

········
PATIENT ASSESSMENT

1. Generally a younger patient population (20–45 years old)
2. Usually no radicular symptoms
3. Advanced imaging studies initially unnecessary

········
NOT TO BE MISSED

- Disc herniations
- Neoplasms
- Infection
- Gynecologic or gastroenterologic problems
- Cauda equina syndrome
- Urologic problems

········
WHEN TO REFER

- Progressive neurologic deficit
- Neoplasm or infection
- Patient not responding to conservative treatment after 4 to 6 months

way in the legs on strength testing, which may affect more than one muscle group, and true weakness secondary to neurologic dysfunction.

Straight-leg testing may provoke back pain but will not cause radicular leg pain and is therefore considered negative in these patients. Other root tension signs will be absent as well, as will long tract signs (such as Babinski).

Studies (Labs, X-rays)

In general, laboratory studies are of no benefit in evaluating the patient suspected of having a lumbosacral sprain, except in cases when a systemic disorder is suspected.

Advanced imaging studies have no role in the early evaluation of a suspected lumbar sprain; these studies are routinely negative and, barring a suspicious warning sign in the history of physical examination, do not contribute to the diagnosis or treatment of the patient.

The timing of ordering plain x-rays of the lumbar spine is somewhat controversial. Some authors have suggested that in the absence of symptoms suggestive of infection, neoplasm, fracture, or neural compression (with or without neural deficit) and those of relatively short duration (<4 weeks), x-rays are not necessary and provide no significant benefit in treating and diagnosing the patient. However, in clinical practice, it is common to order x-rays early in a patient's disability, in an attempt to more definitively exclude more ominous pathology. If x-rays are ordered, they should include AP, lateral, and L5-S1 spot lateral views.

Treatment and Clinical Course

1. NSAIDs
2. Physiotherapy
3. No surgical role

Barring the presence of warning signs, treatment is primarily supportive. A short course of bed rest (up to 4 days) may be of some benefit, as are analgesics, including NSAIDs, acetaminophen, muscle relaxants, and opioids, none of which has been shown to be superior to the others. Braces, such as a lumbosacral corset, may provide some relief as well. The roles of physiotherapy and chiropractic manipulation are poorly understood; however, both of these interventions have been shown in some studies to hasten a patient's recovery, particularly if performed within the first 4 weeks. Epidural steroid injections, or trigger point injections, are probably not indicated for conditions of acute lumbar sprain.

 Refer to Patient Education

 Refer to Physical Therapy

> *ICD9*
>
> *847.2 Lumbar sprain*

References

1. Andersson GBJ, Graziano GP, Kang JD, et al. Lumbar degenerative disorders. In: Beaty JH, ed. *Orthopaedic Knowledge Update 6*. Rosemont, IL: American Academy of Orthopaedic Surgeons; 1999:685–698.
2. Bigos SJ, Bowyer OR, Braen GR, et al. *Acute Low Back Problems in Adults: Assessment and Treatment. Quick Reference Guide for Clinicians No. 14*. AHCPR Publication No. 95-0643. Rockville, MD: Agency for Health Care Policy and Research, U.S. Department of Health and Human Services; 1994.
3. Van Tulder MW, Koes BW, Bouter LM. Conservative treatment of treatment of acute and nonspecific low back pain: a systematic review of randomized controlled trials of the most common interventions. *Spine* 1997;22:2128–2156.

4 Spinal Stenosis

Christian I. Fras

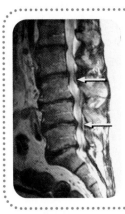

A 71-year-old man complains of pain that starts in the buttocks and radiates down the leg. Patient notes that leaning forward on a shopping cart at the supermarket helps the pain. (Figure from Koval KJ, Zuckerman JD. Atlas of Orthopaedic Surgery: A Multimedia Reference. *Philadelphia: Lippincott Williams & Wilkins; 2004.)*

CLINICAL POINTS

- Narrowing of the spinal canal is a common disorder that usually develops over time.
- Many patients have some back pain, which varies in severity, as well as some numbness or tingling in the legs.
- Not all patients have symptoms.

Clinical Presentation

Lumbar spinal stenosis is a common condition, predominantly affecting the aging spine. It may be defined as any process that narrows the spinal canal or the neural foramina. Occasionally, this narrowing may be of a congenital nature; indeed, some subsets of patients are predisposed to this congenital narrowing (such as achondroplastic dwarfs). More commonly, the narrowing develops over time as a consequence of degenerative processes affecting the spine. The exact etiology of these changes is not perfectly understood; however, it is thought that chronic disc degeneration induces secondary spinal instability, and the body's attempts to control these phenomena ultimately result in narrowing of the spinal canal. As instability develops, facet joint hypertrophy develops in an attempt to stabilize the spine; osteophytes may similarly develop from the facet joints as well as the dorsal aspect of the vertebral bodies.

Not every patient with spinal stenosis noted on imaging studies will have symptoms; indeed, some patients will have radiographically severe stenosis with modest and sometimes no symptoms. However, the typical patient presenting with symptomatic lumbar spinal stenosis will be middle aged or older; usually, the symptoms do not begin before the fifth or six decade of life. Classic symptoms relating to compression of the neural elements are those of "neurogenic claudication": Patients will complain of pain that starts in the buttocks and radiates down the leg (or legs) in a pattern consistent with the distribution of the nerves involved. Most commonly, this will manifest as pain and numbness going down the back of the thighs, into the calves, and sometimes into the ankles and feet; typically, the radiation will be from proximal to distal. Walking commonly provokes the pain, and many patients will be unable to walk even a city block before having to stop because of the pain. Most patients find that sitting down helps the pain, and many find that leaning forward helps as well; conversely, some find that extension of the lumbar spine provokes the pain. Mechanically, it is thought that leaning forward opens the spinal canal, relieving the pressure on the nerves and improving a patient's symptoms, while extending the lumbar spine closes off the canal, exacerbating the symptoms. A classic suggestion of lumbar stenosis is the "shopping-cart sign": Patients will admit to (and sometimes volunteer) leaning forward on a shopping cart when at the grocery store, supporting themselves on their elbows as they do their shopping.

Many patients will have at least some component of low back pain. For some patients, this pain is modest; for others, it is quite significant. There exists a small subset of patients who have only back pain with no leg pain; the etiology of this back pain may be related to the chronic degenerative changes in the spine or might possibly be compounded by chronic muscular fatigue by continually leaning forward to open the spinal canal.

While many patients will report associated numbness or tingling in their legs, very few will complain of true weakness in the legs. While still possible, even fewer patients will complain of symptoms suggestive of cauda equina syndrome, with disturbance of normal bowel or bladder function.

Physical Findings

A thorough neurologic and physical examination is important in these patients. Many will exhibit no evidence of gross motor dysfunction, and few will show any long-tract signs (such as Babinski); however, many will show subtle sensory changes, and some may show reflex changes. Typically, nerve root tension signs, such as the straight-leg-raise test, are negative or only mildly positive. Many patients will find that extending their lumbar spine in the office and then keeping it in an extended position for several moments will provoke their typical pain and that thereafter leaning forward will improve the pain.

Given the age of many of these patients and the potential coexistence of other confounding medical conditions, it is wise to perform a general physical examination as well. Particular attention should be paid to palpation of distal pedal pulses and assessment of skin changes suggestive of diabetes.

Studies (Labs, X-rays)

Further workup of suspected lumbar spinal stenosis beyond the aforementioned history and physical examination is based primarily on radiographic imaging studies.

Plain x-rays of the lumbar spine are an important part of the evaluation: While they cannot directly evaluate neural compression, they can assist in excluding more ominous diagnoses such as tumor, infection, or fracture. Additionally, they are indispensable in evaluating for scoliosis, spondylolisthesis, or overt instability. X-rays should include the following views: AP, lateral, L5-S1 spot lateral, and flexion–extension lateral; on occasion, oblique views are helpful as well.

PATIENT ASSESSMENT

1. Symptoms do not begin until the fifth or sixth decade of life.
2. Pain and numbness are present in the buttock regions and down the legs.
3. Sitting or leaning forward while walking helps the pain.
4. Consider vascular causes of symptoms in differential diagnosis.
5. MRI is helpful in assessing neural compression.

NOT TO BE MISSED

- *Vascular claudication:* May also cause leg pain provoked by walking and relieved by rest. However, these individuals will not report any improvement with leaning forward or worsening of their symptoms with extending their back. Classic signs of vascular claudication, such as the desire of the patient to lay the leg over the side of the bed at night, or diminished pedal pulses should indicate vascular insufficiency.

- *Peripheral neuropathy:* Common among diabetics. It typically affects both legs and causes numbness and dysesthesias in the feet that gradually progresses up the legs. An EMG-NCS can be helpful. Patients with no history of diabetes who are suspected of suffering from peripheral neuropathy should be investigated for chronic progressive neurologic diseases.

- *Arthritis in the hip or knee:* Typically causes localized pain in these areas; however, radiation of the pain down the leg can occur, especially in the case of hip arthritis, where radiation down the anterior thigh is common.

- *Other diagnoses:* Not to be missed are those of malignancy, infection, cauda equina syndrome, progressive neurologic deficit, or aortic aneurysm, among others.

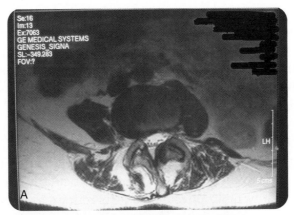

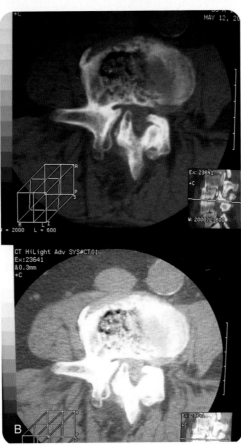

Figure 4.1 A: Axial T2 MRI of lumbar stenosis; note facet joint hypertrophy and encroachment of spinal canal. **B:** Postmyelogram CT scan (with bone and soft tissue windows) of patient with lumbar stenosis; note large osteophytes projecting into the spinal canal from the facet joints. The dye within the spinal canal is poorly visualized because of complete block of the flow of the dye, secondary to the stenosis at this and other levels.

MRI of the lumbar spine has become the imaging modality of choice in evaluating for neural compression, as it allows excellent visualization of the neural and other soft tissue structures and can thoroughly evaluate for infection or malignancy. Furthermore, it is noninvasive (Fig. 4.1A). However, it is not as accurate in evaluating osseous structures and can miss spondylolisthesis and even scoliosis on occasion. If a patient has had previous spine surgery, the MRI should be performed with gadolinium; if not, no such contrast agent needs to be ordered.

If a patient cannot have an MRI (e.g., because of a cardiac pacemaker), a myelogram followed by CT scan of the lumbar spine is an excellent alternative (Fig. 4.1B). Such a study has better visualization of the osseous structures of the spine than that found in MRI and may give other information not available by MRI; for this reason, some spine surgeons will routinely order a myelogram–CT scan preoperatively on all patients who are about to undergo surgery for stenosis. However, its sensitivity for malignancy or infection is not as good as MRI; furthermore, the test is invasive, involving a lumbar puncture for instillation of dye in the spinal canal.

Neurophysiologic tests (e.g., EMG-NCS) are controversial in the evaluation of lumbar stenosis. Many spine surgeons feel that such tests lack sufficient sensitivity and specificity in clinical practice to be of much value; others routinely order them, particularly in the preoperative setting. Certainly, neurophysiologic tests remain a valuable tool in cases where the diagnosis is in doubt despite adequate imaging studies.

Treatment and Clinical Course

1. NSAIDs and analgesia
2. Oral steroids versus epidural injections
3. Spinal decompression for continued symptoms that fail nonoperative measures

Treatment depends greatly on the severity of symptoms and disability of the patient. Absolute indications for surgery are similar as for lumbar disc herniations: progressive neurologic deficit or cauda equina syndrome. Both situations are quite rare in the setting of lumbar stenosis. A patient with overwhelmingly severe symptoms and profound radiographic changes that correspond appropriately to their symptoms may also be treated with early surgical intervention.

However, the majority of patients with lumbar stenosis can be well treated with nonsurgical measures. NSAIDs (if medically appropriate), physical therapy, occasionally wearing a brace or lumbosacral corset, and epidural steroid injections can bring many patients significant relief. During periods of a severe flare-up of pain, especially radiculopathy, a short course of oral steroids may be helpful, as can a short period of bed rest. If the patient can wait long enough, the pain may spontaneously resolve as well, without any measures being taken. The exact efficacy of nonoperative measures is debated; some authors suggest that in the long run, it is no better than simply waiting. However, even if these measures do not ultimately change the prospect for long-term relief, they may hasten a patient's recovery from his symptoms, allowing a return to regular activities more rapidly than if he were simply left to his own devices.

Surgery can be considered in patients who do not respond to conservative measures and in those who are incapacitated by their condition. The surgeon must be mindful of the overall health of patients and their ability to withstand surgery, as many patients suffering from symptomatic lumbar stenosis are elderly. Nonetheless, age itself is not an absolute contraindication to surgery; rather, a patient's "physiologic age" is of far greater importance. To assist in determining a patient's ability to withstand surgery, a clearance from the primary care physician can be most useful; additional evaluations may be necessary, such as a cardiac stress test, as the situation warrants.

A detailed discussion regarding the surgical treatment of lumbar stenosis is beyond the scope of this chapter; however, for cases with only neural compression (i.e., stenosis) and no evidence of instability or deformity in the spine, a lumbar laminectomy is the surgical gold standard. In this procedure, the lamina of the affected area is removed with specialized instruments, thereby opening the spinal canal and decompressing the neural elements. Care must be taken to remove enough bone to adequately relieve the pressure on nerves but not so much bone as to destabilize the spine and cause further difficulties. Such a balance is often difficult to strike. The primary risks directly related to the surgery include infection (the most common complication), spinal fluid leak secondary to dural tear, and nerve damage (fortunately, relatively rarely), with subsequent leg pain, numbness, or weakness. Because of the age and medical comorbidities of many of these patients, systemic medical complications may also occur. Paralysis with paraplegia can potentially occur but is exceedingly rare.

WHEN TO REFER

- Progressive neurologic deficit
- Patient not responding to conservative treatment after 4 to 6 months
- Infection or malignancy

 Refer to Physical Therapy

ICD9

724.00 Spinal stenosis of unspecified region
724.02 Spinal stenosis of lumbar region
724.09 Spinal stenosis of other region
724.9 Other unspecified back disorders

References

1. Hansraj K, Cammisa F, O'Leary P, et al. Decompressive surgery for typical lumbar spinal stenosis. *Clin Orthop* 2001;384:10–17.
2. Hansraj, K, O'Leary P, Cammisa F, et al. Decompression, fusion, and instrumentation surgery for complex lumbar spinal stenosis. *Clin Orthop* 2001;384:18–25.
3. Johnsson KE, Rosen I, Uden A. The natural course of lumbar spinal stenosis. *Clin Orthop* 1992;279:82–86.
4. Katz JN, Lipson SJ, Larson MG, et al. The outcome of decompressive laminectomy for degenerative lumbar stenosis. *J Bone Joint Surg Am*1991;73(6):809–816.
5. Sanderson PL, Wood PL. Surgery for lumbar spinal stenosis in old people. *J Bone Joint Surg Br* 1993; 75:393–397.

SECTION 1 Lumbosacral Spine

Thoraco-Lumbar Spine

CHAPTER 5 Scoliosis

Christian I. Fras

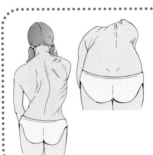

A 44-year-old woman presents with the chief complaint that her shoulders appear asymmetric. (Figure from Weber J, Kelley J. Health Assessment in Nursing*, 2nd ed. Philadelphia: Lippincott Williams & Wilkins; 2003.)*

CLINICAL POINTS

- Adults who seek medical treatment complain of issues related to the spinal curve and/or pain.

- Adults may have typical "S"-shaped or only single curves.

- In general, women seek medical attention more often than do men.

Clinical Presentation

Scoliosis is a three-dimensional deformity of the spine. It is most obviously identified by a curvature in the coronal plane (as seen on an AP radiograph of the spine); however, there will always be a component of rotation of the vertebrae in the curvature. This is an example of a "coupled motion," in which movement in one plane (in this case, the curvature in the coronal plane) will induce an obligatory motion in another plane (in this case, a rotation of the vertebra). Frequently, there is a derangement of the spine in the sagittal plane as well, with decreased, or sometimes increased, thoracic kyphosis and loss of normal lumbar lordosis.

For a spinal curvature to be considered scoliosis, as defined by the Scoliosis Research Society, there must be a lateral curvature (i.e., in the coronal plane) of >10 degrees. The exact prevalence of scoliosis in the adult population is not well known; in the pediatric population, the prevalence of adolescent idiopathic scoliosis is approximately 25 per 1,000 (the vast majority of these curves are minor and require no intervention of any kind).

With the exception of rare types of congenital deformities, the etiology of scoliosis remains unknown. Family studies and studies of twins strongly suggest a genetic component to scoliosis; however, a discrete gene, or the mode of inheritance, has not been clearly established.

Three broad categories of patients with adult scoliosis have been identified: (a) young adults with a known history of scoliosis since adolescence, without significant degenerative changes in the spine (Fig. 5.1); (b) older adults with a history of scoliosis dating back to adolescence, with extensive superimposed degenerative changes (Fig. 5.2); and (c) older adults with no childhood history of scoliosis, with the de novo development of scoliosis and degenerative changes, usually after the age of 40 (Fig. 5.3). Patients in the first two groups typically have S-shaped curves, with one part of the curve in the thoracic spine and another part in the opposite direction in the lumbar spine; patients in the third group often have single curves only

SECTION 2 Thoraco-Lumbar Spine

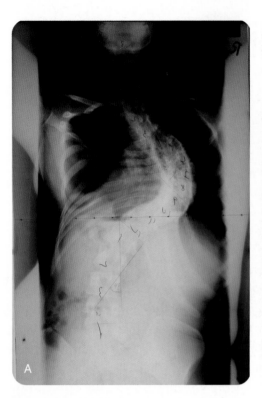
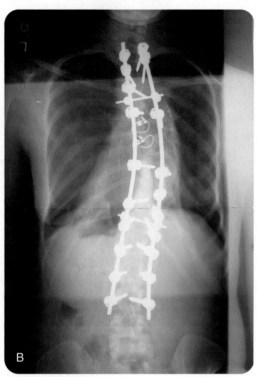

Figure 5.1 A: A 32-year-old woman with 100-degree curvature from untreated scoliosis. **B:** Postoperative x-ray showing T3-L3 posterior spinal fusion with instrumentation. At 4 months postop, she had minimal discomfort and was back to work full-time as a legal secretary.

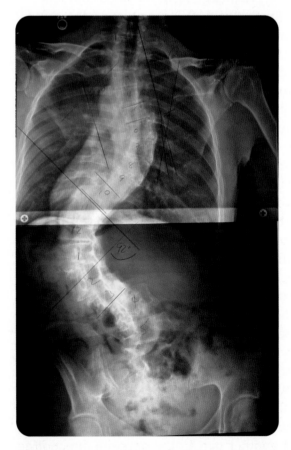

Figure 5.2 A 64-year-old woman with history of scoliosis since childhood, with recently worsening curve and increasing back pain.

in the lumbar spine. While the specific prevalence of each of these groups is not known relative to each other, it appears that the third group may be the most common, at least among those seeking treatment.

Patients with adult scoliosis typically seek medical attention because of issues structurally related to the curve, related to pain, or both. Issues that are structurally related to the curve include the magnitude of their deformity; concerns about their cosmetic appearance; progression of the deformity; and a sense of imbalance, a feeling that they are "tipping" to a side or "pitching" forward. Patients with a history of scoliosis since childhood, who often have substantial thoracic curves, will often complain of asymmetry of the scapulae and excessive prominence of the shoulder blades. Issues relating to pain include back pain (corresponding to the area of the apex of the largest curve but sometimes involving the "entire back") and/or radicular leg pain. Back pain in those with a history of scoliosis since adolescence is often interscapular; back pain in those with a de novo curve (the curve often being confined to the lumbar spine) will typically be in the lower back. Many older patients will complain of their back simply feeling "tired" with prolonged activity. Radicular leg pain is common in those with an adult degenerative curve but is rare in those with a history of scoliosis since adolescence.

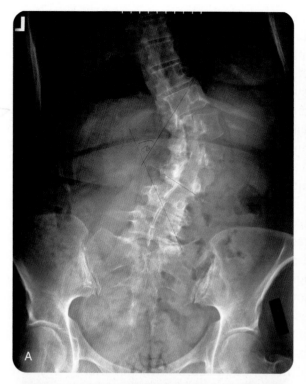

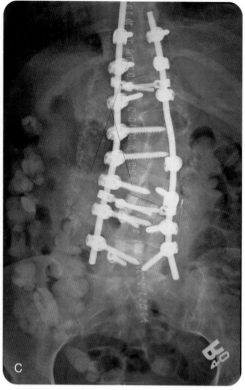

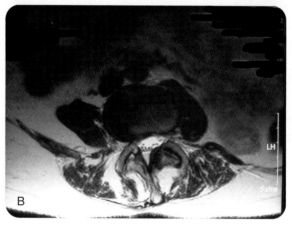

Figure 5.3 A: A 56-year-old woman with back pain, bilateral leg pain, and history of progressive spinal deformity. **B:** Axial T2 MRI showing spinal stenosis. **C:** Treated with anterior and posterior spinal fusion with instrumentation and multiple laminectomies. Patient went back to work as school nurse at 3.5 months postop, with improvement in back and leg pain.

SECTION 2 Thoraco-Lumbar Spine

PATIENT ASSESSMENT

1. The patient describes an imbalance.

2. Generally, the patient is aware of curvature of the spine from childhood.

3. The patient should be examined carefully to assess shoulder/pelvic asymmetry.

4. Generally, the curve is painless and neurologic abnormalities are uncommon.

5. Full-length spine films are helpful in assessing curvature.

While patients with adult scoliosis may present at virtually any age after 18 years, they tend to fall into several clusters, based on the three rough groups of adult scoliosis. Group 1 tends to present in the third to fourth decade of life; group 2 tends to present in the fifth to sixth decade; and those in group 3 tend to present in the sixth to seventh decade. For all groups, women seek medical attention more commonly than men.

Physical Findings

The primary physical findings in adult scoliosis relate to the structural manifestations of the curve itself. These are best appreciated with the patient nearly completely disrobed or in an examination gown. Shoulder asymmetry is common, with one shoulder being higher than the other. Because of the rotation of the spine that occurs concomitantly with the coronal plane deformity, one scapula (and one side of the rib cage) may indeed be more prominent than the other. In adults with a de novo degenerative curve, there is commonly noted a prominence in one side of the thoracolumbar paraspinal musculature; this is also because of the obligatory rotation of the spine that occurs with the spinal deformity. These areas of asymmetry are typically accentuated by having the patient bend forward. In children, these rotational deformities can be reasonably accurately measured with an inclinometer ("scoliometer"), and the subsequent angle of trunk rotation can be correlated with severity of spinal deformity; unfortunately, such measurements are less useful in the adult patient. Pelvic obliquity (in the coronal plane) may rarely also be observed.

Overall sagittal and coronal balance should be assessed with the patient standing upright; abnormalities in these areas essentially involve the trunk being shifted off to the left or right relative to the pelvis (in cases of coronal plane imbalance) or the trunk tipping forward relative to the pelvis (in cases of sagittal plane imbalance). In the latter situation, patients will often try to compensate by bending their knees and hips when standing erect.

There is typically no significant tenderness to palpation anywhere in the back of these patients. Flexibility of the curve is difficult to assess in the adult patient, particularly in the coronal plane; this is because of the natural stiffness that occurs with advancing age and also because of issues of body habitus.

A careful neurologic evaluation should be performed, including assessment of strength, sensation, and reflexes, particularly in the lower extremities. In patients with de novo degenerative scoliosis and severe accompanying spinal stenosis and associated radicular leg pain, abnormalities in the neurologic examination may become evident and should be noted. Neurologic abnormalities are otherwise rare, particularly in patients with scoliosis known since adolescence.

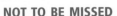

NOT TO BE MISSED

- Intraspinal tumor
- Neurologic deficit

Studies (Labs, X-rays)

The most useful study in evaluating adult scoliosis remains the plain x-ray. While AP and lateral views of the lumbar and thoracic spine can give a useful idea about the overall severity of the deformity, the gold standard test for evaluating scoliosis remains AP and lateral x-rays of the entire spine performed on a single cassette (i.e., 36-inch-long films). With the advent of digital radiography, other (digital) methods of obtaining these films may be developed that are equally as accurate; however, this has yet to be firmly established.

Other studies, such as CT, myelogram followed by CT, and MRI, are all useful in assessing issues of neural compromise, particularly in the setting of radiculopathy as well as in the rare cases of suspected congenital abnormalities. MRI is particularly useful to evaluate preoperatively for the presence of intraspinal abnormalities, such as spinal cord tumor, spinal cord syrinx, or a tethered spinal cord. However, these studies are inferior to 36-inch x-rays in assessing the overall structural characteristics of the curve.

EMG-NCS studies may be of use in evaluating the patient with radicular leg symptoms; however, their accuracy, sensitivity, specificity, and diagnostic and prognostic roles remain somewhat limited.

Treatment and Clinical Course

1. Serial full-length spine films are recommended.
2. Newly diagnosed curves should be assessed by an orthopaedic surgeon.

Treatment of adult scoliosis is aimed at two related but ultimately separate areas: issues directly related to structural aspects of the deformity and pain. In the adult, change of the deformity itself can be achieved only through surgical intervention. There is no data to support the role of physiotherapy, chiropractic therapy, bracing, exercise, traction, or multiple other proposed modalities in effecting a change in the curve itself. Thus, if a patient's complaints are primarily structural (e.g., imbalance in the coronal or sagittal planes, deformity progression, cosmetic concerns, etc.), ultimately a surgical remedy may be necessary.

In contrast, treatment of pain associated with adult scoliosis has many potential nonoperative options in addition to operative solutions. Physical therapy may be of immense value, particularly in situations of a predominance of back pain; other options include various injections into the spine, including epidural steroid injections and facet blocks. Bracing may be of benefit in some patients, particularly on a short-term basis, to help relieve a flare-up of pain. The role of chiropractic manipulation in adult scoliosis is poorly understood, but it appears to have very low chances of causing harm, especially in the lumbar spine. NSAIDs may be of benefit, but their use must be balanced against their potential associated side effects.

The only absolute indications for surgery in adult scoliosis are documented progression of the deformity, as demonstrated by serial x-ray studies, and (rarely) a progressive neurologic deficit. Relative indications for surgery include intolerable pain refractory to conservative treatment, a patient's perception of progression of the deformity, cosmetic concerns, difficulties with activities of daily living because of the severity of the deformity, pulmonary compromise because of the severity of a thoracic deformity, and a curve pattern of sufficient magnitude that strongly predicts future progression of the deformity.

If surgery is pursued, the surgical procedure recommended varies depending on the specific curvature; technical aspects of all the different surgical procedures and the decision-making process whereby a particular plan is selected is exceedingly complex, varies widely between surgeons (and, indeed, from region to region in the country), and is beyond the scope of this chapter.

WHEN TO REFER

- Progressive neurologic deficit
- Patient with severe curvatures
- Pulmonary dysfunction secondary to progressive curve
- Severe pain
- Pain that does not respond to conservative measures

SECTION 2 Thoraco-Lumbar Spine

ICD9

737.30 Scoliosis (and kyphoscoliosis), idiopathic
737.31 Resolving infantile idiopathic scoliosis
737.32 Progressive infantile idiopathic scoliosis
737.33 Scoliosis due to radiation
737.34 Thoracogenic scoliosis
737.39 Other kyphoscoliosis and scoliosis
754.2 Congenital musculoskeletal deformities of spine

References

1. Bradford DS. Adult scoliosis: current concepts of treatment. *Clin Orthop* 1988;229:70–87.
2. Dickson JH, Mirkovic S, Noble PC, et al. Results of operative treatment of idiopathic scoliosis in adults. *J Bone Joint Surg Am* 1995;77(4):513–523.
3. Kostuik JP. Adult scoliosis. In: Bridwell KH, Dewald RL, eds. *The Textbook of Spinal Surgery*, Vol. 1. Philadelphia: JB Lippincott; 1991:249–278.
4. Kostuik JP. Decision making in adult scoliosis. *Spine* 1979;4:521–525.
5. Shapiro GS, Taira G, Boachie-Adjei O. Results of surgical treatment of adult idiopathic scoliosis with low back pain and spinal stenosis: a study of long-term clinical radiographic outcomes. *Spine* 2003;28(4):358–363.
6. Tribus CB. Degenerative lumbar scoliosis: evaluation and management. *J Am Acad Orthop Surg* 2003;11(3):174–183.
7. Weinstein SL, Ponsetti IV. Curve progression in idiopathic scoliosis. *J Bone Joint Surg Am* 1983;65(4):447–455.

CHAPTER 6 Compression Fracture

Christian I. Fras

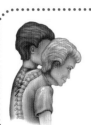

A 72-year-old woman presents with new-onset severe back pain after lifting a box. Patient denies any associated neurologic compromise. (Figure provided by Anatomical Chart Co.)

CLINICAL POINTS

- Many women have no symptoms.
- Some women may have acute back pain, the severity of which varies widely.
- Seemingly insignificant trauma may cause fractures.

Clinical Presentation

Approximately 700,000 vertebral body compression fractures occur each year (twice the rate of hip fractures). It has been estimated that 25% of women reaching menopause will experience at least one osteoporotic vertebral compression fracture (OVCF) in their lifetime.

Typically, the patient affected by an OVCF is a postmenopausal white woman who likely is older than 50 years of age. While current recommendations of organizations such as the American Academy of Orthopaedic Surgeons recommend that all women over age 65 have a screening dual-energy x-ray absorptiometry (DEXA) scan, many will not have had this study and will be unaware of their osteoporosis status.

It has been stated that the majority of OCVFs are asymptomatic and found incidentally during radiographic examinations for other reasons. When symptomatic, they present with sudden or acute back pain. Comparatively, trivial trauma may provoke the fracture, such as falling off a chair or even lifting a mildly heavy object; sometimes, there is no history of trauma at all. Although the pain is often in the area of the fracture, fractures at the thoracolumbar junction may at times cause lower back pain but no mid back pain.

The severity of the pain can vary widely and bears little relationship to the apparent severity of the fracture on subsequent radiographs. Most patients (who have symptoms) find the pain to be moderately severe; there is a subset of patients, however, who have incapacitating pain such that parenteral narcotics are necessary for its control.

Most patients do not complain of any radicular pain, numbness, or weakness; nor do they complain of any disturbance in bowel or bladder habits (excepting constipation that may be related to use of narcotic medication for treatment of the pain). The pain may wake them from sleep at night as they change position. Most patients find that lying down improves their pain and that activity of any kind worsens it. Patient should be asked about generalized constitutional symptoms (fever, chills,

SECTION 2 Thoraco-Lumbr Spine

31

night sweats, weight loss, etc.), as they can signify a more ominous process, such as infection or tumor.

Physical Findings

Many patients with an OVCF will exhibit tenderness about the spinous process of the vertebra that is fractured; some patients will note an exacerbation of their symptoms with leaning forward and improvement in their symptoms with extension of their back.

Otherwise, the physical examination of most patients with an OVCF is relatively unremarkable. There is rarely any neurologic deficit, although some patients will have diminished effort on strength testing of their lower extremities secondary to pain; elderly patients may exhibit global weakness in their legs, but this is most often related to generalized deconditioning. Reflexes, while often absent in the elderly patient, will usually be symmetric. Sensation (either in the legs or in the chest in the case of a thoracic compression fracture) is typically unaffected. Root tension and long tract signs are typically absent; if present, they should alert the physician to potential neural compression from bone fragments (which is quite rare).

Assessment of the patient's general medical condition is important to help indicate if other general medical conditions might be complicating the situation.

Studies (Labs, X-rays)

In the setting of an acute OVCF, laboratory workup is important only to exclude pathology more ominous than a benign compression fracture; this can include CBC, ESR, CRP, SPEP, and UPEP as well as various other tumor markers as clinically indicated. Lab studies for workup of metabolic bone disorders and osteoporosis, while not unimportant, do not directly contribute to the diagnosis and management of the acute OVCF itself.

X-rays will often show a typical wedge-shaped fracture; however, this is not universally visible, particularly early in the course of the OVCF. If none is noted on x-ray, consideration should be given to a bone scan, MRI, or both. A bone scan (Fig. 6.1) is less expensive and can identify abnormalities in other areas of the body than just the particular area of the spine being investigated; however, a bone scan may take several days to become positive after the acute development of an OVCF. Furthermore, some malignancies are not "hot" on bone scan and could, therefore, be missed. MRI (Fig. 6.2) is more expensive and, for some patients, more uncomfortable than a bone scan; yet, an MRI will reliably show an acute OVCF, even immediately after its occurrence, and can help to distinguish between a benign OVCF and a more ominous process such as malignancy and infection. It should be noted, though, that particularly early in the development of a tumor or infection involving a vertebral body, it may be quite difficult to distinguish from a benign OVCF, even on MRI, as there may not yet be obvious soft tissue extension of the process that would act as a telltale sign of such pathology.

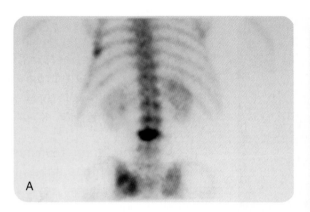

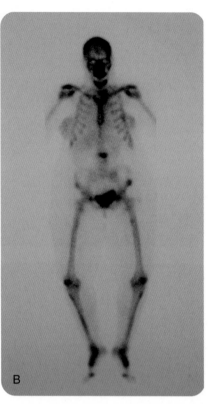

Figure 6.1 A: Bone scan of lumbar spine showing increased uptake of tracer in L3 vertebral body. **B:** Bone scan of entire body showing increased uptake in L3 vertebral body, but not significantly elsewhere.

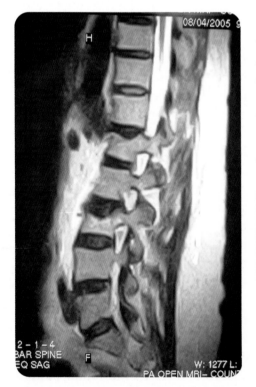

Figure 6.2 Sagittal T2 MRI showing vertebral body fracture in L3 as well as old fracture in L1. Note slight increased signal in L3 just below the superior endplate, indicating that this is a relatively new fracture that has not yet completely healed.

Typically, the age of the fracture cannot be determined by the plain x-ray appearance of the OVCF; in contrast, increased edema within the vertebral body on MRI, or increased uptake on bone scan, can strongly indicate an acute fracture. The absence of these signs on MRI/bone scan strongly indicates that the fracture is old and has healed.

Treatment and Clinical Course

1. Activity modification and analgesics are beneficial for most patients.
2. Rule out a pathological fracture.
3. The role for vertebroplasty and kyphoplasty is evolving.

Most OVCFs, when symptomatic, respond well to conservative treatment. A short course of bed rest (not more than 4 days, as elderly patients can rapidly become deconditioned under such circumstances) combined with judicious use of analgesics (both opioids and NSAIDs) and in some circumstances brace treatment results in a highly acceptable outcome for most patients. Some may require a short hospitalization in the acute phase of the injury to allow adequate pain control. Care must be taken in the use of narcotics in order to avoid side effects

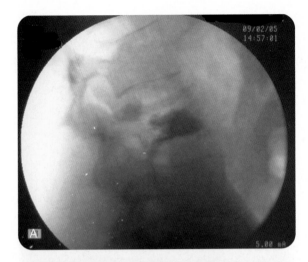

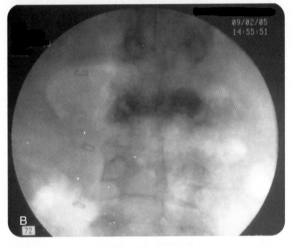

Figure 6.3 A: Lateral intraoperative fluoroscopy view immediately after kyphoplasty, with injection of cement into L3 vertebral body. Note restoration of vertebral body height. **B:** AP intraoperative fluoroscopy view immediately after kyphoplasty of L3 vertebral body.

WHEN TO REFER

• Progressive neurologic deficit

• Metastatic disease

• Infection

of confusion and loss of coordination in the elderly patient; such events may predispose the patient to further falls and further fractures, including hip fractures. With such a treatment program, most patients note complete resolution of their symptoms by about 3 months, with the severe, acute pain resolving after 2 to 4 weeks.

Recently, minimally invasive techniques have been introduced for cement augmentation of OVCF; these include vertebroplasty, involving the percutaneous injection of cement into the fractured vertebral body, which, when hardened, will give immediate stability to the fracture; and kyphoplasty (Fig. 6.3), which involves inflation of a percutaneously introduced balloon into the vertebral body in an attempt to restore vertebral body height and prevent kyphosis, followed by instillation of cement as in vertebroplasty. Both techniques are comparatively new in the United States, with kyphoplasty having been introduced from France in 1994 and kyphoplasty being developed several years thereafter. Clinical outcomes of the two procedures appear to be roughly equivalent; the majority of patients undergoing these procedures experience significant, rapid reduction in their pain. Additionally, a biopsy of the bone may be performed at the time of the procedure, allowing an evaluation for malignancy or infection (it should be noted, though, that absence of these findings in the biopsy material does not completely rule out their presence secondary to sampling error. The statistical risk associated with these treatments is low; however, significant complications can rarely result, including paralysis and even death. Furthermore, the instillation of very rigid cement in a vertebral column that is essentially composed of weak bone may predispose adjacent vertebrae to fracture.

Very rarely, open surgery is indicated for an OVCF, primarily in the case of severe spinal cord injury or progressive neurologic deficit. Surgery typically involves decompression of the spinal canal and concomitant fusion to address any instability. However, such surgery should be undertaken with caution, as the complication rates associated with it are exceedingly high.

Although not part of the acute treatment of the fracture itself, patients with OVCFs should be studied with a DEXA scan to establish a baseline and should be treated for their osteoporosis. The exact nature of the treatment of the metabolic disorder depends on a variety of different factors and is beyond the scope of this section; nonetheless, its importance should not be minimized and, in some ways, it is more important than the treatment of the fracture itself.

ICD9

733.10 Pathologic fracture, unspecified site
733.11 Pathologic fracture of humerus
733.12 Pathologic fracture of distal radius and ulna
733.13 Pathologic fracture of vertebrae
733.14 Pathologic fracture of neck of femur
733.15 Pathologic fracture of other specified part of femur
733.16 Pathologic fracture of tibia or fibula
733.19 Pathologic fracture of other specified site

References

1. Alvarez L Alcaraz M, Perez-Higueras A, et al. Percutaneous vertebroplasty: functional improvement in patients with osteoporotic compression fractures. *Spine* 2006;31(10):1113–1118.
2. Kim DH, Vaccaro AR. Osteoporotic compression fractures of the spine; current options and considerations for treatment. *Spine J* 2006;6(5):479–487.
3. Nevaiser A, Toro-Arbelaez JB, Lane JM. Is kyphoplasty the standard of care for compression fractures of the spine, especially in the elderly? *Am J Orthopaedics* 2005;9:425–429.
4. Taylor RS, Taylor RJ, Fritzell P. Balloon kyphoplasty and vertebroplasty for vertebral compression fractures: a comparative systematic review of efficacy and safety. *Spine* 2006;31(23):2747–2755.

SECTION 2 Thoraco-Lumbr Spine

Cervical Spine

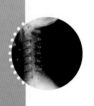

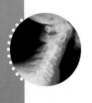

7 Cervical Strain: Whiplash

Jaehon M. Kim, Andrea L. Bowers, and Kingsley R. Chin

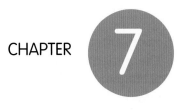

A 36-year-old man presents with neck pain, stiffness, and recurrent headaches since being tackled in a weekend football game. (Figure from *Dean D, Herbener TE.* Cross-Sectional Human Anatomy. *Baltimore: Lippincott Williams & Wilkins; 2000.*)

Clinical Presentation

More than 13 million patients annually are evaluated for cervical spine injury at emergency facilities in the United States and Canada. The charge of the treating physician is to rule out morbid conditions, such as bony fracture and cord injury, from among the large majority of common cervical strain. Known in layman's terms as *whiplash*, cervical strain is the result of sudden hyperextension followed by hyperflexion of the neck (Fig. 7.1). Common mechanisms of cervical strain injury include rear-end automobile collisions, sports trauma (e.g., football), and repetitive occupational injuries. Muscular and ligamentous structures of the cervical spine are stretched beyond their physiologic capacity, generating inflammation within the local soft tissues. Patients with cervical strain may present with a constellation of symptoms including neck pain, persistent stiffness, trapezial pain, back pain, muscle spasm, headache, and limited range of motion. These symptoms often begin acutely, hours after the injury.

Initially, cervical strain may be the cause of much distress to patients, but generally it has a benign course with minimal long-term sequelae. The principle concern is to identify patients with bone and neurologic pathology such as fractures, dislocations, and spinal cord injury. Other more rare diseases that may mimic the symptoms of cervical strain include primary or metastatic neoplasms, vertebral osteomyelitis, and epidural abscess. Persistent axial neck pain over several weeks and/or neurologic abnormalities may warrant closer evaluation for serious underlying pathology.

Physical Findings

When initially evaluating the patient with neck injury, the physician should presume dangerous underlying pathology and consider cervical

CLINICAL POINTS

- Tissue inflammation is seen as a result of whiplash.
- Although such injury may seem serious, the course is generally benign and the prognosis is good.
- Identification of patients with bone and neurologic conditions is important.

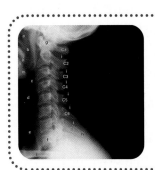

PATIENT ASSESSMENT

1. Cervical strain is a result of sudden hyperextension followed by hyperflexion.
2. Patients complain of stiffness and pain.
3. A detailed neurologic exam is indicated.
4. A cervical x-ray or CT may be indicated.

Hyperextension

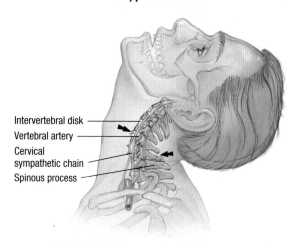

Intervertebral disk

Vertebral artery

Cervical
sympathetic chain

Spinous process

Figure 7.1 Whiplash injuries of the head and neck. Hyperextension. (Provided by Anatomical Chart Co.)

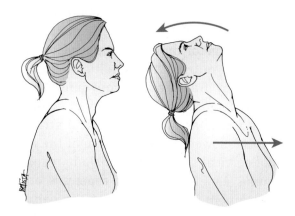

Figure 7.2 Loss of lordosis of the cervical spine in a patient with a whiplash injury. This is nonpathologic. (*From Oatis CA. Kinesiology: The Mechanics and Pathomechanics of Human Movement*. Baltimore: Lippincott Williams & Wilkins; 2004.)

NOT TO BE MISSED

- Cervical fractures
- Cervical instability
- Ankylosing spondylitis
- Klippel-Feil syndrome
- Spinal cord injury
- Cervical dislocation
- Carotid artery dissection
- Meningitis
- Neoplasm
- Vertebral osteomyelitis
- Epidural abscess

strain only as a diagnosis of exclusion. Often, the patient will present in a cervical collar. The patient should first be assessed for alertness, sobriety, cooperativity, and the presence or absence of distracting injury. The neck should be inspected for skin integrity, edema, ecchymosis, or asymmetry. Tenderness or bony step off is assessed by palpation of the spinous processes followed by palpation of the paraspinal soft tissues. A detailed neurologic examination should be performed in both the upper and lower extremities. In the setting of a normal neurologic exam in a reliable patient, cervical range of motion may be tested. Common physical findings in cervical strain include palpable bogginess of the posterior neck musculature, cervical tissue edema (but not pitting), and limited range of motion secondary to muscle spasm.

Studies (Labs, X-rays)

Cervical strain is a clinical diagnosis. Radiographic images are typically utilized to exclude more severe injuries. Although some authors advocate a low threshold for radiographic evaluation, a preponderance of evidence in the literature indicates that its use has not been efficient, since few of these patients actually have cervical fractures (Fig. 7.2). Furthermore, cervical radiographs have proven to be a substantial burden on health care costs due to their high-volume use and have been associated with unnecessary discomfort to patients from prolonged immobilization and delayed management. Nonetheless, some authors report as high as 30% of patients with partial or full paralysis due to missed diagnosis,[1] and physicians should err on the side of precaution.

Therefore, clinical decision guidelines for the judicious use of cervical radiography have been developed based on history, physical examination, and simple tests. Two decision-making tools were developed independently: the National Emergency X-Radiography Utilization Study (NEXUS) Low-Risk Criteria (NLC) and the Canadian C-Spine Rule (CCR).

First described in 1992, NLC is based on five low-risk measures (Table 7.1) with >90% sensitivity and 35% specificity for cervical spine injury. NLC state that trauma patients should undergo radiographic evaluation unless they meet *all* of the following five criteria[2,3] (Table 7.1): (a) no posterior midline cervical spine tenderness, (b) no evidence of intoxication, (c) a normal level of alertness, (d) no focal neurologic deficit, and (e) no painful distracting injuries. NLC was subsequently recommended for use by the emergency department physicians as a decision algorithm for ordering cervical radiography.

More recently, the CCR was developed based on three high-risk criteria, five low-risk criteria, and the patients' ability to rotate their neck (Table 7.2).[4] CCR incorporated various levels of risk factors into the

Table 7.1 The National Emergency X-Radiography Utilization Study Low-Risk Criteria: Cervical spine radiography is indicated for patients with trauma unless they meet all of the following five criteria.[a]

CRITERIA	DESCRIPTIONS
1. No posterior midline cervical spine tenderness.	1. Bony midline cervical spine tenderness on palpation from nuchal ridge to prominence of the first cervical thoracic vertebra or evidence of pain with direct palpation of any cervical spinous process.
2. No evidence of intoxication.	2. Based on history, or an observer of intoxication or intoxicating ingestion, or evidence of intoxication on physical examination (i.e., odor, slurred speech, ataxia, dysmetria, or other cerebellar findings), or behavior consistent with intoxication, or bodily secretion positive for alcohol or drugs that affect the level of alertness.
3. A normal level of alertness.	3. Abnormal results include any of the following: a Glasgow Coma Scale of 14 or less, disorientation to any of the person/time/place/event, inability to recall three objects in 5 minutes, delayed or inappropriate response to external stimuli, or other findings.
4. No focal neurologic deficit.	4. Any neurologic finding on motor and sensory examination.
5. No painful distracting injuries.	5. Any condition thought by clinician to be producing pain sufficient to distract patient away from the neck injury such as long bone fracture, visceral injury, large laceration, degloving injury, crushing injury, large burns, or any other injury causing acute functional impairment.

[a] Hoffman JR, Mower WR, Wolfson AB, et al. Validity of a set of clinical criteria to rule out injury to the cervical spine in patients with blunt trauma. *N Engl J Med* 2000;343:94–99.

SECTION 3 Cervical Spine

decision-making tree to evaluate the need for cervical radiography. Based on a prospective cohort study, CCR demonstrated 99.4% sensitivity and 45.1% specificity.[4] Both NCL and CCR are proven effective guidelines for screening patients, demonstrating overall high sensitivity and excellent negative predictive values[4] (Table 7.3).

Traditionally, when indicated, three-view plain film radiography or helical CT scan is performed. Although flexion extension lateral radiographs are useful for detecting pathologic instability (>3.5 mm of movement between vertebrae or >11 degrees of angulation), these may not be beneficial in the acute setting, since patients are unable to fully cooperate to flex their necks enough due to pain. Although the institutional cost has limited its use, helical CT has been shown to be faster with better sensitivity (>95%) and specificity (>95%) for detecting fractures compared with plain radiography (44%–84% sensitivity, 72%–89% specificity).[5] MRI is more effective for the evaluation of soft tissues, including the spinal cord, muscular, and ligamentous

Table 7.2 The Canadian C-Spine Rule: For patients with trauma who are alert (as indicated by a score of 15 on the Glasgow Coma Scale) and in stable condition and in whom cervical spine injury is a concern.[a]

Any high-risk factor that mandates radiography?

Age ≥65 y or dangerous mechanism[b] or paresthesias in extremities

☐ No   ☐ Yes ⟶ **Radiography**
↓

Any low-risk factor that allows safe assessment of range of motion?

Simple rear-end motor vehicle collision,[b] or sitting position in the emergency department, or ambulatory at any time, or delayed onset of neck pain, or absence of midline cervical spine tenderness

☐ Yes   ☐ No ⟶ **Radiography**
↓

Able to rotate neck actively?

45 degrees left and right

☐ Yes   ☐ Unable ⟶ **Radiography**
↓

No radiography

---

[a] Stiell IG, Clement CM, McKnight RD, et al. The Canadian C-Spine Rule versus the NEXUS Low-Risk Criteria in patients with trauma. *N Engl J Med* 2003;349:2510–2518.

[b] Considered to be a fall from an elevation ≥3 feet or 5 stairs, an axial load to the head, a motor vehicle collision at high speed (>100 km/h) or with rollover or ejection, a collision involving a motorized recreational vehicle, or a bicycle collision.

[c] Excludes being pushed into oncoming traffic, being hit by a bus or a large truck, a rollover, and being hit by a high-speed vehicle.

structures. In patients with multiple injuries and/or neurologic deficits, MRI is indicated in the setting of negative plain film and CT scan results.

Special consideration must also be given to the patient with presumed baseline cervical pathology, as seen in rheumatoid arthritis, ankylosing spondylitis, diffuse idiopathic skeletal hyperostosis, Down syndrome, or other. In these patients, the added insult of "cervical strain" may herald new fracture or instability that must be ruled out, preferably by CT, MRI, or both.

Table 7.3 Sensitivity, Specificity, and Negative Predictive Value of the Canadian C-Spine Rule and Low-Risk Criteria[a]

RESULT OF ASSESSMENT	CCR[b]	NCL[b]
Sensitivity (%)	99.4 (96–100)	90.7 (85–94)
Specificity (%)	45.1 (44–46)	36.8 (36–38)
Negative predictive value (%)	100.0	99.4

CCR, Canadian C-Spine Rule; NCL, Low-Risk Criteria.

[a] Hoffman JR, Mower WR, Wolfson AB, et al. Validity of a set of clinical criteria to rule out injury to the cervical spine in patients with blunt trauma. *N Engl J Med* 2000;343:94–99.

[b] 95% confidence interval values are in parentheses.

Treatment and Clinical Course

1. NSAIDs and analgesia as necessary
2. Encourage normal use as tolerated
3. Physical therapy

The clinical course of cervical strain is benign, and most patients should be able to return to normal daily function within 1 to 2 weeks. The literature currently lacks consensus recommendations or guidelines for optimal management of cervical strain. Many patients find heat and/or ice packs beneficial. NSAIDs or acetaminophen are often used for pain control, and the severe case complicated by muscle spasms may benefit from the judicious use of oral antispasmodics such as diazepan (Valium) or cyclobenzaprine (Flexeril).

An important decision is whether or not to apply a soft collar and/or recommend immobilization. Presently, there is stronger evidence favoring early mobilization with instruction to "self-train" neck movements. Patients who underwent supervised physiotherapy and/or immobilization of the neck for 10 to 14 days had worse outcomes than patients who were instructed to self-exercise their neck daily. Furthermore, a prospective randomized trial indicated that the "act-as-usual" treatment group who received no soft collar and no sick leave of absence had a significant reduction of symptoms 24 weeks after the injury.[6] Significant improvements in these patients were reflected in subjective pain scores, neck stiffness, memory, and concentration. Therefore, soft collar immobilization and time off from work are not recommended for cervical strain injury. The patients should be encouraged to return to their normal daily activities on the first day of treatment.

SECTION 3 Cervical Spine

WHEN TO REFER

- Persistent pain over several weeks
- Neurologic abnormalities
- Abnormal radiologic findings

 Refer to Patient Education

 Refer to Physical Therapy

ICD9
847.0 Neck sprain

References

1. Reid DC, Henderson R, Saboe L, et al. Etiology and clinical course of missed spine fractures. *J Trauma* 1987;27:980–986.
2. Hoffman JR, Schriger DL, Mower W, et al. Low-risk criteria for cervical-spine radiography in blunt trauma: a prospective study. *Ann Emerg Med* 1992;21:1454–1460.
3. Hoffman JR, Mower WR, Wolfson AB, et al. Validity of a set of clinical criteria to rule out injury to the cervical spine in patients with blunt trauma. *N Engl J Med* 2000;343:94–99.
4. Stiell IG, Clement CM, McKnight RD, et al. The Canadian C-Spine Rule versus the NEXUS Low-Risk Criteria in patients with trauma. *N Engl J Med* 2003;349:2510–2518.
5. Grogan EL, Morris JA Jr, Dittus RS, et al. Cervical spine evaluation in urban trauma centers: lowering institutional costs and complications through helical CT scan. *J Am Coll Surg* 2005;200:160–165.
6. Borchgrevink GE, Kaasa A, McDonagh D, et al. Acute treatment of whiplash neck sprain injuries: a randomized trial of treatment during the first 14 days after a car accident. *Spine* 1998;23:25–31.

CHAPTER **8** Cervical Disc Degeneration

Rocco Bassora

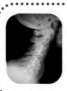 *A 60-year-old woman presents with a 6-month history of neck stiffness, shoulder pain, and headaches.*

Clinical Presentation

Cervical degenerative disc disease is a common cause of neck pain in the elderly, typically causing neck pain, stiffness, and a decreased range of motion. It is much less common than degeneration in the lumbar spine because the neck is generally subjected to much less forces. Nevertheless, degeneration progresses due to the accumulated wear and tear that occurs over a long period of time.

Physical Findings

Patients with cervical degenerative disc disease often complain of low-grade neck pain with stiffness and inflexibility.[1] During the exam, patients should be asked to perform flexion, extension (Fig. 8.1), and rotational movements and report whether the neck pain increases or decreases.[2,3] Additional symptoms may consist of numbness, tingling, or even weakness in the neck, arms, or shoulders as a result of nerves in the cervical area becoming irritated or pinched. Cervical degeneration can become so severe that surrounding osteophytes may encroach on the spinal canal, leading to spinal stenosis and myelopathy. Symptoms of myelopathy include awkward or stumbling gait, difficulty with fine motor skills in the hands and arms, and tingling or shock-type feelings down the torso or into the legs.[4,5] These symptoms are worrisome, and the general practitioner should refer these patients to a spine specialist immediately.

Studies (Labs, X-rays)

Although lab studies are not very useful in the diagnosis of cervical degenerative disc disease, they may be helpful in identifying other disease processes such as rheumatoid arthritis (RA), Reiter's syndrome, and ankylosing spondylitis (AS). RF is often elevated in patients with RA, and HLA-B27 is often elevated in patients with AS. Lab tests such as ESR and CRP are markers for infection and can be used to help diagnose or monitor an infectious process.

CLINICAL POINTS

- In older patients, cervical degenerative disc disease is a frequent cause of neck pain.
- Disc degeneration is much less common in the cervical spine than in the lumbar spine.
- Degeneration results from the "wear and tear" that occurs over time.

Patients who present with neurologic symptoms can be evaluated with studies such as NCS and EMG. These tests can help to determine whether symptoms are due to lesions that are occurring proximally (i.e., cervical nerve root compression, cervical stenosis) or those that are occurring in a more distal location (i.e., cubital tunnel syndrome, carpal tunnel syndrome).

RADIOGRAPHIC EVALUATION

Imaging studies are very helpful in the diagnosis of cervical degenerative disc disease. X-rays of the cervical spine often reveal a decrease in intervertebral disc space, osteophyte formation, and the loss of normal cervical lordosis (Fig. 8.2). Flexion–extension views (Fig. 8.3) can help to determine if cervical instability exists; an AP view can help to identify tumors or fractures; a lateral view helps to define anterior osteophytes and disc space narrowing.

MRI can be utilized to determine whether there is nerve root compression or cervical stenosis in patients who present with neurologic symptoms. Nerve root or spinal cord compression secondary to a herniated nucleus pulposus, abscess, or tumor can be easily identified with MRI.[6,7]

Provocative cervical discography (Fig. 8.4) is an imaging procedure that involves the injection of fluid into the intervertebral disc. If the

SECTION 3 Cervical Spine

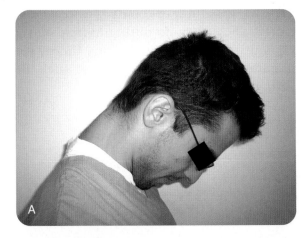
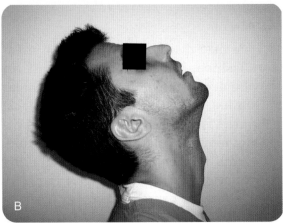

Figure 8.1 A, B: Patient demonstrating flexion and extension of the cervical spine during physical exam.

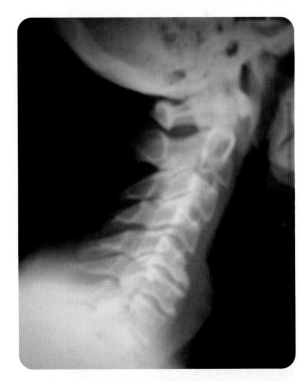

Figure 8.2 Lateral x-ray of the cervical spine. X-ray reveals loss of lordosis, osteophyte formation, and a decrease in disc space.

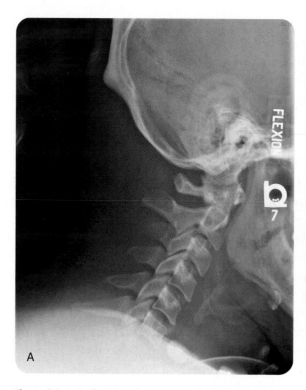
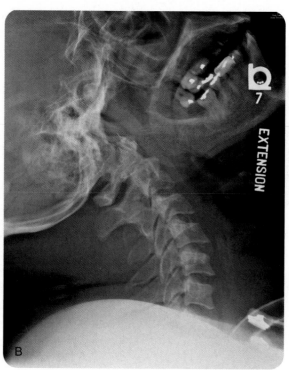

Figure 8.3 A, B: Flexion and extension radiographs.

intervertebral disc is the actual pain generator, patients will have the same exact pain pattern after injection as they do during normal activities of daily living. Discomfort and invasiveness make this procedure less desirable than noninvasive imaging studies, such as x-rays and cervical MRI.[8]

Treatment and Clinical Course

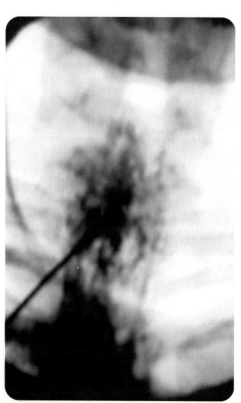

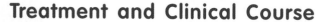

1. NSAIDs
2. Physical therapy, freestyle swimming with snorkel gear
3. Epidural steroids, if needed

NONSURGICAL TREATMENT

Patients with degenerative disc disease can usually be managed in a conservative fashion. Conservative treatment for patients with symptomatic degenerative disc disease includes rest, pain medication, NSAIDs, and physical therapy. The goal of physical therapy is to increase cervical spine flexibility, postural training, and strengthening of paraspinal musculature. Restoring flexibility prevents further repetitive microtrauma from poor movement patterning. Most patients have improvement in symptoms after a 6-week course of physical therapy and NSAIDs.[9]

Other conservative modes of therapy include intermittent cervical traction and epidural injections.[10–13] Cervical traction

Figure 8.4 Cervical discogram.

may relieve radicular pain from nerve root compression by applying enough force to separate the vertebral segments. Light-weight continuous home traction is cost-effective and provides the patient more autonomy.

Epidural corticosteroid injections provide long-lasting relief, allowing patients the opportunity to undergo more aggressive physical therapy. The epidural space is injected to decrease inflammation of the nerve roots, thereby reducing neck and extremity pain. This is typically performed under fluoroscopic guidance, and a mixture of steroid and local anesthetic is typically used.

SURGICAL TREATMENT

Spine surgery is performed if a course of conservative treatment has failed. Surgery consists of disc removal, placement of an intervertebral bone graft, and fusion. Plate fixation is generally used for multiple levels of involvement. Patients are placed in a soft collar postoperatively for comfort and are generally discharged the following day.[14–17]

In conclusion, cervical degenerative disc disease is a long-standing progressive disease that typically affects elderly individuals. Most patients do well with conservative treatment, and surgery is generally reserved for patients who have either failed conservative treatment or have concomitant neurologic symptoms that are progressive in nature.

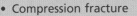

WHEN TO REFER

- Compression fracture
- Cervical myelopathy
- Progressive neurologic symptoms
- Fevers, chills, or other signs of infection
- Failed conservative treatment

 Refer to Patient Education

 Refer to Physical Therapy

ICD9
722.4 Degeneration of cervical intervertebral disc

SECTION 3 Cervical Spine

References

1. Chen TY. The clinical presentation of uppermost cervical disc protrusion. *Spine* 2000;25(4):439–442.
2. Ellenberg MR, Honet JC, Treanor WJ. Cervical radiculopathy. *Arch Phys Med Rehabil* 1994;75(3):342–352.
3. Dwyer A, Aprill C, Bogduk N. Cervical zygapophyseal joint pain patterns. I: A study in normal volunteers. *Spine* 1990;15(6):453–457.
4. Cooper PR. Cervical spondylotic myelopathy. *J Neurosurg Spine* 2005;3(3):253–254; author reply 254.
5. Chagas H, Domingues F, Aversa A, et al. Cervical spondylotic myelopathy: 10 years of prospective outcome analysis of anterior decompression and fusion. *Surg Neurol* 2005;64(Suppl 1):S1:30–35; discussion S1:35–36.
6. Krakenes J, Kaale BR. Magnetic resonance imaging assessment of craniovertebral ligaments and membranes after whiplash trauma. *Spine* 2006;31(24):2820–2826.
7. Noebauer-Huhmann IM, Glaser C, Dietrich O, et al. MR imaging of the cervical spine: assessment of image quality with parallel imaging compared to non-accelerated MR measurements. *Eur Radiol* 2007;17(5):1147–1155.
8. Slipman C, Plastaras C, Patel R, et al. Provocative cervical discography symptom mapping. *Spine J* 2005;5(4):381–388.
9. Slipman C, Lipetz R, Herzog E, et al. Nonsurgical treatment for radicular of pain of zygoapophyseal joint cyst origin: therapeutic selective nerve root block. *Arch Phys Med Rehabil* 2000;81(8):1119–1122.
10. Bush K, Hillier S. Outcome of cervical radiculopathy treated with periradicular/epidural corticosteroid injections: a prospective study with independent clinical review. *Eur Spine J* 1996;5(5):319–325.
11. Slipman CW, Lipetz JS, Jackson HB, et al. Therapeutic selective nerve root block in the nonsurgical treatment of atraumatic cervical spondylotic radicular pain: a retrospective analysis with independent clinical review. *Arch Phys Med Rehabil* 2000;81(6):741–746.
12. Slipman CW, Chow DW. Therapeutic spinal corticosteroid injections for the management of radiculopathies. *Phys Med Rehabil Clin N Am* 2002;13(3):697–711.

13. Slipman CW, Lipetz JS, Plastaras CT, et al. Therapeutic zygapophyseal joint injections for headaches emanating from the C2-3 joint. *Am J Phys Med Rehabil* 2001;80(3):182–188.
14. Boakye M, Mummaneni PV, Garrett M, et al. Anterior cervical discectomy and fusion involving a poly-etheretherketone spacer and bone morphogenetic protein. *J Neurosurg Spine* 2005;2(5):521–525.
15. Yue WM, Brodner W, Highland TR. Long-term results after anterior cervical discectomy and fusion with allograft and plating: a 5- to 11-year radiologic and clinical follow-up study. *Spine* 2005;30(19): 2138–2144.
16. Kwon B, Kim DH, Marvin A, et al. Outcomes following anterior cervical discectomy and fusion: the role of interbody disc height, angulation, and spinous process distance. *J Spinal Disord Tech* 2005;18(4): 304–308.
17. White BD, Fitzgerald JJ. To graft or not to graft: rationalizing choice in anterior cervical discectomy. *Br J Neurosurg* 2005;19(2):148–154.

9 Cervical Disc Herniation

Rocco Bassora

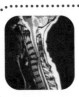 *A 33-year-old man presents with a 1-month history of headaches, neck pain, and right-hand numbness and tingling.*

CLINICAL POINTS

- In young adults, cervical disc herniation often causes neck and arm pain.

- Traumatic episodes may lead to disc herniation.

- Spinal cord (not nerve root) compression requires more aggressive treatment.

PATIENT ASSESSMENT

1. Patients typically complain of frequent headaches and pain/numbness that radiates down an upper extremity.

2. A thorough neurologic exam is necessary.

3. Cervical range of motion typically is limited.

4. MRI is the imaging study of choice.

Clinical Presentation

Cervical disc herniation is a common cause of neck and arm pain in young adults. Disc herniations are often caused by traumatic events, although many cases occur spontaneously. Patients typically complain of frequent headaches, with pain that originates around the paraspinal muscles and radiates down one of the upper extremities. Symptoms of finger numbness and tingling typically occur in conjunction with neck and arm pain.[1,2] In some patients, a cervical herniated disc can cause spinal cord compression (as opposed to just nerve root compression) where disc material pushes directly on the spinal cord. This is a much more serious condition and may require a more aggressive treatment plan. Spinal cord compression symptoms include awkward or stumbling gait, difficulty with fine motor skills in the hands and arms, and tingling or shock-type feelings down the torso or into the legs.[3,4]

Physical Findings

The clinical presentation of a cervical herniated disc can be mistaken for shoulder or forearm pathology. Physicians must therefore perform a careful examination of the shoulder and wrist to rule out shoulder or wrist pathology. Patients often complain of pain, weakness, numbness, and tingling that begins in the shoulder region and extends down into the fingers.[1]

Range of motion is typically limited secondary to pain. The paraspinal muscles may go into spasm, causing great discomfort on palpation. Most herniations occur between C5 and T1, and the most common location is the C5-6 disc space. Patients present with biceps weakness as well as with pain and numbness in the thumb and index fingers.[5] Symptoms vary depending on which nerve root is involved. Table 9.1 lists the different cervical nerve roots with their corresponding sensory and motor disturbances. Symptoms are typically unilateral unless there is a central herniation, which would cause bilateral symptomatology. Pain can often be

Table 9.1	Cervical Nerve Roots and Their Corresponding Sensory and Motor Disturbances	
	NERVE ROOT AFFECTED	**PHYSICAL FINDINGS**
C4-5	C5	• Deltoid muscle weakness • Does not usually cause numbness or tingling • Can cause shoulder pain
C5-6	C6	• Biceps weakness • Numbness and tingling along with pain can radiate to thumb side of hand • Most common level for a cervical disc herniation to occur
C6-7	C7	• Triceps and finger extensor weakness • Numbness and tingling along with pain can radiate down triceps and into middle finger • Second most common level for a cervical disc herniation to occur
C7-T1	C8	• Can cause weakness with handgrip • Numbness and tingling and pain can radiate down arm to small finger

reproduced with the Spurling maneuver (Fig. 9.1). The head is placed into an extended position, and the patient's chin is rotated toward the affected side. A compressive force is then placed onto the patient's head, and symptoms of nerve impingement are reproduced.[6] On the flip side, patients typically get relief of symptoms when asked to place their hands on top of their heads (abduction relief sign).

Patients with myelopathic symptoms complain of weakness and clumsiness of the upper extremities as well as difficulty with maintaining lower extremity balance. Certain physical findings such as clonus, hyperreflexia, and the Babinski sign (Fig. 9.2) are present in patients with myelopathy.[7]

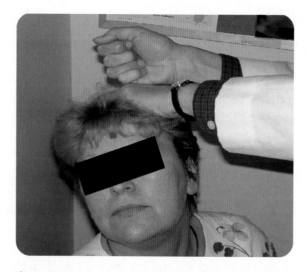

Figure 9.1 Spurling maneuver. The patient's neck is extended and rotated in the direction of symptoms. A compressive force is then applied as shown. This reproduces the symptoms of nerve root compression.

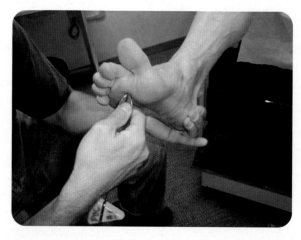

Figure 9.2 Babinski reflex.

Studies (Labs, Nerve, Imaging)

Laboratory studies are generally not helpful in the diagnoses of cervical disc herniation but may identify various disease processes such as rheumatoid arthritis (RA), ankylosing spondylitis, and Reiter syndrome. These tests include RF (elevated in RA), HLA-B27 (positive in ankylosing spondylitis), and ESR (elevated in polymyalgia rheumatica). A WBC count, blood cultures, and ESR rate can also determine whether an infectious process is present.

The neurologic function of the cervical spine can be evaluated with the use of NCS and EMG. The advantages of using these tests include limited expense and low morbitity. NCS-EMG is especially helpful to differentiate cervical radiculopathy from confounding neuropathic conditions such as ulnar nerve entrapment, carpal tunnel syndrome, and peripheral neuropathy.[8]

RADIOGRAPHIC EVALUATION

Imaging studies that are routinely performed include cervical x-rays and MRI. A CT-myelogram is rarely ordered by spine surgeons in patients who had a prior cervical spine surgery and may provide complementary information to an MRI. Plain cervical spine radiographs may reveal sequelae of chronic degenerative disc disease, including a loss of the normal cervical lordosis, osteophytes, and a decrease in disc space (Fig. 9.3). They are generally not helpful in patients with acute herniated discs.

MRI remains the imaging modality of choice to evaluate cervical herniated nucleus pulposus due to its low morbidity, high sensitivity, and high specificity[9] (Fig. 9.4). The advantages include excellent soft tissue definition,

SECTION 3 Cervical Spine

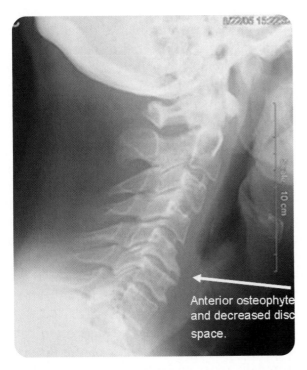

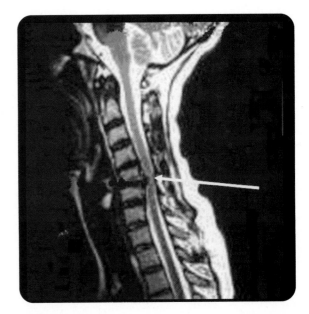

Figure 9.3 Lateral x-ray of the cervical spine. X-ray reveals loss of lordosis, osteophyte formation, and a decrease in disc space.

Figure 9.4 Sagittal MRI. Image reveals a herniated disc protruding into the spinal cord.

cerebral spinal fluid visualization, noninvasiveness, and lack of patient radiation exposure. A herniated disc is readily visualized on the sagittal cut as a soft tissue protrusion into the spinal canal, compressing the involved nerve root. Axial cuts determine in which direction the disc is protruding, helping to correlate radiographic findings with physical exam findings.[6,9–11]

Treatment and Clinical Course

1. NSAIDs and pain medication in conjunction with therapy is highly effective.
2. Cervical epidural steroids can be helpful.
3. Surgical discectomy and fusion are indicated in a minority of cases.

NON-SURGICAL TREATMENT

Most patients do not require surgery. Initially, cold and heat modalities as well as NSAIDs may help to alleviate symptoms. Cold therapy is generally used in the first 48 hours following the onset of pain; it diminishes blood flow to the involved area, which helps to reduce swelling, muscle spasm, and pain. After the first 48 hours, heat therapy can be applied. Heat increases blood flow to warm and relax soft tissues, thereby increasing blood flow and flushing away irritating toxins.[12]

Medications include NSAIDs to reduce swelling, a muscle relaxant to calm spasm, and a painkiller (narcotic) to alleviate intense but acute pain. Physical therapy is an integral part of treating the cervical spine. Physical therapy consists of gentle massage, stretching, and neck traction and is often carried out for several weeks. Most patients have improvement in symptoms after a 6-week course of physical therapy and NSAIDs.

Spinal epidural injections also play a role in the treatment of cervical herniated discs. The epidural space is injected to decrease inflammation of the nerve roots, thereby reducing the pain in the neck, shoulders, and arms. This is usually performed under fluoroscopic guidance, and a mixture of steroid and local anesthetic is typically used.[13,14]

SURGICAL TREATMENT

Spine surgery is considered if nonsurgical treatment does not relieve symptoms or if cervical myelopathy is suspected. To relieve nerve pressure and neck pain, surgery usually involves the removal of the disc through an anterior approach (i.e., an anterior cervical discectomy and fusion with plate [Fig. 9.5] fixation.[7] Bone graft is then placed into the disc space. Either allograft (bone graft from a cadaver) or autograft (bone graft taken from the patient's iliac crest) can be used.

In conclusion, a herniated disc often causes great discomfort in the acute stages of the disease process. Fortunately, most patients become better with conservative management. It is important for the primary care

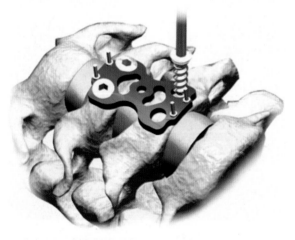

Figure 9.5 Anterior cervical decompression with plate fixation.

WHEN TO REFER

- Cervical myelopathy
- Progressive neurologic symptoms
- Fevers, chills, or other signs of infection
- Failed conservative treatment

physician to recognize more serious processes, such as myelopathy or progressive neurologic deficit, and that the patient is referred to an orthopaedic spine specialist accordingly.

Refer to Physical Therapy

ICD9
722.0 Displacement of cervical intervertebral disc without myelopathy

References

1. Dwyer A, Aprill C, Bogduk N. Cervical zygapophyseal joint pain patterns. I: A study in normal volunteers. *Spine* 1990;15(6):453–457.
2. Aprill C, Dwyer A, Bogduk N. Cervical zygapophyseal joint pain patterns. II: A clinical evaluation. *Spine* 1990;15(6):458–461.
3. Carette S, Fehlings M. Clinical practice. Cervical radiculopathy. *N Engl J Med* 2005;353(4):392–399.
4. Chen TY. The clinical presentation of uppermost cervical disc protrusion. *Spine* 2000;25(4):439–442.
5. Heckmann JG, Lang CJ, Zöbelein I, et al. Herniated cervical intervertebral discs with radiculopathy: an outcome study of conservatively or surgically treated patients. *J Spinal Disord* 1999;12(5):396–401.
6. Rubinstein S, Pool J, Tulder M, et al. A systematic review of the diagnostic accuracy of provocative tests of the neck for diagnosing cervical radiculopathy. *Eur Spine J* 2007;16(3):307–319.
7. Aryan HE, Sanchez-Mejia RO, Ben-Haim S, et al. Successful treatment of cervical myelopathy with minimal morbidity by circumferential decompression and fusion. *Eur Spine J* 2007;16(9):1401–1409.
8. Alrawi MF, Khalil NM, Mitchell P, et al. The value of neurophysiological and imaging studies in predicting outcome in the surgical treatment of cervical radiculopathy. *Eur Spine J* 2007;16(4):495–500.
9. Noebauer-Huhmann IM, Glaser C, Dietrich O, et al. MR imaging of the cervical spine: assessment of image quality with parallel imaging compared to non-accelerated MR measurements. *Eur Radiol* 2007;15(5):1147–1155.
10. Krakenes J, Kaale BR. Magnetic resonance imaging assessment of craniovertebral ligaments and membranes after whiplash trauma. *Spine* 2006;31(24):2820–2826.
11. Peterson CK, Humphreys BK, Pringle TC. Prevalence of Modic degenerative marrow changes in the cervical spine. *J Manipulative Physiol Ther* 2007;30(1):5–10.
12. Murphy DR. Herniated disc with radiculopathy following cervical manipulation: nonsurgical management. *Spine J* 2006;6(4):459–463.
13. Slipman C, Lipetz J, Herzog R, et al. Nonsurgical treatment for radicular of pain of zygoapophyseal joint cyst origin: therapeutic selective nerve root block. *Arch Phys Med Rehabil* 2000;81(8):1119–1122.
14. Slipman CW, Lipetz JS, Jackson HB, et al. Outcomes of therapeutic selective nerve root blocks for whiplash induced cervical radicular pain. *Pain Physician* 2001;4(2):167–174.

CHAPTER 10 Spinal Stenosis

Jaehon M. Kim and Kingsley R. Chin

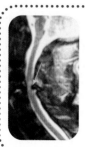

A 74-year-old man presents with neck and shoulder pain and vague complaints of bilateral arm and hand weakness of unknown etiology.

Clinical Presentation

Cervical stenosis refers to narrowing of the spinal canal and in some cases may lead to neural compression and subsequent radiculopathy or myelopathy. Radiculopathy results from root compression and symptoms usually follow a dermatomal pattern, while myelopathy results from cord compression and symptoms are more diffuse. The natural history of cervical myelopathy is characterized by disease progression, usually in a stepwise fashion from subtle early symptoms to more advanced manifestations including bowel and bladder incontinence, but rapid progression can also occur. It is imperative to recognize possible cervical cord compression early to prevent irreversible damage to the cord. Pain alone is not a sensitive predictor of which patients have cervical myelopathy or who will need treatment.

Only about half of the patients with symptomatic cervical stenosis have neck and arm pain. Others present with vague and nonspecific neurologic symptoms. In the upper extremities, patient may complain of feeling clumsy with tendency to drop objects, inability to perform fine motor control, and vague sensory complaints that do not adhere to dermatomal distribution. In the lower extremities, patients may have difficulty walking secondary to imbalance with frequent falls. Subjective weakness, bowel and bladder incontinence, and proprioceptive dysfunctions imply advanced disease. Patients with severe cord compression may demonstrate a positive Lhermitte sign, where an electric-shocklike sensation radiates down the spine or extremities with certain movements of the neck, especially during flexion and extension.

Physical Findings

Physical findings in patients with cervical stenosis and cord compression are often nonspecific and nondiagnostic. However, a full neurologic exam

CLINICAL POINTS

- Patients may have neck and arm pain.

- Others may present with clumsiness or balance problems.

- Nerve compression and radiculopathy or myelopathy may result.

- It is essential to recognize cervical cord compression early to prevent irreversible damage to the spinal cord.

is imperative to apply important findings in conjunction with imaging studies to plan appropriate management (operative vs. nonoperative). Motor testing uncommonly reveals any weakness of the major muscle groups, and if muscle weaknesses are present, they usually manifest as weakness of the intrinsic hand muscles and difficulty of fine motor control. Sensory examinations are nondermatomal in nature, with a variety of symptoms including pain, numbness, and tingling sensation as well as proprioceptive impairment on both upper and lower extremities.

Since cervical stenosis causing cord compression is mainly an upper motor lesion, patients are expected to have hyperreflexia in their upper and lower extremities. Patients may have ankle clonus, which can be elicited by sudden dorsiflexion of the ankle by the examiner and noted for involuntary flexion–extension of the ankle. Some of the earliest signs of cord compression include gait changes and increased knee and ankle reflexes. However, in those patients with cervical stenosis and coexisting lumbar stenosis, brisk upper extremity reflexes can be elicited consistent with upper motor lesion, while the lower extremities may have diminished reflexes secondary to nerve root compression (lower motor neuron). Many patients also have concomitant medical conditions including diabetic peripheral neuropathy and carpal tunnel syndrome, making it difficult to isolate cervical myelopathy.

Several tests are available for evaluating cervical stenosis. Some of the common ones include the Lhermitte sign, Babinski reflex, Hoffmann sign, Spurling sign, and jaw jerk test. The Babinski reflex is a commonly used sign to elucidate upper motor lesion where upward movement of the great toe is considered abnormal in adults when the sole of the foot is stroked. If present, a positive Babinski sign is a poor prognostic indicator in cervical stenosis. The Hoffmann sign is an upper extremity counterpart of the Babinski reflex, and it can be elicited by flicking the volar surface of the third distal phalanx of relaxed and slightly flexed fingers, which results in pathologic flexion of the thumb and index finger (Fig. 10.1). The jaw jerk test is not used to evaluate cervical stenosis but rather to differentiate cervical myelopathy from the lesions in the brain. Tapping the lower jaw leads to abnormal opening of the mouth, which indicate brain pathology.[1] Patients with root compression may have reproduction of their radicular symptoms when the neck is rotated and the examiner's hand presses down on the top of the head (positive Spurling sign) (Fig. 10.2).

The causes of spinal stenosis may be divided according to compression from anterior or posterior structures. Anteriorly, herniated disks; ossification of the posterior longitudinal ligament (OPLL); and osteophytic spurs from the back of the vertebral bodies, endplates, or uncovertebral joints are the common culprits of cord

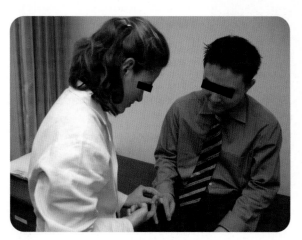

Figure 10.1 The Hoffman sign is elicited by dorsiflexing the distal interphalangeal joint with the phalanx in extension. Extending the neck will narrow the spinal canal and may increase the chances of a positive Hoffman.

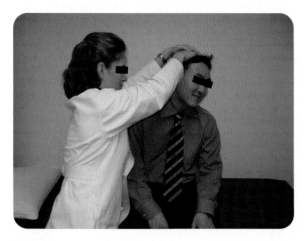

Figure 10.2 The Spurling sign is demonstrated with the examiner's hands applying axial pressure on the head while the patient's neck is rotated and tilted laterally. This maneuver closes down the foramen and may cause nerve root compression by an osteophyte or herniated disc.

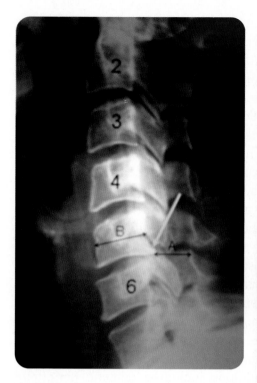

Figure 10.3 A posterior vertebral osteophyte (*yellow arrow*). The Pavlov ratio is calculated as the vertebral body AP length divided by the space available for the spinal cord (A = AP diameter of spinal cord; B = AP diameter of vertebral body).

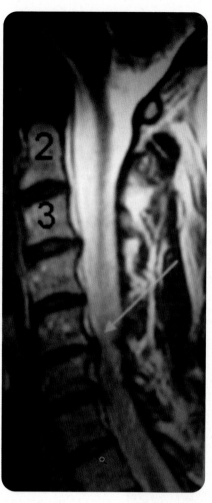

Figure 10.4 Herniated disc–osteophyte complex causing stenosis of the spinal canal.

and root compression (Figs. 10.3, 10.4) Osteophytic spurs develop as a reactive response to hypermobility of the adjacent degenerative disk.[2] The increased stress on the articular cartilage and endplates of the vertebrae stimulates osteophytic spur formation as the body naturally tries to stabilize the spine. OPLL causes cord compression and myelopathy and is more common in Asians and in patients with diffuse idiopathic skeletal hyperostosis. The ligamentum flavum is the main culprit causing posterior compression, losing its tension and buckling into the canal as the disc degenerates anteriorly (Fig. 10.5). The ligamentum flavum may also hypertrophy or ossify to cause more compression to the spinal cord. Anatomically, the spinal cord may stretch over the anterior osteophyte during flexion or be compressed by the ligamentum flavum during extension. In severe spinal stenosis, anterior and posterior compression may exist on the spinal cord even in a neutral spine, causing a pincer effect.

Not all patients have the same degree of symptoms even with similar levels of cervical stenosis. Cervical myelopathy secondary to stenosis often occur in patients with congenital narrowing of the cervical canal. These patients without any cervical pathology may have enough space to provide for the spinal cord. With age, however, degenerative changes cause the canal to become stenotic, with inability to compensate for the narrowing space. Some congenital cervical stenoses are severe, causing symptoms in patients as young as 30 and 40 years old. Other uncommon but important diagnoses to consider include epidural abscess, amyotrophic lateral sclerosis, multiple sclerosis, syringomyelia, primary or metastatic spinal cord tumors, and stroke.[3]

Studies (Labs, X-rays)

MRI AND CT MYELOGRAM

MRI is the diagnostic tool of choice for evaluating cervical stenosis and its associated pathology. It is noninvasive and provides images in multiple

NOT TO BE MISSED

- Epidural abscess
- Multiple sclerosis
- Amyotrophic lateral sclerosis
- Syringomyelia
- Neoplasm
- Rheumatoid arthritis
- Os odontoideum
- Trauma in an ankylosing spondylitic patient

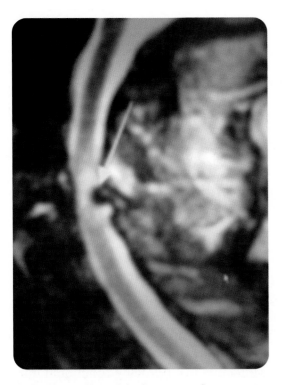

Figure 10.5 Buckling of the ligamentum flavum causing spinal stenosis, cord compression, and myelomalacia. This patient is at risk for central cord syndrome with trauma.

planes, which may elucidate the cause of patient's symptoms. Furthermore, signal changes in the spinal cord and discs can provide valuable information regarding the extent of damage and degeneration. If for various reasons MRI is not feasible, CT scan combined with myelography can be utilized to provide excellent delineation of bony and neural structures of the cervical spine.[4] However, CT myelogram is an invasive procedure and a poor screening test. It should mainly be utilized for surgical planning, especially in patents who have had prior cervical surgery.

CERVICAL X-RAYS

Upright AP, lateral, obliques, flexion, and extension plain radiographs should be obtained in almost all cases before obtaining a MRI or CT myelogram. Flexion–extension views can demonstrate spondylolisthesis and the possibility that a patient is having dynamic compression of the spinal cord with neck movement (Fig. 10.6). Oblique radiographs can demonstrate uncovertebral spurs and foraminal stenosis. A lateral radiograph can be useful for determining the degree of congenital cervical stenosis by assessing the space available for the cord (SAC) (Fig. 10.3). The SAC is the AP diameter of the canal. Patients with a SAC <13 mm are considered stenotic.[5] Another measurement of stenosis is the Pavlov ratio. This is the ratio of the AP diameter of the canal (SAC) divided by the AP diameter of the vertebral body.[6] A nonstenotic spine should have a ratio of approximately 1.0, while a ratio <0.8 is suggestive of congenital stenosis. The Pavlov ratio can be incorrectly low in patients with large vertebral bodies and who are not stenotic, such as athletes. Therefore, the SAC is more reliable. In athletes, a low Pavlov ratio puts the athlete at a higher risk of transient quadriparesis but does not predict who will have permanent quadriplegia and therefore has lost favor as a method to screen players from participating in athletics. EMGs are rarely useful to evaluate spinal cord pathology but may be indicated when peripheral neuropathy is suspected.

Treatment and Clinical Course

1. Use of NSAIDs and physical therapy may be helpful.
2. Serial examination to rule out progression of stenosis is indicated.
3. Epidural steroid injections can moderate symptoms.
4. Surgeon evaluation is recommended in the patient with an abnormal neurologic exam.

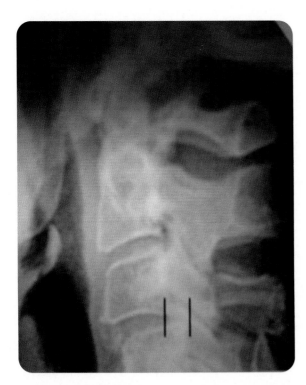

Figure 10.6 Slippage of one vertebra anterior to the adjacent vertebra (spondylolisthesis).

NONOPERATIVE MANAGEMENT

Asymptomatic cervical stenosis or stenosis causing mildly symptomatic myelopathy may be followed but observed closely. Instructions should be given to patients to report any new or worsening symptoms. However, patients with severe cord compression on MRI may be recommended for surgery regardless of any clinical findings. The progression of disease in patients with mild or no symptoms is difficult to predict. Approximately 20% of patients will resolve spontaneously, while 40% will stabilize and the rest will clinically deteriorate.[7] Nonoperative measures such as cervical immobilization and physical therapy so far have been equivocal with varying degree of success.[8]

OPERATIVE MANAGEMENT

The optimal treatment for symptomatic myelopathy is surgery. If left untreated, the risk of worsening compression is high with subsequent neurologic deterioration. The outcome is less predictable if symptoms are left untreated for >6 months. There are a number of surgical options available, and the site of compression usually dictates the approach. Surgical intervention has shown to be effective in improving functional outcome, alleviating pain, and stabilizing neurologic status. It is important to recognize that early operative measures may prevent permanent spinal cord damage.

 Refer to Physical Therapy

> **ICD9**
>
> *723.0 Spinal stenosis in cervical region*
> *724.00 Spinal stenosis of unspecified region*
> *724.09 Spinal stenosis of other region*

WHEN TO REFER

- Abnormal radiologic finding
- Bladder and bowel dysfunction
- Gait instability
- Upper extremity clumsiness
- Symptom progression
- Deteriorating function
- No improvement after conservative treatment for 4 months

References

1. Rhee JM, Riew KD. Cervical spondylotic myelopathy: including ossification of the posterior longitudinal ligament. In: Spivak JM, Connolly PJ, eds. *Orthopaedic Knowledge Update: Spine 3.* Rosemont, IL: AAOS Press; 2006:235–249.
2. Wilkinson M. The morbid anatomy of cervical spondylosis and myelopathy. *Brain* 1960;83:589–616.
3. Young WF. Cervical spondylotic myelopathy: a common cause of spinal cord dysfunction in older persons. *Am Fam Physician* 2000;62:1064–1070.
4. Freeman TB, Martinez CR. Radiological evaluation of cervical spondylotic disease: limitation of magnetic resonance imaging for diagnosis and preoperative assessment. *Perspect Neurol Surg* 1992;3:34–36.
5. Kang JD, Figgie MP, Bohlman HH. Sagittal measurements of the cervical spine in subaxial fractures and dislocations. An analysis of two hundred and eighty-eight patients with and without neurological deficits. *J Bone Joint Surg Am* 1994;76(11):1617–1628.
6. Torg JS, Naranja RJ Jr, Palov H, et al. The relationship of developmental narrowing of the cervical spinal canal to reversible and irreversible injury of the cervical spinal cord in football players. *J Bone Joint Surg Am* 1996;78(9):1308–1314.
7. Kumar VG, Rea GL, Mervis LJ, et al. Cervical spondylotic myelopathy: functional and radiographic long-term outcome after laminectomy and posterior fusion. *Neurosurgery* 1999;44:771–778.
8. Roberts AH. Myelopathy due to cervical spondylosis treated by collar immobilization. *Neurology* 1966; 16:951–954.

Hip

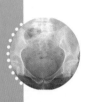
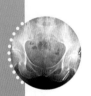

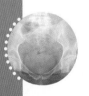

11 Trochanteric Bursitis

Charles L. Nelson and Kristofer J. Jones

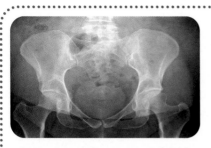

A 42-year-old woman presents with a 4-month history of intermittent left lateral hip pain that extends down into the lateral aspect of the thigh. She describes an intense, sharp pain that it is particularly worse when she attempts to lie on either side. The pain has become greater over the past few months, and she now experiences significant discomfort with routine activities such as climbing stairs and rising out of a chair. She reports that she has been taking four tablets of NSAIDs with mild relief. An AP radiograph of the pelvis is taken.

CLINICAL POINTS

- Inflammation or irritation of the bursae surrounding the hip may lead to symptoms.
- This condition is more common in adults between the fourth and sixth decades of life.
- Women are more likely to have this problem.
- Inflammation triggered by focal trauma is a causal factor.

Clinical Presentation

There are approximately 14 to 21 bursae surrounding the hip joint. It is the aggregate of bursae around the greater trochanter that are responsible for the constellation of symptoms characterized as trochanteric bursitis. Of the four bursae typically found in the area of the greater trochanter, three are constant: (a) gluteus minimus bursa, (b) subgluteus medius bursa, and (c) subgluteus maximus bursa. Ultimately, any inflammation or irritation of these bursae can result in symptoms characteristic of trochanteric bursitis.[1–5]

Various researchers state that trochanteric bursitis is likely often associated with repetitive microtrauma caused by dynamic use of the muscles that insert on the greater trochanter. Consistent active use of these specific muscles can lead to the insidious degeneration of tendons, muscles, and fibrous tissue in the area secondary to localized inflammation. In fact, the inflammatory processes incited by focal trauma have been clearly shown to be a cause of trochanteric bursitis.[6] Additional identifiable causes include any condition that creates alterations in the regular biomechanics of the hip that potentially lead to abnormal stresses and shear forces of the tendons gliding over these bursae. Such predisposing conditions include osteoarthritis, lumbar spine disease, leg-length inequalities, and ipsilateral knee and quadriceps weakness.[7] Occasionally, localized calcification in the area of involvement can be observed, and it is still unclear if these calcifications are related to degenerative changes of the tendons and bursae secondary to trauma and inflammation or biomechanical alterations at the hip. Currently, many researchers believe that bursal inflammation associated with tendinous calcifications is most likely a secondary phenomenon.[8]

The majority of patients with trochanteric bursitis present with complaints of chronic or subacute symptoms of aching pain in the lateral hip localized to the area overlying the greater trochanter. The pain is classically described as a sharp and intense pain. In a small number of patients, the initial symptoms may be experienced in the area of the lumbar back or near the knee; however, the typical distribution of pain usually becomes apparent as time progresses.[8] Occasionally, patients may report that the pain radiates along the lateral thigh toward the knee but rarely beyond the insertion site of the iliotibial tract.[9] Frequently, patients may experience numbness and paresthesias that do not follow a dermatomal distribution in the proximal thigh. The incidence of trochanteric bursitis peaks between the fourth and sixth decades of life, with a female-to-male preponderance of 4:1.[8,10] Further diagnostic clues include exacerbation of pain while lying on the affected side or while climbing stairs.

Physical Findings

Findings consistent with trochanteric bursitis on physical examination include localized tenderness to palpation over the tip of the lateral or posterior aspects of the greater trochanter. While the patient is lying in the lateral decubitus position with the affected hip up, the clinician should palpate the hip in a cephalad direction, beginning below the greater trochanteric eminence until the area of maximal tenderness is localized.[11] The area of extreme sensitivity is usually found near the gluteus medius insertion site on the greater trochanter.[11] In three separate series evaluating physical signs in patients with confirmed diagnoses, focal tenderness was present in over 90% of patients.[12–14] Painful symptoms typically increase with specific maneuvers at the hip, namely extreme hip abduction and external rotation. The majority of patients demonstrate pain on Patrick-fabere testing of the affected leg. With this test, the patient lies supine and places the foot of his or her affected side on the contralateral knee, actively flexing, abducting, and externally rotating the lower extremity.[8] The patient should be carefully assessed for any evidence of associated conditions such as osteoarthritis, leg-length inequality, and degenerative disc disease, as treatment of these disorders can potentially lead to resolution of symptoms. Ege Rasmussen and Fano[15] suggested a modified set of criteria, which include many of the aforementioned signs and symptoms, to establish the clinical diagnosis of trochanteric bursitis (Table 11.1).

Studies

IMAGING

While the diagnosis of trochanteric bursitis primarily relies on clinical findings, there are many reports detailing various findings on imaging studies that are associated with the condition. As mentioned previously, local calcifications can be identified in the region of the trochanteric bursa with the use of plain radiographs; these are thought to be a result of local inflammatory processes. These calcifications are extremely variable in size

PATIENT ASSESSMENT

1. Common problem
2. Well-localized tenderness over trochanter
3. Pain on flexion, external rotation, and abduction
4. X-rays negative, rule out stress fractures and avascular necrosis
5. May be persistent

NOT TO BE MISSED

- *Femoral neck stress fracture:* Patient has localized hip pain that worsens with activity and typically improves with rest. Radiographs of stress fractures are often negative, just as plain radiographs of a patient with trochanteric bursitis. The diagnosis can be established with a bone scan, MRI, or diagnostic injection with local anesthetic into the bursa. It is important to distinguish these diagnoses to prevent fracture displacement.

- *Avascular necrosis:* Patient rarely presents with lateral hip pain; instead, the pain is typically localized to the groin. There is no local tenderness.

- *Labral tear:* Patient present with complaints of painful clicking in the hip and pain with passive motion. Typically, there is no point tenderness. If the diagnosis is unclear, MR arthrography can help to elucidate the labral tear.

Table 11.1 List of Signs and Symptoms Necessary for Clinical Diagnosis of Trochanteric Bursitis[a,b]

1. Pain over the area of the lateral hip
2. Focal tenderness in the area overlying the greater trochanter
3. Pain with passive hip rotation, abduction, or adduction (also includes pain with positive Patrick-fabere test)
4. Pain with resisted hip abduction.
5. Presence of pain radiating down the lateral thigh

---

[a] From Ege Rasmussen KJ, Fano N. Trochanteric bursitis: treatment by corticosteroid injection. *Scand J Rheumatol* 1985;14:417–420.
[b] Three of five criteria must be present to make clinical diagnosis, with two of the three signs/symptoms constituting numbers 1 and 2.

and appear as linear or small, rounded masses that can be separated or gathered together. The frequency of these calcifications ranges from 27% to 40%.[12,13] Radiographs of the hip, pelvis, and surrounding areas may reveal associated musculoskeletal conditions, thereby allowing an optimal treatment plan to be devised.

MRI can be helpful in both confirming the diagnosis of trochanteric bursitis and ruling out more serious diagnoses of lateral hip pain. A study by Caruso and Toney[16] found that an abnormal increased signal in the greater trochanteric bursa on T2-weighted images, representative of increased fluid, is common in trochanteric bursitis. These researchers further demonstrated that bone scan imaging could be used to elucidate the large inflammatory process involved in this condition, as early scan images showed increased tracer uptake in the affected area. Overall, these advanced imaging studies can help to confirm the diagnosis of trochanteric bursitis, but they are unnecessary if a careful clinical history and physical are performed.

DIAGNOSTIC INJECTION

The most useful and definitive test in establishing the diagnosis of trochanteric bursitis is a diagnostic injection of the greater trochanteric bursa with a local anesthetic and corticosteroid. If the patient experiences significant relief following administration of these medications, the diagnosis is confirmed.[7]

Treatment

1. NSAIDs
2. Injection with intrabursal cortisone and local anesthetic
3. May be persistent; occasional surgery required for chronic and recurrent pain

Most cases of trochanteric bursitis are relatively mild and can be effectively treated with conservative therapy. An initial treatment protocol should consist of NSAIDs and focused physical therapy directed at strengthening and stretching the muscles around the hip. A study by Krout and Anderson[17] investigating the efficacy of conservative management of trochanteric bursitis revealed that when the pathologic process is secondary to an associated musculoskeletal condition such as surrounding muscle atrophy or leg-length discrepancy, focused treatment of the underlying problem can lead to prompt resolution of symptoms.

If conservative measures fail and symptoms of pain and functional limitations persist, the clinician may resort to local administration of a combined anesthetic and corticosteroid solution. A study by Schapira and colleagues[18] demonstrated resolution of symptoms in all 59 patients treated with a local anesthetic/corticosteroid solution.

INJECTION TECHNIQUE

When an injection is indicated, the point of maximal tenderness is identified by palpation on physical examination. The injection site is then prepped in a sterile manner. The size of the needle that is used is dependent on the patient's body habitus. The clinician should direct the needle toward the greater trochanter until contact is made with the bone to serve as confirmation of appropriate depth and position. Once bony contact is established, the needle should be withdrawn approximately 5 to 10 mm to ensure that the tip of the needle is in the bursa. Betamethasone or methylprednisolone can be combined with lidocaine and injected at the site. About half of the mixture is injected directly into the bursa, and the remaining solution should be administered in the surrounding area.

Occasionally, some patients may experience intractable symptoms that do not respond to conservative measures. Surgery should be considered for patients who do not demonstrate adequate symptomatic relief following an extensive nonoperative treatment regimen. Prior to considering surgery, a repeated diagnostic injection should demonstrate a transient response to a local anesthetic and corticosteroid but fail to provide a satisfactory long-term response.[7] Furthermore, other potential sources of pain in the area should be ruled out with a complete diagnostic workup to reaffirm the diagnosis of trochanteric bursitis. Overall, there are myriad available surgical techniques to treat refractory trochanteric bursitis, and the majority of them involve the same basic principles of local débridement, removal of local calcifications, and an iliotibial band release.[7]

 Refer to Patient Education

 Refer to Physical Therapy

Clinical Course

According to Roberts and Williams,[19] trochanteric bursitis is the second most common cause of lateral hip pain, after osteoarthritis.[19] The primary criteria utilized to make the diagnosis are marked tenderness to deep palpation immediately over the greater trochanter and relief of pain following

WHEN TO REFER

- If an adequate trial of conservative therapy (6 months duration) fails

- Diagnostic injection demonstrates a short-lived response; surgical referral should occur when these conditions have been satisfied, and the patient should be encouraged that several operations are available and that the majority of them have proved to be efficacious.[7]

diagnostic injection with corticosteroids and local anesthetics. Once the diagnosis is established, conservative therapy should be utilized to manage the patient. This form of therapeutic management is typically successful in facilitating resolution of symptoms. In a study by Gordon,[13] 54 of 61 patients (89%) experienced good or excellent results without any surgical intervention. On rare occasion, patients may require surgery for definitive relief.

ICD9
726.5 Enthesopathy of hip region

References

1. Leonard MH. Trochanteric syndrome. *JAMA* 1958;168:175–177.
2. Bywaters EGL. The bursae of the body (editorial). *Ann Rheum Dis* 1965;24:215–218.
3. Cloyd WL. Bursitis of the hip. *Mississippi Valley Med J* 1954;76:219–220.
4. Slawski DP, Howard RF. Surgical management of refractory trochanteric bursitis. *Am J Sports Med* 1997;25:86–89.
5. Swezey RL. Pseudoradiculopathy in subacute trochanteric bursitis of the subgluteus maximus bursa. *Arch Phys Med Rehab* 1976;57:387–390.
6. Haller CC, Coleman PA, Estes NC, et al. Traumatic trochanteric bursitis. *Kans Med* 1989;90:17–18.
7. Berry DJ. Soft tissue disorders. In: Callaghan JJ, Rosenberg AG, Rubash HE, eds. *The Adult Hip*, Vol. 1. Philadelphia: Lippincott–Raven Publishers; 1998:593–601.
8. Shbeeb MI, Matteson EL. Trochanteric bursitis (greater trochanter pain syndrome). *Mayo Clin Proc* 1996;71:565–569.
9. Hays MB. The trochanteric syndrome. *J Bone Joint Surg Am* 1963;45:657.
10. Bird PA, Oakley SP, Shnier R, et al. Prospective evaluation of magnetic resonance imaging and physical examination findings in patients with greater trochanteric pain syndrome. *Arthritis Rheum* 2001;44(9):2138–2145.
11. Little H. Trochanteric bursitis: A common cause of pelvic girdle pain. *Can Med Assoc J* 1979;120:456–458.
12. Anderson TP. Trochanteric bursitis: Diagnostic criteria and clinical significance. *Arch Phys Med Rehab* 1958;39:617–622.
13. Gordon EJ. Trochanteric bursitis and tendinitis. *Clin Orthop* 1961;20:193–202.
14. Spear IM, Lipscomb PR. Noninfectious trochanteric bursitis and peritendinitis. *Surg Clin North Am* 1952;32:1217–1224.
15. Ege Rasmussen KJ, Fano N. Trochanteric bursitis: Treatment by corticosteroid injection. *Scand J Rheumatol* 1985;14:417–420.
16. Caruso FA, Toney MAO. Trochanteric bursitis: a case report of plain film, scintigraphic, and MRI correlation. *Clin Nucl Med* 1994;19(5):393–395.
17. Krout RM, Anderson TP. Trochanteric bursitis: management. *Arch Phys Med Rehab* 1959;40:8–14.
18. Schapira D, Nahir M, Scharf Y. Trochanteric bursitis: a common clinical problem. *Arch Phys Med Rehab* 1986;67:815–817.
19. Roberts WN, Williams RB. Hip pain. *Prim Care* 1988;15:783–793.

CHAPTER 12

Osteoarthritis of the Hip

Charles L. Nelson and Kristofer J. Jones

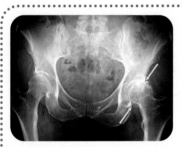

A 62-year-old obese woman reports left lateral hip pain of gradual onset during the past 12 months that has significantly limited her activities. She reports that the pain is particularly bad following activities and denies any morning stiffness or pain in other joints. She cannot recall any preceding traumatic injury to the area and states that she has been taking six to eight ibuprofen tablets per day, which has provided mild relief. AP radiographs of both hips were obtained.

CLINICAL POINTS

- Many people older than 60 years have this condition.
- Changes in quality of life may result, especially in people who are active.
- Clinical course is quite variable.
- Onset of symptoms is gradual.

Clinical Presentation

Osteoarthritis is the most prevalent form of arthritis and is a leading cause of impaired mobility in the elderly. The clinical course of osteoarthritis of the hip is highly variable, as associated symptoms can temporarily improve in some patients, remain stable for many patients, or progressively become worse in many. Arthritic disease of the hip can hinder lifestyle choices in the active aging population, thereby significantly affecting an individual's quality of life. Unfortunately, many patients with arthritis of the hip have significant functional limitations that prevent them from participating in their usual daily activities. To this end, the societal burden of this condition, both in terms of personal suffering and utilization of health resources, is expected to rise with the increasing prevalence of obesity and the increased life expectancy of the general population.[1]

Approximately 16 million people in the United States have osteoarthritis, and one in three people over the age of 60 suffer from the disease. The risk factors for osteoarthritis of the hip can be divided into those that are secondary to a generalized predisposition to the disorder and those that reflect abnormal biomechanical loading at the hip. Generalized susceptibility is characterized by increasing age, a positive family history, diabetes, and hypertension. While epidemiologic studies have demonstrated a large genetic contribution to the development of this disease that is most likely polygenic, the specific genes responsible have not yet been identified.[2] Any abnormalities in joint shape can contribute to local biomechanical factors that ultimately lead to increased stress forces at the joint and eventual joint deterioration. These abnormalities could be the result of congenital or acquired abnormalities of the hip, including Legg-Calve-Perthes disease, slipped capital femoral epiphysis, or developmental dysplasia of the hip.

A complete history should include questions directed at finding out if any of these conditions were present during childhood. More recently, acetabular labral tears and femoroacetabular impingement have been reported as etiologies of premature osteoarthritis.[3]

Osteoarthritis of the hip typically involves the joint in a focal manner, as localized areas of hyaline articular cartilage loss can increase focal stress across the joint, thereby leading to further joint damage. As hyaline articular cartilage is lost, bony remodeling occurs with resultant capsular stretching. In some patients, synovitis may be present and ligamentous laxity may develop. Ultimately, a vicious cycle of hip joint damage leads to joint failure when progressive focal cartilage loss leads to bony remodeling and potential alterations in stress forces across the joint. Researchers have shown that the presence of local inflammation in the synovium and cartilage may contribute to significant pain and structural deterioration.[4,5]

Patients with osteoarthritis of the hip typically present with complaints of insidious pain in the groin or inguinal region and, on occasion, may report pain on the side of the buttock or upper thigh. The joint pain of osteoarthritis is typically exacerbated with varied amounts of activity and is usually relieved with rest. In more advanced cases, it is not uncommon for patients to experience pain at rest or even at night. It is important to note that while symptoms of pain at night can represent severe symptomatic disease, it can also point to causes other than osteoarthritis, such as inflammatory arthritis, tumors, infection, or crystal disease. For osteoarthritis of the hip, activities such as walking long distances or even putting on shoes and socks can bring on pain. The pain tends to be more pronounced in the morning, as patients complain of "stiffness" when they wake up. This morning stiffness tends to last no more than 30 minutes and gradually resolves as the patient mobilizes the joint.[5] The precise source of pain is not well understood at this time. Of the various inflammatory events localized to the hip joint, researchers postulate that the subchondral bone, periosteum, synovium, and joint capsule could be the source of nociceptive stimuli, as they are all densely innervated structures in contrast to articular cartilage, which is actively destroyed throughout the progression of the disease but aneural.[6] Given the potential development of capsular stretching, ligamentous laxity, or even weakness of periarticular muscles that support the joint, some patients may also describe symptoms of joint instability.

PATIENT ASSESSMENT

1. Stiffness, especially after prolonged activity
2. Stiffness after sitting
3. Groin pain occasionally radiating into the knee
4. Limited motion, especially internal rotation
5. X-rays document progression of disease

Physical Findings

Physical examination of the patient should begin with an initial assessment of body weight and height to establish the patient's body mass index, as obesity is a significant contributing factor to arthritic disease. The patient should then be adequately undressed for proper inspection of the hips and pelvis. Careful assessment should reveal a level pelvis, and the presence of pelvic obliquity suggests a leg-length discrepancy or spinal deformity. Clinical leg-length discrepancy is not uncommon in patients with osteoarthritis, as the loss of joint space at the hip can cause

SECTION 4 Hip

significant shortening on the involved side. Range of motion of the spine and careful comparison of leg lengths while lying supine can help to differentiate the exact source of leg-length discrepancy. A Trendelenburg test should be assessed by having the patient stand on one leg and lift the other leg with the hip and knee flexed to a 90-degree angle. Patients with deficient abductor muscles or pain on contraction of these muscles secondary to arthritis demonstrate an impairment of this normal mechanism. Consequently, these patients will allow the pelvis to drop contralateral to the stance-phase side or may even shift their center of gravity over the stance phase in order to reduce the muscular demand of the involved leg. Examination of the hip consists of testing of both passive and active range of motion at the hip. Patients typically display limitations in passive external and internal rotation of the hip secondary to pain and/or mechanical difficulties (i.e., osteophyte formation). Abduction and internal rotation are typically more restricted than adduction and external rotation. Occasionally, crepitus can be felt on passive range of motion. This crackling sensation is due to the irregularity of opposing cartilage surfaces and is a frequent sign of osteoarthritis.

Studies

IMAGING

Plain Radiography

The plain radiograph remains the standard imaging modality used in the diagnosis of osteoarthritis. The basic radiographic series obtained in a patient with suspected hip osteoarthritis includes an AP pelvis view and frog-leg lateral views of the hip. Typical radiographic findings consist of joint space narrowing, which often begins in the superolateral direction (Table 12.1). Apical (up and into the pelvis) and medial (toward the center of the body) directed narrowing also occurs. Subchondral bone cysts and areas of sclerosis, represented by increased density on the radiograph, develop as the cartilage loss becomes more severe. In order to compensate for the cartilage loss and narrowed joint space, osteophyte (bone spurs) formation gradually occurs on the side opposite to the direction of narrowing to help stabilize the joint. In patients with hip osteoarthritis, the radiographic findings can correlate poorly with the severity of pain, and radiographs occasionally may even be normal in patients with this disease. Researchers have shown that standard radiographs are an insensitive indicator of joint pathology, as the presence of osteoarthritis can

NOT TO BE MISSED

- *Septic arthritis:* Acute pain on any motion is typical in patients with this condition. The standard workup should involve routine laboratory tests, blood cultures, and joint aspiration, which should establish the diagnosis.

- *Rheumatoid arthritis:* A chronic inflammatory disorder that causes progressive disability. Early presentation is similar to osteoarthritis, as the initial dysfunction is usually achy groin or thigh discomfort and/or difficulty putting on a sock or shoe. Typically,

Table 12.1 Typical Radiographic Changes Observed in Osteoarthritis of the Hip
Bony sclerosis of the femoral head and neck
Subchondral bone cysts
Joint space narrowing
Osteophyte formation

other joints are affected, and this may help to differentiate this disorder from osteoarthritis.

- *Gout or pseudogout (crystalline arthropathies):* Occurs rarely in the hip. Symptoms may be subtle or acute and may mimic those of a patient with osteo- or septic arthritis. The presence of crystals or a positive culture on synovial fluid analysis can easily help to differentiate these disorders.

- *Lyme disease:* A multisystem illness. Suspicion for this disorder should be high based on geographic exposure. Patients typically complain of migratory joint pain, and a characteristic red, annular skin rash (erythema migrans) can help to identify the disease. Early diagnosis is important.

- *Avascular necrosis (AVN):* Patients typically present with pain localized to the groin, although radiation of symptoms to the knee or buttock is not uncommon. The pain is usually deep and throbbing. It is important for the physician to carefully identify any risk factors that may predispose the patient to AVN (i.e., young age, steroid use, renal failure, alcoholism, blood coagulopathies).

- *Bone tumors:* Such tumors should always be considered in patients complaining of persistent hip or pelvic pain. Any complaints of pain at night should be a red flag. Radiographic evaluation of the affected area is important. The management of these pathologic lesions should be undertaken by an experienced orthopaedic physician.

occasionally be detected on oblique or lateral views, causing missed diagnoses when radiographic evaluation is completed only by utilizing an AP view.[7] Thus, additional views may be necessary on occasion to detect subtle arthritic changes. Signs of femoroacetabular impingement, a cause of early arthritis, can be noticed on traditional AP pelvis and frog-leg lateral views. A crossover sign on the AP pelvis view indicates relative retroversion of the acetabulum, which can cause early arthritic damage. Impingement can also be suspected when a bony spur is observed on the anterolateral femoral neck on the frog-leg lateral view.[3]

Magnetic Resonance

Given the fact that clinical signs of osteoarthritis may be evident before they are observed on standard radiographic views, MRI can be used in certain instances to help detect early arthritis. MRI is extremely sensitive to subtle bony and soft tissue changes and can be helpful in the imaging of early degenerative changes of articular cartilage. Typical MRI findings can demonstrate reactive bone edema and soft tissue swelling as well as small cartilage or loose bone fragments within the joint.[8,9] When there is objective evidence of articular cartilage wear, an appropriate treatment plan can be devised to prevent or delay further progression. MRI is even more valuable in assessing other potential occult sources of hip pain such as osteonecrosis, stress fractures, or transient osteoporosis.

Computed Tomography

While rarely useful, CT is an excellent imaging modality for demonstrating the degree of osteophyte formation and its relationship to adjacent soft tissue structures. Furthermore, CT scans can also be used to evaluate the radiographic joint space.[8,9] CT scans are primarily indicated to look for occult fractures, particularly in patients who are not candidates for MRI. Lastly, CT scans may be useful in the setting of preoperative planning to evaluate the acetabular bone stock prior to osteotomy or total hip arthroplasty in the setting of posttraumatic arthritis following acetabular fracture or complex hip deformity. Overall, CT can provide guidance for therapeutic and diagnostic procedures, but it should be reserved for specific cases in which fine osseous detail is required.

Radionuclide Bone Scan

Bone scintigraphy is a sensitive but relatively nonspecific way of detecting osteoarthritis. One common feature of osteoarthritis is increased regional blood flow, which may be evident on flow images of a technetium-99m phosphate or diphosphate bone scan. Given the fact that destructive and productive changes take place in adjacent bones, static images from bone scintigraphy can reveal increased uptake of radionuclide tracer in periarticular regions. For this reason, scintigraphic abnormalities can precede changes on standard radiographic imaging and aid in early identification of disease, although the findings are very nonspecific.[8–10] Furthermore, bone scans can provide the clinician with helpful information in patients who may have multiple sites of arthritic involvement. The authors do not routinely recommend bone scintigraphy in the evaluation of osteoarthritis.

SECTION 4 Hip

LABORATORY

Routine blood tests are not generally indicated in the workup of a patient suspected to have osteoarthritis, and the clinician should not rely on laboratory testing to establish the diagnosis. However, if inflammatory arthritis is a possibility, evaluation for inflammatory arthritic conditions may be appropriate (i.e., Lyme titer, RF, ANA, HLA B-27). Because osteoarthritis is a noninflammatory condition, laboratory findings are expected to be within normal range. If the diagnosis is not clear given the history, physical, and radiographic findings, certain blood tests could prove useful in ruling out other potential diagnoses.

ESR and CRP values can indicate whether an inflammatory component of disease is present. The American College of Rheumatology (ACR) has developed descriptive criteria that help to distinguish osteoarthritis of the hip from other rheumatic disorders. A low ESR value in conjunction with the hallmark physical and radiographic findings can help in establishing the diagnosis[11] (Table 12.2).

Joint aspiration with examination of synovial fluid is indicated if inflammatory arthritides, gout, pseudogout, or septic arthritis are suspected. If the WBC count from the aspirate reveals <1,000 WBCs per cubic millimeter, osteoarthritis is likely; if the count is higher, further laboratory evaluation is indicated to establish a diagnosis.[12] Given the systemic side effects of certain medications, the clinician should consider obtaining a baseline hemoglobin level, creatinine concentration, and liver function tests before initiating treatment with medications, particularly NSAIDs.

Table 12.2 **American College of Rheumatology Classification Criteria for Osteoarthritis of the Hip**

Clinical Criteria

  1. Hip pain+

2a. Internal rotation <15+

2b. ESR <44 mm/h

      OR

3a. Internal rotation >15+

3b. Morning stiffness <60 min+

3c. Age >50 y+

3d. Pain on internal rotation

Clinical and Radiographic Criteria

  1. Hip pain and at least two of the following:

2a. ESR <20 mm/h

2b. Radiographic osteophytes

2c. Radiographic joint space narrowing

ESR, erythrocyte sedimentation rate.
Adapted from Altman R, Alarcon G, Appelrouth D, et al. The American College of Rheumatology criteria for the classification and reporting of osteoarthritis of the hip. *Arthritis Rheum* 1991;34:505–514.

Treatment

1. Conservative
2. Activity modification
3. NSAIDs
4. Intra-articular injection
5. Total hip replacement

The optimal treatment of osteoarthritis continues to evolve as knowledge of the underlying pathogenesis improves and novel therapeutic modalities are discovered. In 1995, an ad hoc committee of the ACR published specific guidelines outlining the recommended treatment of patients with osteoarthritis of the hip and knee.[13,14] The primary goals of treatment identified by the aggregate group included pain control, limitation of disability, maintenance of joint mobility, and patient education and awareness. Ultimately, these guidelines highlighted the value and primary position of nonpharmacologic interventions as a foundation of therapy that could be augmented with pharmacologic therapy. In light of new therapies and data supporting their efficacy, an updated approach to the appropriate management of patients with osteoarthritis was developed in 2000.[15] These new guidelines propose a spectrum of available treatment options for clinicians and emphasize individual therapy based on patient characteristics as well as sound clinical judgment.

Nonpharmacologic therapy remains the mainstay of osteoarthritis of the hip and serves as a base on which other treatments may be added.[15] Obesity is a significant risk factor for the development of osteoarthritis and has been associated with radiologic progression of the disease and disability.[16] To this end, weight reduction should be a key goal. Considerable data have supported this approach and confirmed the efficacy and cost-effectiveness when used appropriately in patients with knee and hip osteoarthritis.[17–21] Exercise increases aerobic capacity, muscle strength, and endurance, thereby facilitating weight loss, and all patients capable of participating in a low-impact aerobic exercise program (walking, biking, swimming) should be encouraged to do so. Participation in physical therapy can facilitate resolution of symptoms and improve functional deficits if the patient has symptomatic disease. Although there is no current data supporting the proposed benefits of mechanical aids, such as canes, that help decrease weight-bearing forces, they are widely recommended.[15] For patients with advanced disease, nonpharmacologic interventions alone do not provide sufficient control of symptoms. Pain and disability can continue and preclude them from making significant functional gains. In these particular cases, pharmacologic intervention is an important and essential next step.

Pharmacologic management should augment exercise and physical therapy. Furthermore, it should be individualized following a careful assessment of symptom severity, comorbid conditions, drug side effects, cost of therapy, and patient preferences. Acetaminophen remains the drug of choice in patients who require pharmacologic therapy, based on research

SECTION 4 Hip

demonstrating effective relief of pain and its relatively safe side effect profile in a wide spectrum of patients.[15] Several researchers have demonstrated that NSAIDs and cyclooxygenase-2-specific (COX-2) inhibitors provide superior efficacy relative to acetaminophen.[22–24] These drugs may be more useful in the small aggregate of patients demonstrating an inflammatory component (effusion) to their disease. Clinicians now have a choice between conventional NSAIDs and COX-2 inhibitors, as they demonstrate similar analgesic effects; however, COX-2 inhibitors are the preferred drug in patients at high risk for developing gastrointestinal toxicity or bleeding. Individual patient factors that may be associated with an increased risk of adverse gastrointestinal events include age ≥65 years, comorbid medical conditions, concomitant use of anticoagulants or oral glucocorticoids, and a past history of peptic ulcer disease or upper gastrointestinal bleeding.[15] Aside from gastrointestinal side effects, some COX-2 inhibitors may be associated with an increased potential risk of cardiovascular events. A recent study comparing rofecoxib and naproxen found a fourfold increase in the rate of myocardial infarction in patients using rofecoxib.[25] To this end, patients with cardiovascular risk factors should also be counseled prior to using these drugs. For patients with renal insufficiency, both NSAIDs and COX-2 inhibitors should only be prescribed after careful consideration, as these drugs may worsen renal function.

The dietary supplements glucosamine and chondroitin sulfate have been advocated, particularly in the media, as safe and effective options for the management of symptoms of osteoarthritis. These supplements are derivatives of glycosaminoglycans that are naturally found in articular cartilage. A recent meta-analysis concluded that these compounds may have a small analgesic effect; however, issues of study quality and publication bias confounded several of the studies that were included in the analysis.[26] Ultimately, patients with advanced disease and higher reported pain scores do not seem to benefit from these supplements.

Unlike osteoarthritis of the knee, topical analgesic agents have not been studied for the hip; however, the increased amount of soft tissue at the hip joint suggests that this type of therapy would not be useful. Intraarticular steroid injections of the hip have not been extensively studied, and if they are performed, they should be done so by an experienced clinician under fluoroscopic guidance. To date, intra-articular hyaluronic acid injections have not been approved for treatment of osteoarthritis of the hip.

 Refer to Patient Education

 Refer to Physical Therapy

Clinical Course

The natural history of hip osteoarthritis is extremely variable. Some radiographic studies have demonstrated that some patients are able to demonstrate clear-cut radiologic and clinical recovery, while other individuals demonstrate rapid progression of symptomatic and radiographic disease.[27,28] There have been several explanations for pathologic improvements in hip osteoarthritis. First, some propose that the joint space may be protected by large osteophytes that unload stress on affected areas. Another explanation is that the joint may lose motion, permitting restitution of the joint space with the growth of fibrocartilage.[29] Overall, it is difficult to predict the individual course of patients with osteoarthritis of the hip. Patients with suspected disease should be counseled early to prevent potential progression of disease.

> ### ICD9
>
> *715.35 Osteoarthrosis, localized, not specified whether primary or secondary, involving pelvic region and thigh*
> *715.95 Osteoarthrosis, unspecified whether generalized or localized, involving pelvic region and thigh*

References

1. Hunter DJ, Felson DT. Osteoarthritis. *BMJ* 2006;332:639–642.
2. Peach CA, Carr AJ, Loughlin J. Recent advances in the genetic investigation of osteoarthritis. *Trends Mol Med* 2005;11:186–191.
3. Beck M, Kalhor M, Leunig M, et al. Hip morphology influences the pattern of damage to the acetabular cartilage: femoroacetabular impingement as a cause of early osteoarthritis of the hip. *J Bone Joint Surg Br* 2005;87(7):1012–1018.
4. Pelletier JP, Martel-Pelletier J, Abramson SB. Osteoarthritis, an inflammatory disease: potential implication for the selection of new therapeutic targets. *Arthritis Rheum* 2001;44:1237–1247.
5. Arai KI, Lee F, Miyajima A, et al. Cytokines: coordinators of immune and inflammatory response. *Annu Rev Immunol* 1990;59:783–836.
6. Altman R, Asch E, Bloch D, et al. Development of criteria for the classification and reporting of osteoarthritis. *Arthritis Rheum* 1986;29:1039–1049.
7. Dieppe PA, Lohmander LS. Pathogenesis and management of pain in osteoarthritis. *Lancet* 2005;365: 965–973.
8. Summers MN, Haley WE, Reveille JD, et al. Radiographic assessment and psychologic variables as predictors of pain and functional impairment in osteoarthritis of the knee or hip. *Arthritis Rheum* 1988; 31:204–209.
9. Martel W, Adler RS, Chan K, et al. Overview: new methods in imaging osteoarthritis. *J Rheumatol Suppl* 1991;27:32–37.
10. Kaye JJ. Radiologic assessment of osteoarthritis. New techniques. *Rheum Dis Clin North Am* 1993;19(3): 659–672.
11. Altman R, Alarcon G, Appelrouth D, et al. The American College of Rheumatology criteria for the classification and reporting of osteoarthritis of the hip. *Arthritis Rheum* 1991;34:505–514.
12. Puett DW, Griffin MR. Published trials of nonmedicinal and noninvasive therapies for hip and knee osteoarthritis. *Ann Intern Med* 1994;121:133–140.
13. Hochberg MC, Altman RD, Brandt KD, et al. Guidelines for the medical management of osteoarthritis, part I: osteoarthritis of the hip. *Arthritis Rheum* 1995;38:1535–1540.
14. Hochberg MC, Altman RD, Brandt KD, et al. Guidelines for the medical management of osteoarthritis, part II: osteoarthritis of the hip. *Arthritis Rheum* 1995;38:1541–1546.
15. Altman RD, Hochberg MC, Moskowitz RW, et al. Recommendations for the medical management of osteoarthritis of the hip and knee. American College of Rheumatology Subcommittee on Osteoarthritis Guidelines. *Arthritis Rheum* 2000;43:1905–1915.
16. Felson DT, Lawrence RC, Dieppe PA, et al. Osteoarthritis: new insights. Part I: The disease and its risk factors. *Ann Intern Med* 2000;133:635–646.
17. Ettinger WH Jr, Burns R, Messier SP, et al. A randomized trial comparing aerobic exercise and resistance exercise with a health education program in older adults with knee osteoarthritis: the Fitness Arthritis and Seniors Trial (FAST). *JAMA* 1997;277:25–31.
18. Hurley MV, Scott DL. Improvements in quadriceps sensorimotor function and disability of patients with knee osteoarthritis following a clinically practicable exercise regime. *Br J Rheumatol* 1998;37: 1181–1187.
19. Martin K, Nicklas BJ, Bunyard LB, et al. Weight loss and walking improve symptoms of knee osteoarthritis [abstract]. *Arthritis Rheum* 1996;39(suppl):S225.
20. Toda Y, Toda T, Takemura S, et al. Change in body fat but not body weight or metabolic correlates of obesity, is related to symptomatic relief of obese patients with knee osteoarthritis after a weight control program. *J Rheumatol* 1998;25:2181–2186.
21. Van Baar ME, Dekker J, Oostendorp RAB, et al. The effectiveness of exercise therapy in patients with osteoarthritis of the hip or knee: a randomized clinical trial. *J Rheumatol* 1998;25:2432–2439.

SECTION 4 Hip

22. Pincus T, Swearingen C, Cummins P, et al. Preference for non-steroidal anti-inflammatory drugs versus acetaminophen and concomitant use of both types of drugs in patients with osteoarthritis. *J Rheumatol* 2000;27:1020–1027.

23. Pincus T, Callahan LF, Wolfe F, et al. Arthrotec compared to acetaminophen (ACTA): a clinical trial in patients with osteoarthritis of the hip or knee [abstract]. *Arthritis Rheum* 1999;42(suppl):S404.

24. Geba GP, Weaver AL, Schnitzer TJ, et al. A comparison of rofecoxib to celecoxib and acetaminophen in the treatment of osteoarthritis [abstract]. *Arthritis Rheum* 2000;43(Suppl 9):S384.

25. The Australian COX-2 Specific Inhibitor (CSI) Prescribing Group. Considerations for the safe prescribing and use of the COX-2-specific inhibitors. *Med J Aust* 2002;176:328–331.

26. McAlindon TE, LaValley MP, Gulin JP, et al. Glucosamine and chondroitin for treatment of osteoarthritis. A systematic quality assessment and meta-analysis. *JAMA* 2000;283:1469–1475.

27. Danielsson LG. Incidence and prognosis of coxarthrosis. *Acta Orthop Scand* 1964;66:9–87.

28. Bland JH. The reversibility of osteoarthritis: A review. *Am J Med* 1983;75(suppl):16–26.

29. Felson DT. The course of osteoarthritis and factors that affect it. *Rheum Dis Clin North Am* 1993;19(3):607–615.

30. Harris W, Sledge C. Total hip and knee replacement. *N Engl J Med* 1990;323:725–731.

13 Coxa Saltans: The Snapping Hip

Charles L. Nelson and Kristofer J. Jones

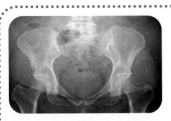

A 28-year-old woman presents complaining of right lateral hip pain associated with a loud "click." She reports that she is an avid cross-country runner and that the pain has prevented her from participating in running activities for the last 3 weeks. She denies any inciting traumatic event that may have caused injury to the area. Review of systems is negative, and her past medical history is significant for asthma. She has had no prior surgeries. Physical examination reveals no localized area of tenderness to palpation in the area; however, an audible snap can be voluntarily reproduced with active extension of the flexed, abducted, and externally rotated right lower extremity. AP radiograph of the pelvis is unremarkable.

CLINICAL POINTS

- Patients frequently complain of hip pain associated with an audible snap or pop.
- Symptoms are common in younger adults.
- Affected individuals participate in activities that involve repetitive motions of the hip.
- Actual cause relates to the anatomic location of the unstable structure (e.g., internal, external, intra-articular).

Clinical Presentation

Athletic injuries about the hip and groin have been shown to occur at a low rate relative to injuries that are sustained in more distal areas of the lower extremity. Various epidemiologic studies have defined the frequency of hip injury in high school athletes, as they have found that distinct injuries to the hip comprise 5% to 9% of all injuries sustained.[1–3] Given the complex anatomy and biomechanics of the hip region, the diagnosis and management of musculoskeletal problems can be extremely challenging.

Coxa saltans, or *snapping hip syndrome*, is characterized by an audible snap or pop that typically occurs with flexion and extension of the hip during exercise; however, given the severity of the pathologic cause, it can occur with activities of daily living. The condition is commonly found in patients in their late teens to early 20s. Patients often report that the audible sound is felt on the lateral aspect of the hip and is associated with pain as the hip is placed through repetitive flexion, extension, and abduction. The pain may occasionally radiate down to the knee. These symptoms are commonly seen in distance runners or other individuals who place their hips through these repetitive motions.

Several causes of this clinical entity have been implicated, and all are related to the anatomic location of the offending structure: external, internal, and intra-articular (Table 13.1).

EXTERNAL ETIOLOGY

The external form of coxa saltans is the most common cause of snapping hip. In cases of external etiology, the history can be extremely helpful in

Table 13.1 Various Etiologies of Snapping Hip

EXTERNAL ETIOLOGY	INTERNAL ETIOLOGY	INTRA-ARTICULAR ETIOLOGY
Iliotibial band snapping over the greater trochanter	Iliopsoas tendon snapping over femoral head	Labral tear
Gluteus maximus tendon snapping over the greater trochanter	Iliopsoas tendon snapping over pelvic brim	Loose bodies
—	Iliopsoas tendon snapping over lesser trochanter	Osteochondral lesion
—	Tendinitis of the femoris iliopsoas or rectus muscles	Synovial chondromatosis
—	—	Hip subluxation

establishing the diagnosis. Patients will explain a "snapping, painful" sensation over the lateral hip and will point to the greater trochanter when asked to identify the area of maximal tenderness. Traditionally, the external snapping hip has been associated with a thickened posterior border of the iliotibial band or anterior border of the gluteus maximus, which predisposes the band to slipping back-and-forth over the greater trochanter.[4–8] Ultimately, the thickened iliotibial band lies posterior to the greater trochanter as the hip sits in extension. As the hip is flexed, the band forcefully slides anteriorly over the trochanter, producing pain and an audible sound. Anatomically, there is no laxity present at any time within band as the hip is placed through flexion and extension. Both the tensor fascia lata and the gluteus maximus—the two major proximal musculotendinous attachments of the iliotibial band—pull on the band, making it taut in flexion and extension. Given the fact that it remains tight throughout motion of the hip, any slight anatomic changes or swelling in the area may lead to snapping over the greater trochanter.[9] The greater trochanteric bursa, which lies between the iliotibial band and the greater trochanter, can become inflamed as the band continuously slides over the bursa, leading to inflammation and contributing to the patient's painful symptoms.

INTERNAL ETIOLOGY

Confusion regarding the diagnosis can occur when the snapping hip cannot be attributed to an external etiology. Patients report the classic symptoms of pain with an audible click and usually point to the anterolateral region of the hip or groin when asked to identify the area of maximal pain and tenderness. The first internal etiology of coxa saltans was postulated by Nunziata in 1951, as he believed that the source of pain and audible snapping came from the iliopsoas tendon sliding over the iliopectineal eminence.[10] Further studies have shown that another possible cause of internal coxa saltans results from the conjoined iliopsoas tendon moving from the lateral to the medial side of the femoral head when

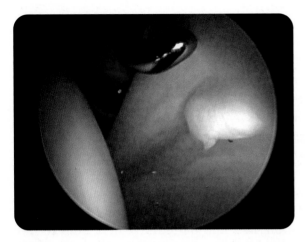

Figure 13.1 Intraoperative arthroscopic picture demonstrating a large acetabular labral tear. Note that the torn labrum is being lifted away from the acetabular bone with the probe.

the hip moves from extension to flexion.[9] It is this back-and-forth motion of the tendon over the femoral head that causes the majority of symptomatic cases of internal coxa saltans.[9] Additional areas known to cause snapping of the tendon are a bony prominence of the iliopectineal ridge and the lesser trochanter. A significant source of pain found in patients with an internal snapping hip can be related to the iliopsoas bursa, which is the largest synovial bursa in the body. The iliopsoas bursa is found between the iliopsoas tendon and anterior hip capsule, with a communication between the two existing in approximately 15% of adult hips.[11] Significant inflammation of this structure from repetitive sliding of the tendon can be extremely painful for patients with this condition.

INTRA-ARTICULAR ETIOLOGY

The majority of causes of intra-articular coxa saltans have a distinct presentation, thereby allowing the clinician to easily distinguish this type from the internal and external forms. These patients classically describe a clicking sensation rather than a distinct feeling of snapping, and pain is usually the chief complaint. The intra-articular form can be caused by an intracapsular lesion as well as the result of hip instability, loose bodies, a labral tear (Fig. 13.1), or synovial chondromatosis.[12] A careful history can reveal possible inciting events that may have led to intra-articular pathology, such as hip trauma leading to small fracture fragments within the joint. Patients with loose bodies typically complain of intermittent clicking, as the loose body can lodge and dislodge within the foveal region of the acetabulum or within large synovial tissue folds.[9] Despite the presence of persistent clicking in the hip, patients with acetabular labral tears primarily complain of significant pain. They may also demonstrate symptoms of catching or giving away on the affected side. A history of hip dysplasia or hip dislocation should prompt further investigation for a possible tear of the labrum.

Physical Findings

EXTERNAL TYPE

As mentioned previously, the most common type of coxa saltans is the external form, where the thickened posterior border of the iliotibial band or the anterior border of the gluteus maximus slides over the greater trochanter. On physical examination, the diagnosis can be established by reproducing the snapping motion of the tendon over the greater trochanter. In order to test properly, the patient should lie on her side with the affected leg up. On flexion of the involved leg at the hip, it should be easy to palpate the area of snapping over the greater trochanter. Ultimately, the diagnosis can be substantiated if the tendon snapping can be prevented by direct manual pressure applied over the greater trochanter by the clinician.

INTERNAL TYPE

The actual snapping mechanism associated with the internal form of coxa saltans is poorly understood compared with that of the external type. However, the pain with internal coxa saltans is generally believed to be due to the movement of the iliopsoas tendon over the pelvic pectineal eminence, femoral head, or lesser trochanter. Gruen et al.[12] have found that patients with this particular form of coxa saltans typically identify the largest source of pain over the area of the pectineal eminence, a finding attributed to the iliopsoas tendon being most taut over the pelvic brim. In order to examine these patients, they should be placed in the supine position. The involved hip should then be flexed and extended to reproduce the snapping sensation. In some patients, it may help to flex and abduct the hip and then subsequently extend and adduct it to feel the snapping tendon.[9] If direct pressure over the iliopsoas tendon at the level of the femoral head prevents the snapping sensation, the diagnosis of internal coxa saltans can be made with clinical confidence. Occasionally, patients with iliopsoas bursitis, secondary to repetitive back-and-forth motion of the tendon over the bursa, will exhibit point tenderness inferior to the inguinal ligament and 2 cm lateral to the femoral artery, and a palpable mass may be noticeable.

INTRA-ARTICULAR TYPE

There are various pathologic etiologies of the intra-articular form of coxa saltans. The two primary causes in presenting patients include loose cartilage or bony fragments within the joint space or labral tear. In patients with symptoms consistent with a labral tear, clicking in the inguinal area is common. On physical examination, the painful click can be reproduced with the McCarthy test (with the opposite hip fully flexed, the affected hip is extended, first in external rotation and then in internal rotation). Loose intra-articular bodies can be due to several pathologic processes, such as avascular necrosis of the femoral head or even a traumatic injury. The characteristic clicking can usually be reproduced on examination with passive range of motion at the hip; however, the definitive diagnosis must be made with appropriate imaging studies.

Studies

IMAGING

While the evaluation of snapping hip syndrome with diagnostic imaging can be extremely useful, there is no clear consensus on the optimal imaging tests that should be used to establish the diagnosis. Various researchers have not found plain radiographs to be useful in the diagnosis, except to exclude intra-articular conditions such as synovial chondromatosis and loose bodies.[9] Studies investigating the utility of standard radiographic measurements have reported that coxa vara is associated with snapping hip syndrome.[13] Conversely, another radiographic study found that a reduced bi-iliac width is associated with an increased degree of valgus angulation at the hip. The researchers propose that the resultant imbalance

---

NOT TO BE MISSED

- *Avascular necrosis:* The early phase of this disease is segmental necrosis of the femoral head, which may have occasional snapping sensations. Imaging studies of the involved area can prove useful in the initial distinction between these two conditions, as plain radiographs can help to identify the necrotic bone lesion.

- *Femoral head stress fracture:* A stress fracture should be considered in a patient population similar to that observed in snapping hip syndrome (chronic repetitive motion such as running, dancing, rowing). Patients present with persistent groin pain and complain of decreased range of motion. A careful physical examination should be able to easily distinguish snapping hip from a femoral stress fracture.

- *Labral tear:* A torn acetabular labrum can produce symptoms of pain, clicking, and catching on the involved side; patients can also have negative radiographic findings. High resolution MRI or MR arthrography are the best imaging modalities to identify labral tears.

between hip abductors and adductors can lead to snapping hip; however, this hypothesis has not been confirmed with further studies.[14,15]

MRI can be helpful in delineating intra-articular lesions, particularly the presence of loose bodies within the joint. Conventional MRI is limited in evaluating the labral pathology as a potential cause of intra-articular coxa saltans due to the variability in labral size and shape. MR arthrography can be more useful, as the principle of the procedure relies on capsular distension, thereby outlining the labrum with contrast and highlighting any tears that may be present (Fig. 13.2). Iliopsoas bursography, typically used for internal coxa saltans, also utilizes contrast material to highlight the snapping iliopsoas tendon. This imaging modality is the definitive and single most useful procedure in the diagnosis of internal snapping hip syndrome. During this procedure, the patient is prepped and draped in a supine position, and under fluoroscopic guidance, an 18-gauge spinal needle is placed over the superomedial quadrant of the femoral head. The needle is advanced until bony contact is achieved, and it is then retracted approximately 5 mm. Contrast material is injected to define the occupying space of the bursa. The hip is subsequently placed through a full range of motion, and any sudden jerking of the iliopsoas tendon (identified as a filling defect adjacent to the bursa) with a lateral to medial motion is diagnostic of internal coxa saltans.[9,16,17]

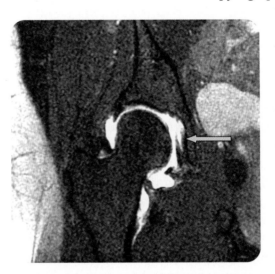

Figure 13.2 Coronal T1 fat-saturated MR arthrogram of the hip following intra-articular injection of dilute gadolinium demonstrates contrast extending through the base of the anterior labrum, consistent with an acetabular labral tear. The contrast is able to leak beneath the labrum when it becomes detached from the underlying acetabular bone.

Treatment

1. Identify etiology of snapping
2. NSAIDs and/or injection into trochanteric bursa
3. Occasional surgery to relax the iliotibial band or remove loose bodies and the like

Asymptomatic snapping hip should be considered a benign and normal occurrence, especially in young, athletic patients. For these individuals, the snapping should be viewed as a normal occurrence, and no definitive treatment should be sought unless the condition becomes symptomatic and functionally limiting to the patient.

Symptomatic snapping hip usually develops over an extended period of time, and the patient presents with complaints that his or her "hip feels like it's dislocating in and out of the joint." If the patient has been experiencing the symptoms for a short period of time (no more than 6 months), occurs sporadically with activity, and an external or internal etiology can be definitively diagnosed, the optimal treatment consists of conservative measures. However, if there are findings suggesting intra-articular pathology, referral to an orthopaedic surgeon is appropriate to minimize potential articular cartilage damage.

Conservative therapy for such a patient often consists of icing the affected area to reduce any inflammation, NSAIDs, rest, and avoidance of all activities that reproduce the pain. For patients who experience severe

SECTION 4 Hip

symptoms such as pain with normal ambulation and other activities of daily living, an appropriate treatment protocol should consist of ice, rest, and hydrocortisone injection into the affected area. Of note, the clinician should never inject corticosteroid into an area that appears infected. Steroid treatment should be followed by a detailed physical therapy program that consists of stretching the tensor fascia lata and gluteus muscles. Ultimately, conservative therapy is the mainstay of treatment in this disorder because most patients improve with a dedicated treatment regimen.[18–20]

Surgical intervention is rarely necessary and should only be considered following an extensive course of conservative modalities. There are myriad effective surgical procedures that have been described for refractory cases of coxa saltans, and appropriate selection depends on the underlying pathologic process (external, internal, or intra-articular). In the setting of intra-articular pathology, arthroscopic surgical intervention may be necessary.

 Refer to Physical Therapy

Clinical Course

Although the specific prevalence of snapping hip has not been reported relative to other hip disorders, the reasonably low frequency in the general population and variable causes of snapping hip syndrome can cause considerable difficulties in creating optimal treatment plans. The majority of patients with snapping hip syndrome are asymptomatic; however, repetitive motion in sports such as running, dancing, and rowing may additionally incite pain and disability. Overall, asymptomatic snapping hip syndrome is a benign condition, and the patient should be reassured that the majority of these cases are amenable to stretching, physical therapy, activity modification, a course of NSAIDs, and selective injections into the trochanteric bursa. Steroid injections may complement the conservative treatment regimen, and more than one injection may be necessary. A study investigating the efficacy of steroid injections found that in a series of 51 patients, 49 had good or excellent results with an average of 1.5 (steroid or anesthetic) to 1.8 injections (anesthetic only).[21] If the patient does not demonstrate significant symptomatic relief following 6 months of extensive conservative therapy, it may be necessary to explore surgical options.

> *ICD9*
>
> *719.65 Other symptoms referable to joint of pelvic region and thigh*

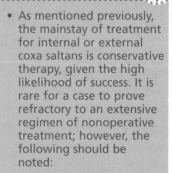

WHEN TO REFER

- As mentioned previously, the mainstay of treatment for internal or external coxa saltans is conservative therapy, given the high likelihood of success. It is rare for a case to prove refractory to an extensive regimen of nonoperative treatment; however, the following should be noted:

- If intractable pain and functional limitations remain despite the clinician and patient's best efforts, it is best to consider surgical alternatives of therapy.

References

1. Anderson K, Strickland SM, Warren R. Hip and groin injuries in athletes. *Am J Sports Med* 2001;29(4): 521–533.
2. DeLee JC, Farney WC. Incidence of injury in Texas high school football. *Am J Sports Med* 1992;20:575–580.
3. Gomez E, DeLee JC, Farney WC. Incidence of injury in Texas girl's high school basketball. *Am J Sports Med* 1996;24:684–687.
4. Jacobson T, Allen WC. Surgical correction of the snapping iliopsoas tendon. *Am J Sports Med* 1990;18:470–474.

- All cases in which intra-articular pathology is suspected should be referred to an orthopaedic surgeon. The authors currently recommend a 6-month trial of conservative treatment, and if there is no improvement beyond this time, referral to an orthopaedic surgeon is appropriate.

5. Binnie JF. Snapping hip. *Ann Surg* 1913;58:59–66.
6. Schaberg JE, Harper MC, Allen WC. The snapping hip syndrome. *Am J Sports Med* 1984;12:361–365.
7. Mayer L. Snapping hip. *Surg Gynecol Obstet* 1919;29:425–428.
8. Staple TW, Jung D, Mork A. Snapping tendon syndrome: hip tenography with fluoroscopic monitoring. *Radiology* 1988;166:873–874.
9. Allen WC, Cope R. Coxa saltans: the snapping hip revisited. *J Am Acad Orthop Surg* 1995;3:303–308.
10. Nunziata A, Blumenfeld I. Cadera a resorte: a proposito de una variedad. *Presna Med Argent* 1951;38:1997–2001.
11. Jones FW. The anatomy of snapping hip. *J Orthop Surg* 1920;2:1–3.
12. Gruen GS, Scioscia TN, Lowenstein JE. The surgical treatment of internal snapping hip. *Am J Sports Med* 2002;30(4):607–613.
13. Larsen E, Johansen J. Snapping hip. *Acta Orthop Scand* 1986;57:168–170.
14. Jacobs M, Young R. Snapping hip phenomenon among dancers. *Am Correct Ther J* 1978;32:92–98.
15. Singleton MC, LeVeau BF. The hip joint: structure, stability, and stress—a review. *Phys Ther* 1975;55:957–973.
16. Berry DJ. Soft tissue disorders. In: Callaghan JJ, Rosenberg AG, Rubash HE, eds. *The Adult Hip*, Vol. 1. Philadelphia: Lippincott–Raven Publishers; 1998:593–601.
17. Harper MC, Schaberg JE, Allen WC. Primary iliopsoas bursography in the diagnosis of disorders of the hip. *Clin Orthop* 1987;221:238–241.
18. Brignall CG, Stainsby GD. The snapping hip. *J Bone Joint Surg Br* 1991;73(2):253–254.
19. Beals RK. Painful snapping hip in young adults. *West J Med* 1993;159(4):401–402.
20. Zoltan DJ, Clancy WG, Keene JS. A new operative approach to snapping hip and refractory trochanteric bursitis in athletes. *Am J Sports Med* 1986;14(3):201–204.
21. Gordon EJ. Trochanteric bursitis and tendonitis. *Clin Orthop* 1961;20:193–202.

SECTION 4 Hip

14 Meralgia Paresthetica

Charles L. Nelson and Kristofer J. Jones

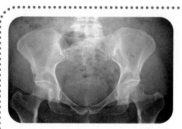

A 48-year-old overweight, diabetic woman presents with a 14-month history of left anterolateral thigh pain. She reports that she has been trying to lose weight through an intense exercise regimen for the past 3 months. Over the last 2 months, she has experienced spontaneous "burning" over the left anterolateral thigh but has had no associated weakness or numbness. She reports that palpating the area typically aggravates the pain. Review of systems is otherwise negative, and her past surgical history is noncontributory. An AP pelvis radiograph is obtained and is unremarkable.

CLINICAL POINTS

- The condition is most commonly seen in middle-aged patients.

- A wide range of complaints is characteristic.

- Diagnosis is largely clinical.

- If diagnosis is missed or delayed, significant disability may occur.

Clinical Presentation

Meralgia paresthetica is a relatively uncommon condition that is characterized by the symptom complex of pain, numbness, tingling, and paresthesias localized to the anterolateral area of the thigh. The condition was first described by Hager in 1885 and more extensively by Bernhardt and Roth in 1895 as an entrapment neuropathy of the lateral femoral cutaneous nerve.[1,2] Today, meralgia paresthetica is recognized as a mononeuropathy that is highly variable in etiology, as more than 80 different etiologic causes have been reported in the literature.[3] Although the condition is widely recognized as a clinical entity, it remains an ambiguous diagnosis and can lead to significant disability when the diagnosis is overlooked or delayed by practicing clinicians.

The diagnosis of meralgia paresthetica is primarily clinical, as it is based on the characteristic location of pain or dysesthesia, sensory oddity on exam, and absence of any other abnormal neurologic findings. The condition can be classified into one of two categories: spontaneous or iatrogenic.[4] Spontaneous meralgia paresthetica takes form in the absence of any previous surgical procedure that may have led to inadvertent injury of the lateral femoral cutaneous nerve along its anatomic course. Anatomic studies of this nerve have detailed its precise pathway in the lower extremity.[5,6] As the nerve appears through the iliopsoas muscle, it runs underneath the iliac fascia and travels along the anterior surface of the iliacus muscle. The nerve traverses the ilium, directed toward the anterior superior iliac spine, and enters the anterior thigh by passing under, through, or above the inguinal ligament. It is this precise area where the nerve is most susceptible to entrapment injury.[4] The spontaneous form can be further categorized as idiopathic or metabolic depending on the etiologic factors involved.[4] Metabolic disorders, most notably diabetes mellitus, have been identified as potential causes of this condition. According to researchers, there are a few possible explanations as to why patients with diabetes may be more susceptible to this neuropathy. First, axoplasmic transport is rendered dysfunctional in patients with high blood glucose, thereby resulting in nerve swelling and an increased probability of entrapment injury.[7] A second hypothesis is that it holds abnormalities in pyruvate, sorbitol, and lipid metabolism responsible for impairments of sodium-potassium adenosine triphosphatase activity, which ultimately causes nerve conduction abnormalities.[8] Alcoholism and lead toxicity have also been implicated as potential causes of metabolic meralgia paresthetica.

Iatrogenic meralgia paresthetica is secondary to mechanical factors, most notably specific surgical procedures in which the patient is positioned in a manner that may cause compression of the nerve. Specific surgical approaches can also predispose the injury to direct trauma or entrapment secondary to postoperative scarring. The site at which the lateral femoral cutaneous nerve exits the pelvis varies, and symptoms of this condition have been reported with each of five known variants identified by Aszmann[9] (Table 14.1). The nerve is most susceptible at superficial areas along its anatomic course, such as those seen in types A, B, and C in the aforementioned classification system. Various reports of external compression via obesity, pregnancy, abdominal ascites, tight garments, seat belts, braces, direct trauma, and pelvic tumors have been documented.[10] The nerve may also be entrapped in a retroperitoneal location or at the precise location where it penetrates the fascia lata.[4]

There is no age predilection for the occurrence of spontaneous meralgia prosthetica, although it is most frequently observed in middle-aged patients. There is no clear consensus on whether there is a male or female predominance. The spontaneous form is relatively uncommon compared with the iatrogenic form. A study by Ecker and Woltman[11] demonstrated that the estimated incidence of disease was 0.03% (3 in 10,000 cases). Patients typically present with a wide array of complaints,

Table 14.1	**Five Variant Locations of the Lateral Femoral Cutaneous Nerve As It Exits the Pelvis**	
ANATOMIC VARIANT	**GENERALIZED OCCURRENCE (%)**	**ANATOMIC LOCATION**
A	4	LFCN overlies iliac crest
B	27	LFCN ensheathed by inguinal ligament
C	23	LFCN covered by sartorius tendon
D	26	LFCN deep to inguinal ligament and medial to sartorius muscle
E	20	LFCN located over iliopsoas

LFCN, lateral femoral cutaneous nerve.
From Aszmann OC, Dellon ES, Dellon AL. Anatomical course of the lateral femoral cutaneous nerve and its susceptibility to compression and injury. *Plast Reconstr Surg* 1997;100:600–604.

PATIENT ASSESSMENT

1. Pain, numbness, tingling anterior lateral thigh

2. Irritation to the lateral femoral cutaneous nerve

3. Rule out lumbar disc radiculopathy

4. Check for tight belts, corsets, excessive panniculus

including burning, coldness, sharp electric pain, deep muscle aches, tingling, numbness, and hair loss in the distribution of the sensory abnormality.

Physical Findings

For the most part, patients with meralgia paresthetica have a benign physical examination except for a few specific, localized physical findings that can help to aid in the diagnosis. Hypersensitivity to touch and dysesthesias are common, and palpating the involved area usually exacerbates the patient's symptoms. Given the anatomic position and course of the nerve, symptomatic irritation of the nerve is typically elicited with passive hip extension movements. The Tinel sign (performed by lightly percussing over the nerve to elicit a sensation of tingling or "pins and needles" in the distribution of the nerve being tested) is frequently positive 1 cm medial and inferior to the anterior superior iliac spine.[4] One particularly helpful diagnostic sign is the absence of hair over the distribution of the sensory abnormality, which is thought to occur secondary to excessive rubbing by the patient to help relieve symptoms. While most studies report that the majority of patients present with unilateral involvement (10%–20%),[11,12] the incidence of bilateral involvement has been shown to be as high as 50%.[13,14]

Studies

DIAGNOSTIC IMAGING

It is important to remember that meralgia paresthetica can be caused by mechanical factors that result in stretch or compression injury of the nerve. In fact, the classic clinical symptoms that are observed in this condition can serve as a harbinger of a more insidious process, including a cecal tumor, appendiceal abscess, retroperitoneal lipofibrosarcoma, and periostitis of the ilium.[15,16] If there are any additional symptoms or signs that lead to suspicion of a mechanical cause for the mononeuropathy, initial standard radiographic imaging of the pelvis should be obtained. Advanced studies such as MRI, CT, or ultrasound may be indicated in certain cases where soft tissue or osseous pelvic tumors are suspected. Definitive confirmation of the diagnosis can be obtained when injection of lidocaine and 80 mg of methylprednisolone in the area of the lateral femoral cutaneous nerve achieves temporary relief.[17]

ELECTRODIAGNOSTIC TESTING

Although meralgia prosthetica is a widely known clinical disorder, the diagnosis is often missed. Subsequently, patients are forced to endure extreme pain and discomfort, given the clinician's inability to appropriately recognize and treat the mononeuropathy in a timely manner. If the diagnosis is unclear following a careful clinical assessment, referral to a physical medicine and rehabilitation physician or neurologist for electrodiagnostic testing may prove useful in establishing the diagnosis.

There are two electrodiagnostic techniques that can be utilized in the evaluation of meralgia prosthetica. Both techniques can use somatosensory

NOT TO BE MISSED

• *Lumbar disc disease:* The clinical entity most commonly mistaken for meralgia paresthetica is lumbar disc disease, given the similarity of presenting radicular symptoms. However, patients with lumbar disc disease do not have sensory symptoms specific to this nerve distribution. Furthermore, patients with lumbar disc disease typically show a mixed picture of sensory and motor deficits. While clinical examination should be sufficient to differentiate these two disorders, MRI can prove valuable to establishing a definitive diagnosis.

evoked potentials (SSEPs) or nerve conduction measurement to evaluate the function of the lateral femoral cutaneous nerve; however, they differ in the selected locations of stimulation and measurement. In one technique, the lateral femoral cutaneous nerve is stimulated near the anterior superior iliac spine, and the resultant potentials are measured at a distal location on the thigh. Conversely, the second form of testing occurs as the nerve is stimulated at a site distal to the pelvis, and the response is recorded proximally near the anterior superior iliac spine.[4] Both SSEPs and nerve conduction studies have been shown to be accurate in the diagnosis of meralgia prosthetica if performed in the hands of an experienced neurophysiologist.[18,19] One study demonstrated that sensory nerve action potential amplitude comparison between the affected and unaffected side in unilateral presentation may be more useful than sensory nerve conduction velocity or SSEP latency comparisons for the diagnosis.[20] Most importantly, electrodiagnostic studies may help to rule out other serious underlying neurologic abnormalities.

LABORATORY

There are no specific laboratory tests that can help in establishing the diagnosis of meralgia paresthetica, as it is a clinical disease that is diagnosed given the specific constellation of signs and symptoms that have been discussed. Any patient who presents with neurologic abnormalities outside of sensory defects in the distribution of the lateral femoral cutaneous nerve should be evaluated for other conditions. Motor deficits, abnormal reflexes, and sensory defects not specific to the area of the lateral femoral cutaneous nerve are not observed in meralgia paresthetica. Given the fact that metabolic disorders such as diabetes, lead poisoning, vitamin B deficiency, alcoholism, and hypothyroidism can potentially cause neuropathy, it is important to rule out these causes by obtaining a complete workup for patients with a history or at risk for these particular diseases.[21]

Treatment

1. Conservative measures after identifying source of nerve irritation
2. Local injection in the site of nerve with xylocaine and corticoid steroid
3. Surgical relief rarely indicated

The majority of patients with meralgia paresthetica respond well to conservative management alone. A recent study revealed that conservative treatment was successful in relieving symptoms in 91% of patients who were treated.[22] A careful history can reveal a recent increase in weight or even a predilection toward wearing tight clothing. Subsequent counseling on weight loss and avoidance of compression to the area along with protective padding for a brief period of time can cause resolution of symptoms. Pregnant women can be reassured that the symptoms typically resolve following childbirth.[23] In patients who do not have an identifiable external cause, pharmacologic therapy may provide relief. NSAIDs are the drug of choice,[4] as they are relatively inexpensive and have a relatively low side effect profile. NSAIDs can reduce inflammation in the area of involvement, which may subsequently lead to release of compression at the site of entrapment. Similar effects on inflammation can be achieved with injection of Xylocaine and methylprednisolone. This local injection can be performed by directing the needle 1 cm medial to the anterior superior iliac spine or in the region of maximal tenderness to palpation, which typically represents the area of nerve compression.[4] Additional pharmacologic agents that have shown some benefit include tricyclic antidepressants and anticonvulsants (gabapentin and carbamazepine) to reduce symptoms of neuropathic pain.[24] Topical anesthetic agents such as capsaicin and lidocaine-prilocaine cream may provide symptomatic relief by reducing tactile hypersensitivity. For refractory cases, surgical decompression, neurolysis of constricting tissue, or transection with partial excision of the lateral femoral cutaneous nerve can provide long-lasting relief. Surgery should be reserved only for when the complaints become fixed and disabling and numerous attempts at nonoperative treatment have failed. Treatment with spinal cord stimulation for refractory cases has shown promising results, as implanted spinal cord stimulators can modulate the disinhibition of descending analgesia pathways.[21] Researchers believe that this novel therapy could prove extremely beneficial given the fact that it is not inherently destructive to the nerve and can be performed as a temporary percutaneous trial to predict successful permanent implantation. Furthermore, it can always be explanted without significant permanent adverse effects. Ultimately, this form of therapy currently is experimental, and further large-scale clinical studies are needed to establish the true efficacy.

 Refer to Physical Therapy

Clinical Course

Although historically recognized, the diagnosis of meralgia paresthetica is often delayed, and definitive treatment may be refractory. A comprehensive history and physical examination should provide the necessary information to make an accurate diagnosis. All attempts at treating the patient with conservative measures should be exhausted prior to considering surgical therapy, as most cases respond to patient education about avoiding risk factors, weight loss, pharmacologic therapy, and local nerve block injections. In select cases, the condition may be persistent despite adequate attempts at avoiding surgery; therefore, neurolysis, surgical decompression, or nerve transaction with partial excision must be considered. While there are no specific guidelines on when conservative therapy should be abandoned in favor of surgical treatments, a recent study suggested that surgical options should begin to be explored when patients demonstrate persistent symptoms along with a clearly defined sensory loss for at least 1 year.[25]

WHEN TO REFER

- Intractable persistent symptoms lasting for at least 1 year[25]
- Immediate surgery for patients with an obvious mechanical cause that can be remedied surgically (i.e., tumor resection)

ICD9

355.1 Meralgia paresthetica

References

1. Wilson SAK. *Neurology*, 2nd ed. Baltimore: Williams & Wilkins; 1955:369.
2. Lee FC. Meralgia paresthetica. *Int Clin* 1936;1:216–229.
3. Ulkar B, Yildiz Y, Kunduracioglu B. Meralgia paresthetica: a long standing performance limiting cause of anterior thigh pain in a soccer player. *Am J Sports Med* 2003;31:787–789.
4. Grossman MG, Ducey SA, Nadler SS, et al. Meralgia paresthetica: diagnosis and treatment. *J Am Acad Orthop Surg* 2001;9:336–344.
5. Keegan JJ, Holyoke EA. Meralgia paresthetica: an anatomical and surgical study. *J Neurosurg* 1962;19: 341–345.
6. Hospodar PP, Ashman ES, Traub JA. Anatomic study of the lateral femoral cutaneous nerve with respect to the ilioinguinal surgical dissection. *J Orthop Trauma* 1999;13:17–19.
7. Nahabedian MY, Dellon AL. Meralgia paresthetica: etiology, diagnosis, and outcome of surgical decompression. *Ann Plast Surg* 1995;35:590–594.
8. Kim J, Kyriazi H, Greene DA. Normalization of Na(+)-K(+)-ATPase activity in isolated membrane fraction from sciatic nerves of streptozocin-induced diabetic rats by dietary myo-inositol supplementation in vivo or protein kinase C agonists in vitro. *Diabetes* 1991;40:558–567.
9. Aszmann OC, Dellon ES, Dellon AL. Anatomical course of the lateral femoral cutaneous nerve and its susceptibility to compression and injury. *Plast Reconstr Surg* 1997;100:600–604.
10. Ivins GK. Meralgia paresthetica: the elusive diagnosis—clinical experience with 14 adult patients. *Ann Surg* 2000;232(2):281–286.
11. Ecker AD, Woltman HW. Meralgia paresthetica: a report of one hundred and fifty cases. *JAMA* 1938;110: 1650–1652.
12. Kitchen D, Simpson J. Meralgia paresthetica, a review of sixty-seven patients. *Acta Neurol Scand* 1972;48: 547–555.
13. Rosencheck C. Meralgia paresthetica—its relation to osteoarthritis of the spinal vertebrae. *JAMA* 1925; 85:416.
14. Edelson R, Stevens P. Meralgia paresthetica in children. *J Bone Joint Surg Am* 1994;76:993–999.
15. Atkinson FRB. Meralgia paresthetica. *Med Press* 1938;197:177.
16. Pecina M, Kimpotic-Nemanic J, Markiewitz A. *Tunnel Syndromes*. Boca Raton, FL: CRC Press; 1991:105–111.
17. Benini A. Meralgia paresthetica: pathogenesis, clinical aspects and therapy of compression of the lateral cutaneous nerve of the thigh. *Schweiz Rundsch Med Prax* 1992;18:215–221.
18. Wiezer MJ, Franssen H, Rinkel GJ, et al. Meralgia paresthetica: differential diagnosis and follow-up. *Muscle Nerve* 1996;19:522–524.
19. Seror P. Lateral femoral cutaneous nerve conduction vs somatosensory evoked potentials for electrodiagnosis of meralgia paresthetica. *Am J Phys Med Rehabil* 1999;78:313–316.
20. Collins VJ. Blocks of nerves of lower extremities. In: Rovenstine EA, ed. *Fundamentals of Nerve Blocking*. Philadelphia: Lea & Febiger; 1960:266.
21. Barna SA, Hu MM, Buxo C, et al. Spinal cord stimulation for treatment of meralgia paresthetica. *Pain Physician* 2005;8:315–318.
22. Eubanks S, Newman L, Goehring L, et al. Meralgia paresthetica: a complication of laparoscopic herniorrhaphy. *Surg Laparosc Endosc* 1993;3:381–385.
23. Massey EW. Sensory mononeuropathies. *Semin Neurol* 1998;18:177–183.
24. Ghent WR. Further studies on meralgia paresthetica. *Can Med Assoc J* 1961;85:871–872.
25. Macnicol MF, Thompson WJ. Idiopathic meralgia paresthetica. *Clin Orthop* 1990;254:270–274.

15 Nontraumatic Osteonecrosis of the Femoral Head

Charles L. Nelson and Kristofer J. Jones

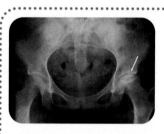 *A 32-year-old woman with systemic lupus erythematosus (SLE) presents with complaints of intermittent left groin pain that radiates to the posterior buttock. She describes the pain as deep and throbbing, stating that it has gradually become worse over the past 8 months. She cannot recall any associated trauma to the area and states that she has been taking six to eight tablets of acetaminophen (500 mg) daily without any significant relief. Of note, the patient has been on systemic prednisone for management of her SLE over the past 10 months. Radiographs and an MRI scan were obtained (Figs. 15.1, 15.2).*

CLINICAL POINTS

- Middle-aged individuals may have considerable hip damage.
- Men are more likely to be affected.
- A combination of disorders may lead to a common pathology.
- Onset may be gradual or sudden.

Clinical Presentation

Osteonecrosis, also referred to as *avascular necrosis*, of the femoral head is a potentially debilitating disease that typically causes significant hip joint destruction in patients who are in their third to fifth decade of life. While the incidence and prevalence of osteonecrosis of the femoral head varies with the populations from which the data are derived, it has been estimated to develop in 10,000 to 20,000 new patients each year in the United States, with an approximated male-to-female ratio of 4:1.[1,2] The condition is characterized by inconsistent areas of necrotic trabecular bone and bone marrow that can extend deep into and include the subchondral plate.[3] The pathogenesis of osteonecrosis is still poorly understood, and there is no current consensus regarding a specific pathologic event that causes cellular death. At present, the most commonly accepted mechanism of cellular death is impairment of circulation to the affected areas of bone, with potential underlying causes including intravascular coagulation, increased intraosseous pressure, hyperviscosity, venous stasis, or fatty emboli occlusion.[4,5] Many researchers have observed an association between osteonecrosis and radiation and chemotherapy, which implies that there may be a direct cytotoxic cellular effect in patients receiving these therapies. Ultimately, necrosis of the femoral head may be due to extrinsic pathophysiologic events as well as intrinsic cellular insults. Given the wide array of etiologic factors contributing to osteonecrosis, it may be appropriate to not think of the condition as a distinct disease, but rather as a multifactorial, heterogenous group of disorders that lead to an irrevocable common pathology typified by mechanical collapse of the femoral head.[6]

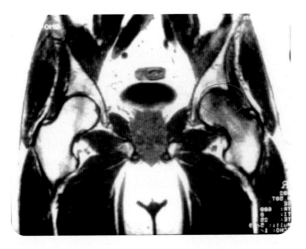

Figure 15.1 Coronal T1-weighted MRI scan of both the left and right hips demonstrates an area of low signal intensity consistent with osteonecrosis in the superior aspect of the left hip.

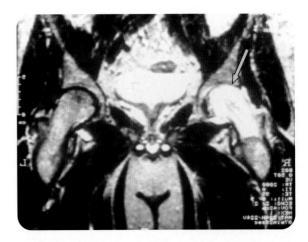

Figure 15.2 Coronal T2-weighted MRI scan of both hips demonstrates a diffuse, high signal intensity in the left femoral head consistent with osteonecrosis.

Patients with osteonecrosis typically present with pain localized to the groin, although occasional radiation of symptoms to the knee or buttock is not uncommon. The pain is usually characterized as deep and throbbing and may be insidious in nature but then may become more severe. Occasionally, the pain may present suddenly without any previous warning signs. Patients frequently report that the pain is exacerbated with ambulation, and they frequently describe a "catching" or "popping" sensation with motion. When taking the history, it is important for the physician to carefully identify any risk factors that may predispose the patient to osteonecrosis (Table 15.1).

Table 15.1 Common Clinical Risk Factors for Nontraumatic Osteonecrosis

Chronic alcohol abuse

Corticosteroid use

SLE

Sickle cell disease or trait

Pancreatitis

Renal failure

Hyperlipidemia

Hematologic disorders/Coagulopathies

Irradiation

Cytotoxic therapy

Idiopathic osteonecrosis

Pregnancy or oral contraceptive use

Smoking

HIV/AIDS or HIV therapy

SLE, systemic lupus erythematosus.

Physical Findings

Physical examination of patients with osteonecrosis should focus on a complete examination of their lower extremities. Both passive and active range of motion should be assessed with the involved leg in both flexion and extension. Gait examination is also of paramount importance. Physical exam findings typically reveal pain with passive and active range of motion at the hip as well as with ambulation. Limitation of internal rotation in both flexion and extension is common, and most patients demonstrate tremendous pain with passive internal rotation in extension. It is also common to notice a Trendelenburg gait while observing the patient walk. The contralateral hip of patients who have unilateral involvement should be carefully evaluated because the prevalence of bilateral involvement has been reported to be as high as 80%.[7–9]

Studies

IMAGING

Plain Radiography

Initial imaging of the patient suspected to have osteonecrosis of the hip should begin with AP and frog-leg lateral radiographs of the involved hip. Unfortunately, because plain radiography is designed to identify bone density changes related to remodeling, clear evidence of areas of necrosis may not be noticed for months to years after the initial development of the disorder. The AP radiographs typically demonstrate the affected area; however, it is important to note that because the anterior and posterior acetabular walls are superimposed on the superior margin of the femoral head, small areas of sclerotic or cystic changes in the subchondral regions can be missed. Frog-leg lateral radiographs can aid in the detection of any pathology in this area. Some researchers have demonstrated that the lateral radiograph can be helpful for staging purposes because the anterior segment of the femoral head, which is clearly displayed on this view, is the first area to exhibit early collapse or the crescent sign.[10] If radiographic evaluation shows changes consistent with osteonecrosis, no additional tests are necessary; however, as mentioned previously, radiographs may not reveal any abnormality in the early phase of the disease. Ultimately, there must be a high index of suspicion for osteonecrosis in any patient who complains of pain in the hip or has negative radiographic findings and any identifiable risk factors.

Magnetic Resonance

MRI has been shown to be the most sensitive imaging modality for the diagnosis of osteonecrosis.[11,12] Several studies have demonstrated a single density line of low-intensity signal on T1-weighted images that represents the early separation of normal and ischemic bone. When T2-weighted images of the affected area are examined, a second high signal intensity line can be found within this line, which is believed to represent hypervascular granulation tissue. This second line is referred to as the *double-line sign.*[13,14] MRI can easily outline the area of necrotic bone and

Table 15.2 Ficat and Arlet Radiographic Classification of Osteonecrosis of the Femoral Head	
STAGE	**DESCRIPTION OF RADIOGRAPHIC FINDINGS**
I	Normal
II	Sclerotic or cystic lesions without subchondral fracture
III	Crescent sign (subchondral collapse) and/or step-off in contour of subchondral bone
IV	Osteoarthritis with decreased presence of articular cartilage and presence of osteophytes

help the clinician to differentiate active repair from both normal and necrotic bone. This differentiation is important in staging of the disease as well as in treatment planning. Currently, there are five primary staging systems available to help classify the extent of osteonecrotic involvement. The most descriptive classification system is the University of Pennsylvania system, which incorporates findings on bone scan or MRI as well as stage and size of the lesion.[15] Another commonly used system is the Ficat and Arlet system, which consists of four distinct stages[16] (Table 15.2).

Computed Tomography

Because of the superb diagnostic quality of MRI, CT is not typically used in the diagnosis and management of osteonecrosis. CT scans can be useful in the assessment of subtle subchondral collapse, as bony collapse may be better appreciated on CT than on MRI.

Radionuclide Bone Scan

Bone scanning can be a useful technique for the detection of osteonecrosis, as this modality identifies areas of increased vascularity by relying on the incorporation of a tracer (technetium Tc 99m–labeled phosphate) into the surface of hydroxyapatite crystals during osteogenesis.[17] However, it is important to note that the sensitivity of bone scanning is reduced during the ischemic phase, as increased vascularity is only observed during the reparative phase. Furthermore, this imaging modality has been shown to be less sensitive in the detection of osteonecrosis in the early stages or when both hips are symmetrically involved, because the results of the study are based on asymmetric findings.[6] Lastly, increased uptake alone can be observed in several pathologic conditions, and there are no specific changes on radionuclide scanning that are specific to osteonecrosis, making a definitive diagnosis utilizing this modality difficult to establish. For these reasons, the authors do not currently advocate use of this modality in the available collection of diagnostic tools unless the patient has a pacemaker or is unable to undergo evaluation with MRI.

LABORATORY

Laboratory tests have limited utility in the diagnosis of osteonecrosis, as there are no available systemic markers specific to the condition. There

SECTION 4 Hip

are a few lab tests that could prove useful if osteonecrosis is suspected in a patient with hip pain and identifiable risk factors. For example, genetic testing for sickle cell disease or trait could prove useful in young black patients at risk for this disease. A lipid profile could help to identify hyperlipidemia in an older adult patient who presents with suspected osteonecrosis of the femoral head. Additionally, screening tests for coagulopathies, including familial thrombophilias and hypofibrinolysis, can prove helpful. These tests include those for protein C, protein S deficiencies, factor V Leiden disease, and a number of genetic markers, which are currently utilized only for experimental purposes due to cost and lack of influence on diagnosis. Ultimately, these diseases act by decreasing circulation to the femoral head, resulting in osteonecrosis.

Treatment

- Decompression of the femoral head with the subcutaneous drilling
- After collapse and persistent pain, total hip replacement

Treatment options can be classified into three groups: nonoperative/ conservative therapy, joint-preserving procedures, and prosthetic replacements. There are a number of nonoperative treatment protocols that have been used in the past. Historically, these treatments have not led to alterations in the natural history of the disease, although a recent study determined that oral alendronate (Fosamax) may be effective in preventing collapse of the femoral head, even with extensive necrosis, presumably by inhibiting bone resorption in the necrotic region.[18] Overall, the choice of treatment is dependent on the size of the necrotic lesion, the stage of the disease at presentation, the amount of femoral head collapse, and the morbidity of the potential treatment. As mentioned previously, the natural history of osteonecrosis still remains unclear. Due to the lack of knowledge concerning the pathogenesis of osteonecrosis, treatment has been limited to the elimination of symptoms, and increased therapeutic efforts have been directed at the result of the disease rather than addressing the actual cause of the problem.

Various methods of treatment exist for patients with this condition; however, individual factors such as patient age and associated medical comorbidities should also be taken into account. Most researchers agree that if left untreated, the disease will quickly progress to secondary end-stage degeneration of the hip.[19,20] Conservative therapies utilize modified weight bearing in attempts to reduce the forces across the hip joint to promote healing before subchondral bone collapse takes place. A meta-analysis of 21 studies involving 819 hips treated with nonoperative treatment helped to shed significant light on the natural history of this condition.[21] Researchers found that of the 819 hips treated conservatively, only 22% had a satisfactory clinical result at a mean follow-up of 34 months (range, 20 months to 10 years). Furthermore, approximately 76% of the hips that were available for follow-up examination were ultimately treated with surgery. These results suggest that nonoperative therapy with modified weight-bearing protocols ranging from full weight bearing as tolerated to partial weight bearing with crutches does not result in favorable clinical outcomes.

Given the fact that the pathogenesis of osteonecrosis can result from several different disorders, available pharmacologic therapy is controversial at this time. Some researchers have attempted to target different potential causes of this disorder. For example, naftidrofuryl has been shown to selectively reduce bone marrow pressure in the body, thereby increasing circulation to the bone.[22] Pharmacologic agents directed toward lowering lipid levels or enhancing fibrinolysis in the circulatory system have also been explored as potential treatments. While the results of some of these studies are promising, these drugs remain experimental for now and have not been approved for clinical use in patients with osteonecrosis.

Electrical stimulation is another investigational method for the treatment of osteonecrosis of the femoral head. Theoretic advantages of this treatment lie in its ability to stimulate osteogenesis and neovascularization in the affected area of necrotic bone, thereby preventing disease progression. An early study investigating electrical stimulation by Aaron and Steinberg[23] supported the notion that inductive coupling with pulsed magnetic fields was a promising technique. A recent retrospective analysis of treatment results with pulsed electromagnetic field stimulation in 66 patients with osteonecrosis of the femoral head was performed. Patients with Ficat stage I, II, or III osteonecrosis were treated with pulsed electromagnetic field stimulation for 8 hours per day for an average of 5 months. The authors found that pulsed electromagnetic field treatment may be indicated in the early stages of osteonecrosis of the femoral head (Ficat stages I and II), as it may be able to either preserve the hip or delay the time until surgery by protecting the articular cartilage from the catabolic effect of inflammation and subchondral bone marrow edema.[24] Additional randomized, prospective clinical trials are needed to definitively conclude whether this form of therapy should be incorporated into routine clinical practice.

Clinical Course

Treatment of osteonecrosis is more successful when it is initiated in the early stages of the disease. The focus of most diagnostic and treatment efforts to date have been directed at prevention of subchondral collapse. Ultimately, revascularization techniques have altered the natural history of this disease in a favorable manner.

Early studies reported an overall clinical progression rate of 77% to 98% and a radiographic progression rate of 68% to 75%, with an average of 3 years follow-up.[25] From these studies, it was concluded that osteonecrosis of the femoral head is generally a progressive disorder and that it typically advances within 2 to 3 years following the initial onset of symptoms. More recent studies have utilized Ficat staging to investigate the natural clinical course of this condition if left untreated. Table 15.3 displays the observed progression of osteonecrosis in each Ficat stage.[25]

Several studies have examined various demographic, clinical, and radiographic features of patients with osteonecrosis in an attempt to identify

SECTION 4 Hip

Table 15.3 Observed Rates of Clinical and Radiographic Progression of Osteonecrosis According to Ficat Stage

FICAT STAGE	CLINICAL FAILURE (%)	RADIOGRAPHIC FAILURE (%)
I	76	92
II	85	64
III	89	87
IV	N/A	N/A

N/A, not available; this end stage of osteonecrotic disease is definitively treated with surgery.

any specific risk factors for more rapid progression of disease. Interestingly, researchers have found that clinical characteristics, including patient age, gender, and etiology do not predict more rapid clinical or radiographic progression. However, Ficat III lesions in older patients (>40 years) did exhibit more rapid clinical and radiographic progression, as did lesions occupying over 50% of the femoral head. Segmental collapse of more than 4 mm on initial radiograph was also associated with more rapid clinical and radiographic failure than hips with initial presenting collapse measuring 0 to 1 mm.[25]

 Refer to Physical Therapy

ICD9

733.42 Aseptic necrosis of head and neck of femur

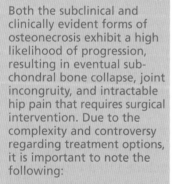

WHEN TO REFER

Both the subclinical and clinically evident forms of osteonecrosis exhibit a high likelihood of progression, resulting in eventual subchondral bone collapse, joint incongruity, and intractable hip pain that requires surgical intervention. Due to the complexity and controversy regarding treatment options, it is important to note the following:

• Early referral to an orthopaedic surgeon is advisable. If collapse is not present, there may be a limited window for joint-preserving surgical alternatives. Even in the presence of collapse, some patients

References

1. Mankin HJ. Nontraumatic necrosis of bone (osteonecrosis). *N Engl J Med* 1992;326:1473–1479.
2. Robinson HJ Jr, Springer JA. Success of core decompression in the management of early stages of avascular necrosis: a four year prospective study. *Orthop Trans* 1992–1993;16:707.
3. Catto M. Pathology of aseptic bone necrosis. In: Davidson JK, ed. *Aseptic Necrosis of Bone.* Amsterdam: Excerpta Medica; 1976.
4. Chang CC, Greenspan A, Gershwin ME. Osteonecrosis: current perspectives on pathogenesis and treatment. *Semin Arthritis Rheum* 1993;23:47–69.
5. Schroer WC. Current concepts on the pathogenesis of osteonecrosis of the femoral head. *Orthop Rev* 1994;23:487–497.
6. Etienne G, Mont MA, Ragland PS. The diagnosis and treatment of nontraumatic osteonecrosis of the femoral head. *Inst Course Lect* 2004;429:131–138.
7. Meyers MH. Osteonecrosis of the femoral head. Pathogenesis and long term results of treatment. *Clin Orthop* 1988;231:51–61.
8. Ohzono K, Saito M, Takaoka K, et al. Natural history of nontraumatic avascular necrosis of the femoral head. *J Bone Joint Surg Br* 1991;73(1):68–72.
9. Zizic TM, Hungerford DS, Stevens MB. Ischemic bone necrosis in systemic lupus erythematosus. The early diagnosis of ischemic necrosis of bone. *Medicine* 1980;59:134–142.
10. Hungerford DS, Jones LC. Diagnosis of osteonecrosis of the femoral head. In: Schoutens A, Arlet J, Gardeniers JWM, et al., eds. *Bone Circulation and Vascularization in Normal and Pathological Conditions.* New York: Plenum Press; 1993:265–275.
11. Takatori Y, Kokubo T, Ninomiya S, et al. Avascular necrosis of the femoral head. Natural history and magnetic resonance imaging. *J Bone Joint Surg Br* 1993;75(2):217–221.
12. Thickman D, Axel L, Kressel HY, et al. Magnetic resonance imaging of avascular necrosis of the femoral head. *Skel Radiol* 1986;15:133–140.
13. Kokubo T, Takatori Y, Ninomiya S, et al. Magnetic resonance imaging and scintigraphy of avascular necrosis of the femoral head. Prediction of subsequent segmental collapse. *Clin Orthop* 1992;277:54–60.

may be candidates for either joint-preserving procedures or hemiarthroplasty (resurfacing only the femoral head) early in the course of the disease. The largest goal of the primary care clinician should be to assess whether precollapse or postcollapse disease is present by standard radiographic imaging or MRI if the extent of disease is not clear.

- If femoral head collapse has occurred at the time of initial presentation, the patient should be immediately referred.

- When subchondral bone integrity is present, there are certain prognostic factors that should influence whether the patient should be referred. The extent of femoral head involvement has been found to be very important, with lesions that involve <15% of the head faring better with all treatment methods than those with a more significant lesion.[21] Ultimately, these patients could do well with an initial attempt at conservative therapy.

- Complicated patients who present with multisystem disease, such as those with organ transplant or those with sickle cell disease, or patients who have poor health in general should be referred to an orthopaedic surgeon for definitive care, as attempts at hip preservation rarely succeed, and these patients often require a total hip replacement.

14. Lang P, Jergesen HE, Moseley ME, et al. Avascular necrosis of the femoral head: high-field strength MR imaging with histologic correlation. *Radiology* 1988;169:517–524.
15. Steinberg ME, Hayken GD, Steinberg DR. A quantitative system for staging avascular necrosis. *J Bone Joint Surg Br* 1995;77(1):34–41.
16. Ficat RP, Arlet J. Functional investigation of bone under normal conditions. In: Hungerford DS, ed. *Ischemia and Necrosis of Bone*. Baltimore: Williams & Wilkins; 1980:29–52.
17. Hedley AK, Kim W. Prosthetic replacement in osteonecrosis of the hip. *Instr Course Lect* 1983;32:265–271.
18. Nishii T, Sugano N, Miki H, et al. Does alendronate prevent collapse in osteonecrosis of the femoral head? *Clin Orthop Relat Res* 2006;443:273–279.
19. Romer LL, Wettstein P. Results of treatment of eighty-one Swiss patients with idiopathic ischemic necrosis of the femoral head. In: Zinn WM, ed. *Idiopathic Ischemic Necrosis of the Femoral Head in Adults*. Baltimore: University Park Press; 1971:205–212.
20. Musso ES, Mitchell SN, Schink-Ascani M, et al. Results of conservative management of osteonecrosis of the femoral head: a retrospective review. *Clin Orthop* 1986;207:209–215.
21. Mont MA, Hungerford DS. Non-traumatic avascular necrosis of the femoral head. *J Bone Joint Surg Am* 1995;77(3):459–474.
22. Arlet J, Mazieres B, Thiechert M, et al. The effect of IV injection of naftidrofuryl (Praxilene). In: Arlet J, Mazieres B, eds. *Intramedullary Pressure in Patients with Osteonecrosis of the Femoral Head. Bone Circulation and Bone Necrosis*. Berlin: Springer; 1990:405–406.
23. Aaron RK, Steinberg ME. Electrical stimulation of osteonecrosis of the femoral head. *Semin Arthroplasty* 1991;2(3):214–221.
24. Massari L, Fini M, Cadossi R, et al. Biophysical stimulation with pulsed electromagnetic fields in osteonecrosis of the femoral head. *J Bone Joint Surg Am* 2006;88(Suppl 3):56–60.
25. Aaron RK, Mont MA, Urbaniak JR, et al. Osteonecrosis of the hip: management in the 21st century. Presented at the 72nd Annual American Academy of Orthopaedic Surgeons conference. Washington, DC, February 23, 2005.

SECTION 4 Hip

Knee

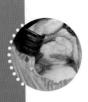
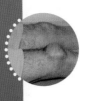

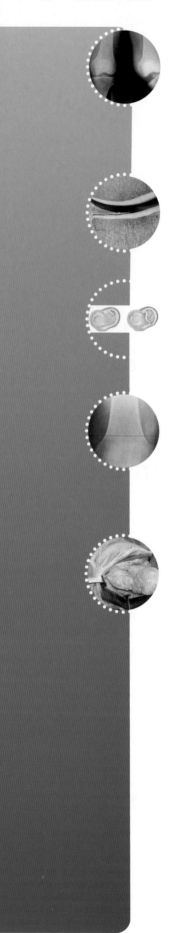

CHAPTER 16 Swollen Knee/Effusion

Sharat Kusuma and Jess H. Lonner

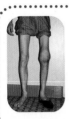 *A 45-year-old male "weekend warrior" athlete presents with a 3-day history of a swollen, painful knee after a minor twisting injury during a pick-up basketball game. He is able to bear weight but with some pain.*

CLINICAL POINTS

- Acute knee problems are generally preceded by significant trauma.

- Somewhat less acute and atraumatic effusions may be due to infection or gout.

- Chronic conditions that develop more gradually may be due to osteoarthritis or rheumatoid arthritis.

PATIENT ASSESSMENT

1. Numerous causes

2. Acute swelling from trauma and overuse most common

3. Chronic knee problems and most swelling commonly related to variable degrees of osteoarthritis

4. Rule out hemarthrosis, sepsis

5. Aspirate for diagnosis and treatment early to help identify cause

6. MRI, if symptoms persist

Clinical Presentation

There are numerous causes, both acute and chronic, of a swollen knee and/or an effusion. The clinical presentation is often dependent on its underlying pathology. The factors in the patient history to consider carefully when formulating a differential diagnosis of the cause of a knee effusion include a history of trauma and the time course over which the effusion has developed. Acute knee trauma often precedes the development of an acute effusion and pain. Occasionally, however, such as with a meniscus tear, the trauma may be relatively innocuous, and the mechanism may be no greater than squatting or pivoting. Atraumatic effusions that develop acutely over the course of hours or a few days may suggest an infectious etiology or acute gouty attack. Additionally, septic arthritis may be accompanied by fevers, chills, or malaise. Those that develop more insidiously and wax and wane in size are more suggestive of chronic causes such as osteoarthritis or rheumatoid arthritis (Fig. 16.1).

Physical Findings

Patients with effusions have anterior knee pain with flexion because of capsular distension and pressure. The source of the effusion may also cause pain. For instance, a medial meniscus tear may cause sharp, stabbing posteromedial pain with deep flexion or joint line palpation. An anterior cruciate ligament (ACL) tear may produce instability on anterior drawer testing; patellar tendon rupture may manifest with a palpable gap in the tendon and profound limitation and weakness in active knee extension.

Studies

The single most useful study in determining the cause of an acute or chronic knee effusion is aspiration and analysis of the joint fluid. Given the easily accessible subcutaneous location of the knee joint space,

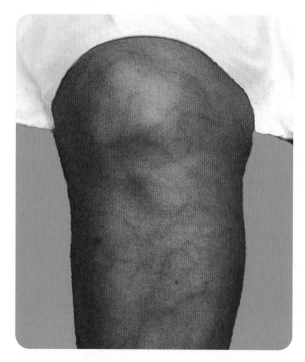

Figure 16.1 This image shows a knee with an effusion. Swelling above and adjacent to the patella suggests synovial thickening or effusion in the knee joint. (From Bickley LS, and Szilagyi P. *Bates' Guide to Physical Examination and History Taking*, 8th ed. Philadelphia: Lippincott Williams & Wilkins; 2003.)

aspiration is a simple procedure that can be performed in the outpatient setting. The gross appearance of the fluid can provide clues regarding the etiology of the effusion. Clear, synovial fluid is most often indicative of osteoarthritis or a torn meniscus. Bloody fluid often indicates trauma (such as an acute ACL rupture or fracture). Cloudy/blood-tinged fluid is suggestive of infection or inflammatory etiology. Turbid fluid is common in gout, chondrocalcinosis, Lyme arthritis, or infection. Fluid analysis should include Gram stain, culture, cell count, and crystal analysis.

Plain x-rays of the knee joint can also be helpful in identifying the cause of effusion. Unless there is concern about a fracture, the painful, swollen knee should be evaluated first with weight-bearing AP, lateral, and sunrise x-rays. Joint space narrowing suggests osteoarthritis or rheumatoid arthritis, while traumatic causes of effusion such as patella fracture, quadriceps tendon rupture (manifest as patella baja), patellar tendon rupture (manifest as patella alta), or tibial plateau fracture will be apparent on plain x-rays. Soft tissue injuries such as meniscus tears or ACL rupture will not be evident on plain x-ray; any suspicion of these should prompt an MRI.

Finally, laboratory studies such as CRP, ESR, serum uric acid levels, and WBC count can also be useful. Septic knee effusions will usually be associated with an elevated CRP and ESR and perhaps elevated WBC count. Gout and other inflammatory arthropathies will have moderately elevated ESR and CRP, although not to the same degree as that seen with septic effusions. Elevated serum uric acid levels are common in gout. RF, HLA-B27, and ANA are helpful in diagnosing or excluding certain types of inflammatory arthritis.

NOT TO BE MISSED

- Septic knee arthritis
- Gout/Pseudogout
- Patella fracture
- Tibial plateau fracture
- ACL rupture
- Acute meniscus tear
- Hemophilic arthropathy
- Lyme disease
- Pigmented villonodular synovitis
- Patellar tendon/quadriceps tendon rupture

Treatment

1. Treatment depends on the etiology.
2. Clear, yellow fluid can be treated with aspiration and intra-articular cortisone injection.
3. Recurrent effusion from degenerative joint disease can be treated with intra-articular cortisone injections.
4. Identify the cause in order to specify treatment.

Sterile aspiration of the painful knee effusion can provide considerable relief of pain. However, the pathology contributing to the effusion, if left alone, can continue to contribute to the formation of effusions. Therefore, treatment of the knee effusion should focus on treating the underlying pathology.

Septic effusions in adults require surgical irrigation, débridement, and long-term intravenous or oral antibiotics. Recurrent effusions from

WHEN TO REFER

- Patients with acute traumatic effusions should be referred for orthopaedic care.

- Acute septic effusions should also be referred for orthopaedic management, as they will usually require surgical management. Additionally, consultation with an infectious diseases specialist can help to guide antibiotic management.

- Patients with chronic effusion related to severe osteoarthritis or rheumatoid arthritis that has failed conservative management may be surgical candidates for joint reconstruction procedures and should also be referred for orthopaedic care.

osteoarthritis or rheumatoid arthritis that are recalcitrant to medical management may require surgery.

Refer to Physical Therapy

Clinical Course

The clinical course of knee effusion often parallels the treatment of the underlying condition. Acute traumatic effusions will gradually subside as the underlying bony or soft tissue trauma heals. With septic effusions, surgical irrigation and débridement should result in resolution; recurrence of the effusion should raise concern for recurrent or persistent septic arthritis. Patients with chronic causes of effusion will have recurrent effusions that will often wax and wane in size.

ICD9
719.06 Effusion of lower leg joint

CHAPTER 17

Chondromalacia Patella: Anterior Knee Pain in the Young Patient

Sharat Kusuma and Jess H. Lonner

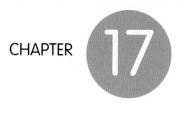

A 17-year-old female basketball player complains of a long history of bilateral knee pain, most pronounced anteriorly. She states that pain is made worse by sports, stair climbing, and prolonged sitting.

CLINICAL POINTS

- The condition is a common problem in young women.
- Anterior knee pain is characteristic.
- Deep knee bending aggravates the pain.

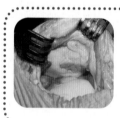

PATIENT ASSESSMENT

1. Predisposed to patella alta, patella dysplasia, and high Q angle
2. Hypermobile patella, significant patella crepitus
3. X-rays generally negative
4. MRI generally negative

Clinical Presentation

The term *chondromalacia patella* is often incorrectly assumed to be synonymous with anterior knee pain, yet it specifically refers to anterior knee pain due to softening and degeneration of the articular cartilage of the patella. Chondromalacia patella causes anterior knee pain with maneuvers such as deep knee flexion, stair and hill ascent and descent, and prolonged sitting. It is more common in young women. Anatomic factors that may predispose a patient to chondromalacia include patella alta (high-riding patella), patellofemoral dysplasia, and a high Q angle.

Physical Findings

Patients with true chondromalacia patella will often demonstrate a knee effusion, tenderness on the undersurface of the patella, and patellar crepitation. Increased Q angle and valgus posture of the leg may be noted. Evidence of hypermobility of the patella with medial or lateral subluxation may be seen. Pain will be elicited with patellar inhibition testing. Prior evidence of trauma to the anterior knee may be present.

Studies

Initial studies that are useful in discerning the cause of anterior knee pain include plain x-rays of the knee. The most helpful views are standing AP, lateral, and Merchant or sunrise views. The latter x-ray is performed with the knee in 45 degrees of flexion with the x-ray beam directed 30 degrees caudad from the horizontal. The Merchant/sunrise

SECTION 5 Knee

views can visualize the patellofemoral articulation and the degree of joint space narrowing.

Advanced studies such as MRI, CT, and bone scan are rarely indicated in the initial evaluation of anterior knee pain.

Treatment

1. Conservative
2. Muscle strengthening activities
3. Occasionally, patella taping helpful
4. Occasionally, patella bracing helpful
5. Occasionally, injections helpful
6. Symptoms may be refracted in therapy, especially in the young, active patient

Most patients with anterior knee pain and/or chondromalacia patella can be treated with isometric exercises and activity modifications. Other interventions that may be helpful include patellar taping (i.e., McConnell taping) or patellar bracing[1] and injections.

 Refer to Patient Education

 Refer to Physical Therapy

Clinical Course

The majority of patients with both anterior knee pain and chondromalacia patella will respond favorably to nonoperative treatment. Data has demonstrated that up to 84% of patients will have decreased pain after 8 weeks of quadriceps stretching and strengthening exercises.[2]

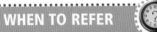

ICD9
717.7 Chondromalacia of patella

References

1. Friederichs MG, Burks RT. Patellofemoral disorders. In: Garrick JG, ed. *Orthopaedic Knowledge Update, Sports 3.* Rosemont, IL: American Academy of Orthopaedic Surgeons; 2004:213–221.
2. Doucette SA, Goble EM. The effect of exercise on patellar tracking in lateral patellar compression syndrome. *Am J Sports Med* 1992;20(4):434–440.

18 Prepatellar Bursitis: Housemaid Knee

Sharat Kusuma and Jess H. Lonner

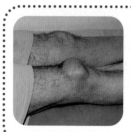

A 45-year-old man who is employed as a plumber spends significant amounts of time working in a kneeling position and presents with complaints of anterior knee pain, swelling, tenderness, and redness.

Clinical Presentation

Prepatellar bursitis is an inflammation, swelling, and enlargement of the prepatellar bursa. This bursa is one of several around the knee (others include the infrapatellar, deep patellar, and pes anserinus bursa) (Fig. 18.1). It can result from frequent kneeling or from acute trauma to the anterior knee (Fig. 18.2). Often, it is only painful when kneeling directly on it.

Aseptic, inflammatory prepatellar bursitis can evolve into pyogenic prepatellar bursitis. The synovial fluid within the prepatellar bursa provides an excellent medium for bacterial growth, and the bursa can be inoculated by direct trauma or abrasions to the overlying skin.

Physical Findings

Focal swelling on the anterior surface of the knee overlying the patella and the patellar tendon is normally seen. Pain is unusual unless infected. Erythema suggests septic bursitis.

Studies

The diagnosis of prepatellar bursitis is mostly clinical, and additional studies are rarely necessary. In cases associated with acute trauma, plain x-rays of the knee may be helpful in ruling out fractures. In cases where there is concern for septic prepatellar bursitis, aspiration of the bursa can be diagnostic. Clear or serosanguineous fluid is indicative of aseptic bursitis, while purulent fluid is diagnostic of pyogenic bursitis.

Treatment and Clinical Course

1. Aspiration and evaluation of fluid to rule out infection
2. Injection of intra-articular cortisone if clear, yellow fluid
3. May recur

CLINICAL POINTS

- Frequent kneeling or trauma to the anterior knee may be causal factors.
- The patient may feel pain only when kneeling directly on the anterior knee.
- Infectious bursitis may develop.

PATIENT ASSESSMENT

1. Swelling over tibial tubercle related to kneeling or acute trauma
2. Usually painless
3. Rule out sepsis
4. X-rays should be negative

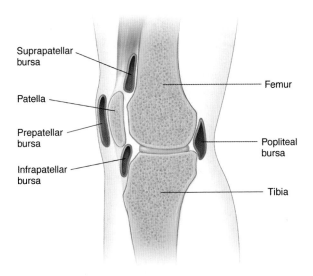

Suprapatellar bursa

Patella

Prepatellar bursa

Infrapatellar bursa

Femur

Popliteal bursa

Tibia

Figure 18.1 Knee joint; *F*, medial aspect of the knee showing the location of bursae. This schematic cross section of the knee shows the location of several bursae around the knee. Note the subcutaneous location of the prepatellar bursa. (From Premkumar K. *The Massage Connection Anatomy and Physiology*. Baltimore: Lippincott Williams & Wilkins; 2004.)

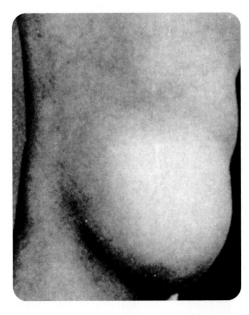

Figure 18.2 Prepatellar bursitis is usually a bursitis caused by friction between the skin and patella. If the inflammation is chronic, the bursa becomes distended with fluid and forms a swelling ("housemaid knee") anterior to the knee. This image of a knee with prepatellar bursitis demonstrates the impressive amount of swelling that can occur.

SECTION 5 Knee

NOT TO BE MISSED

- Septic knee arthritis
- Gout
- Rheumatoid arthritis of the knee
- Osteoarthritis of the knee
- Patella fracture
- Patellar tendon rupture
- Quadriceps tendon rupture
- Osteochondral fracture of the femur

WHEN TO REFER

- Patients with chronic prepatellar bursitis who have failed nonoperative treatment, including aspiration and steroid injection, should be referred to an orthopaedic surgeon.
- Cases of septic bursitis, or cases in which there is concern for patella fracture, patellar/quadriceps tendon rupture, or septic knee arthritis should be referred to an orthopaedist immediately.

Aseptic prepatellar bursitis occasionally resolves with rest, icing, NSAIDs, compression wraps, and avoidance of kneeling. Often, however, aspiration of the bursa and injection with a corticosteroid preparation is necessary. In very rare instances, when the bursitis recurs, surgical excision is necessary. When pyogenic bursitis is present, surgical excision and drainage is required. Often, excision of the chronically infected bursal tissue is also necessary to eradicate infection. Postoperative antibiotics should also be used in this scenario.

 Refer to Patient Education

 Refer to Physical Therapy

ICD9
726.65 Prepatellar bursitis

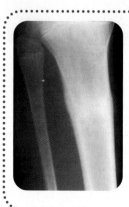
CHAPTER 19 Overuse Syndrome

Sharat Kusuma and Jess H. Lonner

A 45-year-old slightly overweight man who has not participated in vigorous physical activity in several months participates in a pickup 5-on-5 basketball game without warming up and presents 2 days after the game with severe generalized right knee pain and difficulty walking. He denies any discrete history of traumatic injury.

Clinical Presentation

The general terms *overuse syndrome* or *overuse injury* refer to musculoskeletal pain or dysfunction that is the result any physical activity that exceeds the strength of musculoskeletal tissues such as bone, tendons, ligaments, joints, or bursae.[1] Such activity causes microtrauma to these structures and results in pain and dysfunction that can be severe. The knee joint is not immune to this. The diagnosis of overuse syndrome must be entertained in any active individual with knee pain after heavy physical activity with no discrete history of trauma. Overuse can cause tendinitis, capsulitis, periostitis, bursitis, or stress fractures.

Pain is often achy and most pronounced 1 to 2 days after intense physical activity, particularly when the patient has not warmed up or stretched.

CLINICAL POINTS

- Tissue pain and dysfunction may be severe.
- Pain is frequently achy.
- Vigorous physical activity with no distinct history of trauma may trigger the syndrome.

Physical Findings

Physical findings in patients with knee overuse injuries are many and varied. Pain may be vague and poorly localized. However, the underlying structures that have suffered microtrauma will often be tender and inflamed, including the hamstrings, quadriceps, patellar tendon, and the pes anserinus.

Overuse stress fractures may be present in any bony structures about the knee, most commonly the anterior medial tibia. Patients with stress fractures will have focal point tenderness over the affected bone.

Studies

Radiographs are often nondiagnostic, even early in a stress fracture. MRI or bone scan should be obtained if there is suspicion of stress fractures or avascular necrosis (Fig. 19.1).

PATIENT ASSESSMENT

1. Classical overuse with structural problem if a stress fracture
2. More commonly in the middle-aged "weekend warrior"
3. Related to tendinitis, capsulitis, bursitis, or other inflammation around the knee
4. Pain may be vague and poorly localized or may be very well localized
5. X-rays rule out stress fracture or other structural change

NOT TO BE MISSED

- Patellar tendon/ quadriceps tendon rupture (usually acute onset)
- Tibial stress fracture
- Patella fracture
- Anterior cruciate ligament rupture
- Tibial plateau fracture
- Meniscus tear

WHEN TO REFER

- Patients with very severe pain, large effusions, and x-ray evidence of bony trauma or fracture should be referred to an orthopaedic surgeon for definitive management.
- Patients with stress fractures, particularly of the tibia, should be made nonweight bearing immediately and referred to an orthopaedic surgeon.
- Patients whose symptoms do not resolve after 2 to 3 months of conservative care should be referred to an orthopaedist for further workup and diagnostic imaging.

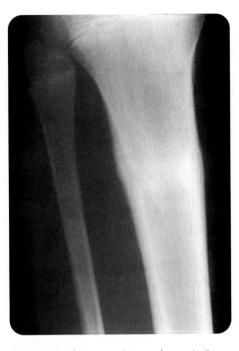

Figure 19.1 Plain x-ray image demonstrating a stress fracture in a young male athlete. Note the sclerosis and widened cortices associated with bone healing.

Treatment

1. Temporarily discontinue excessive activity
2. Rule out structural abnormality
3. Occasional use of steroid injection into area of soft tissue inflammation
4. May be recurrent

There should be a deliberate discontinuation of activities that cause pain and disability. Use of crutches may be prudent, particularly if there is a stress fracture. Ice, rest, compression, elevation, and NSAIDs are very effective in reducing local swelling and inflammation.

After an initial period of rest, physical therapy should be initiated, including stretching, strengthening, and conditioning exercises, which will increase the strength, flexibility, and endurance of the bony and soft tissue structures about the knee, thereby decreasing the probability of repeat overuse injury.

Steroid injections into tendons or ligaments should be avoided because steroids can weaken these structures and increase the risk of rupture. Additionally, corticosteroid injections around a stress fracture can inhibit healing.

 Refer to Physical Therapy

Clinical Course

Most overuse injuries will heal with elimination of the offensive activity and rest. The time frame until resolution can be variable but is often complete within 8 weeks. Pain that persists beyond this time frame should raise concern for diagnoses other than simple overuse syndrome.

ICD9

726.60 Enthesopathy of knee, unspecified
730.36 Periostitis, without mention of osteomyelitis, involving lower leg
733.93 Stress fracture of tibia or fibula
733.95 Stress fracture of other bone
719.46 Pain in joint involving lower leg

Reference

1. Duca MA. Medical care of athletes. In: Vaccaro AR, ed. *Orthopaedic Knowledge Update 8.* Rosemont, IL: American Academy of Orthopaedic Surgeons; 2005:149–158.

20 Medial Collateral Ligament Sprain

Sharat Kusuma and Jess H. Lonner

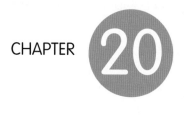

A 20-year-old male football player reports medial knee pain, swelling, and difficulty ambulating after suffering a blow with an audible "pop" to the lateral aspect of the knee during a game.

Clinical Presentation

The MCL is a strong structure located on the medial side of the knee. It originates on the medial femoral epicondyle and inserts on the medial proximal tibia. The ligament is an important stabilizer against valgus stress. Patients with MCL sprain will usually have history of medial knee pain after trauma to the lateral side of the knee or lower leg or a fall with a valgus moment. Patients may also report of history of twisting injury with a "pop" or "snap" heard at the time of injury. Pain may be worse with weight bearing, and an effusion may be present. There may be a sense of knee instability or "giving way" with high-grade MCL sprains.

Physical Findings

Patients will have tenderness and possibly ecchymosis on the medial side of the knee extending from the medial femoral condyle to the proximal tibia. An effusion may be present. Pain will likely be elicited when a valgus stress is applied to the knee. Often, the medial knee laxity with valgus stress is most apparent at 20 to 30 degrees of knee flexion. With complete MCL tears, this laxity will be more pronounced than with partial tears. With isolated MCL tears, the knee will be stable to valgus stress at full extension. It is important when examining patients with suspected MCL sprain to compare the injured extremity to the uninjured one with regard to medial laxity and medial opening with valgus stress (Fig. 20.1).

MCL sprains are graded on a three-point scale based on physical exam findings. A grade I sprain is characterized by medial knee tenderness, minimal swelling and ecchymosis, and no medial gapping when valgus stress is applied to the knee in slight flexion.

A grade II sprain demonstrates more pain and tenderness to palpation that can be localized to either the tibial or femoral insertion of the MCL or along its fibers, depending on where the sprain has taken place.

CLINICAL POINTS

- A history of knee pain after trauma to the side of the knee or lower leg is common.

- The medial collateral ligament (MCL) is a significant stabilizer against valgus stress.

- Knee instability may occur as a result of ligament injury.

PATIENT ASSESSMENT

1. Identifiable trauma with sudden pain along the course of the MCL

2. Local tenderness over the MCL

3. Complete tears lead to laxity from medial side of the knee

4. Marked laxity associated with other ligament injuries within the knee

5. X-rays to rule out structural bone problem

6. MRI for severe injuries to rule out associated ligament injuries

NOT TO BE MISSED

- Combined anterior cruciate ligament/MCL and posteromedial capsule injury

- Medial meniscus tear

- Tibial plateau fracture

- Physeal fracture (in children and adolescents)

- Avascular necrosis of medial femoral condyle

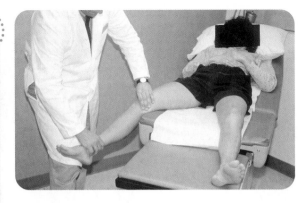

Figure 20.1 The collateral ligaments are tested by stabilizing the femur with one hand and placing a varus or valgus stress on the knee by grasping the ankle. (From Bucholz RW, Heckman JD. *Rockwood and Green's Fractures in Adults*, 5th ed. Philadelphia: Lippincott Williams & Wilkins; 2001.)

Additionally, a discernible difference in the medial knee opening with valgus stress is noted when the injured leg is compared with the uninjured leg, usually gapping between 5 and 10 mm.

Grade III sprains are characterized by complete rupture of the MCL. In such injuries, knee joint swelling and effusion may be minimal, as much of the hemorrhage diffuses into the soft tissues around the knee rather than into the knee joint. These injuries will demonstrate pronounced medial gapping (>10 mm) with valgus stress at 30 degrees of flexion. Isolated MCL sprains should yield a stable knee to valgus stress in full extension. However, if the knee does demonstrate medial gapping with full extension, concern should be raised for a cruciate ligament injury as well.[1]

Studies

Diagnostic studies for suspected MCL injury include plain x-ray AP and lateral views of the affected knee. Patients with complete MCL rupture may have medial gapping of the knee on these views. Additional helpful views include valgus stress views of the affected knee (Fig. 20.2). These plain x-rays are performed with the knee in 15 to 20 degrees of flexion.

The knee is given a valgus stress while the x-ray is performed (Figs. 20.3, 20.4). Pathologic laxity of the MCL will demonstrate a widened medial space of the knee joint.

Patients with a chronic MCL injury may demonstrate a Pellegrini-Stieda lesion on AP plain x-rays of the knee. This radiographic sign appears as an area of calcification on the medial distal aspect of the femur at the insertion site of the MCL and indicates a chronic MCL injury that has undergone some healing with concomitant calcification.

Advanced studies such as MRI may be helpful in the initial stages of the workup of patients with an MCL injury. Particularly, if patients have medial laxity at full extension and at 20 to 30 degrees of flexion, an early MRI may identify an associated cruciate ligament tear (Fig. 20.5). Early identification of such combined injuries can aid in planning possible surgical ligamentous repair or reconstruction that may be necessary.

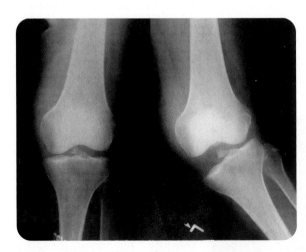

Figure 20.2 Stress radiograph revealing gross medial joint line opening indicating complete tears of the medial collateral, anterior, and posterior cruciate ligaments. (From Bucholz RW, Heckman JD. *Rockwood and Green's Fractures in Adults*, 5th ed. Philadelphia: Lippincott Williams & Wilkins; 2001.)

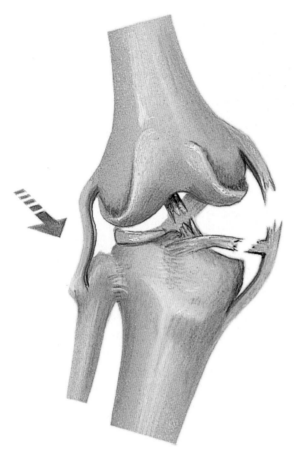

Figure 20.3 This diagram shows a schematic picture of a knee that receives a valgus force and results in an MCL rupture. Hip and knee. "Unhappy triad." (Asset provided by Anatomical Chart Co.)

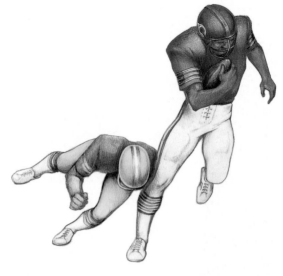

Figure 20.4 Football player receiving valgus injury. Hip and knee. Tackling can result in the "unhappy triad." (Asset provided by Anatomical Chart Co.)

Treatment

1. Grade I sprains require no specific treatment.

2. Grades II and III sprains should be protected for 6 weeks.

3. Grade III or severe instability should be evaluated for reconstruction of the possible associated ligament injury.

WHEN TO REFER

- Patients with grade III MCL injuries with gross laxity at full extension and 30 degrees of flexion likely have combined cruciate and MCL injuries and should be referred for orthopaedic specialty care.

- Patients with persistent valgus laxity after 6 weeks of conservative treatment should also be referred, as they may have an unhealed grade III MCL sprain that may require reconstruction.

- Patients with persistent tenderness to palpation over the medial side of the knee after 3 or 4 weeks may have coexistent medial meniscus tear.

The treatment of most isolated MCL sprains is nonoperative, including an initial and brief course of protected weight bearing with crutches to allow pain and swelling to subside. Range of motion exercises should commence immediately. Motion (flexion and extension) promotes MCL healing. NSAIDs are helpful in reducing pain and inflammation and have not been demonstrated to impair MCL ligament healing.[2] Unlocked, hinged knee braces that shield the knee from valgus stresses should be worn for 6 weeks in patients with grades II and III sprains. If instability persists despite bracing and appropriate nonoperative treatments, surgical repair of the MCL may be necessary. Patients with combined MCL and cruciate or meniscal pathology should initially be treated with immobilization and then referred to an orthopaedic surgeon for definitive management.

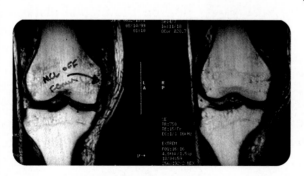

Figure 20.5 Coronal T1-weighted MRI of the knee revealing injury to the femoral origin of the MCL. (From Bucholz RW, Heckman JD. *Rockwood and Green's Fractures in Adults*, 5th ed. Philadelphia: Lippincott Williams & Wilkins; 2001.)

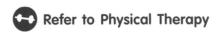 **Refer to Physical Therapy**

Clinical Course

Patients with grades I and II MCL sprains should have resolution of tenderness to palpation on the medial side of the knee within about 6 weeks of their injury. If tenderness persists, a medial meniscus tear should be suspected. As described previously, during the first 1 to 2 weeks, patients can begin ambulation and range-of-motion exercises. Patients with persistent medial laxity and valgus instability may have a grade III injury with insufficient healing that requires surgical repair.

> ### *ICD9*
> *844.1 Sprain of medial collateral ligament of knee*

References

1. Shaffer B. The knee and the leg. In: Wiesel SA, Delahay JN, eds. *Principles of Orthopaedic Medicine and Surgery.* Philadelphia: WB Saunders; 2001:711–766.
2. Ma CB, Rodeo SA. Meniscal injuries. In: Garrick JG, ed. *Orthopaedic Knowledge Update, Sports 3.* Rosemont, IL: American Academy of Orthopaedic Surgeons; 2004.

SECTION 5 Knee

21 Pes Anserinus Bursitis

Sharat Kusuma and Jess H. Lonner

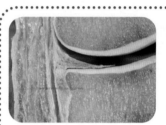

A 22-year-old female competitive college swimmer who specializes in the breaststroke presents with several weeks of medial-sided knee pain that is exacerbated during and after breaststroke swimming sessions. The pain subsides somewhat with rest. There is no history of trauma.

CLINICAL POINTS

- Patients usually give no history of acute trauma.
- A history of overuse is common.
- The onset of pain may be insidious.

PATIENT ASSESSMENT

1. Local tenderness on medial side of the tibia near the joint line
2. Usually associated with increased activity
3. Related to repeated strains to medial side of the knee
4. Rule out stress fracture

Clinical Presentation

The pes anserine bursa is located on the medial side of the knee at the proximal tibia where the pes anserine complex of medial tendons (sartorius, gracilis, and semitendinosus) attach. The function of the pes bursa is to provide cushioning to these tendons during activity. Patients with pes bursitis, like patients with medial collateral ligament (MCL) sprain, will also have medial-sided knee pain. The pain is more often insidious in onset, and there is often no history of trauma; this is in contrast to an MCL sprain, in which there often is a history of distinct trauma. Patients with pes bursitis will report a history of overuse, commonly in sports such as breaststroke swimming or with repeated kicking of ball. Both of these activities place repeated strain on the medial knee tendons and can result in bursitis. Occasionally, a history of direct trauma to the area is reported.

Physical Findings

There is tenderness to palpation at the proximal medial tibia, at the attachment of the pes anserine tendons. This is different from the medial joint line tenderness common with medial meniscus tears.

Studies

Patients with pes bursitis will not demonstrate any radiographic abnormalities, and plain x-ray stress views of the knee will also be normal.

112

Treatment

1. Identify stress etiology
2. NSAIDs
3. Ice
4. Reduced activity
5. Corticoid steroid preparation if symptoms persist

Treatment of pes anserinus bursitis is similar to the treatment of bursitis in other locations. Rest, ice, compression, elevation, and NSAIDs initially will prove effective in most patients. A corticosteroid preparation may also be helpful, but first rule out a stress fracture or spontaneous osteonecrosis.

 Refer to Physical Therapy

Clinical Course

Patients with pes bursitis often have resolution of their symptoms; however, it occasionally becomes a chronic problem.

ICD9
726.61 Pes anserinus tendinitis or bursitis

SECTION 5 Knee

CHAPTER 22 Torn Meniscus

Sharat Kusuma and Jess H. Lonner

A 30-year-old man reports a 1-week history of knee pain and swelling after a twisting injury during a softball game. The patient describes symptoms of the knee catching on occasion, resulting in difficulty straightening.

CLINICAL POINTS

- Acute meniscus tears are more common in younger adults.
- Chronic meniscus tears are often more frequent in older adults.
- The nature of pain is variable.
- Effusion may be present.

Clinical Presentation

Meniscal tears can be acute or chronic degenerative tears. Acute meniscus tears occur most commonly occur in patients between the second and fourth decades of life. With acute meniscal tear, a patient will report a rotational or "twisting" injury to the flexed knee that often results in an audible "pop" with concurrent sharp pain. The pain may be of limited severity such that the individual is able to return to activity relatively soon after the injury. The patient may develop an effusion with mild to moderate knee pain. Patients may also describe mechanical symptoms of the knee catching or locking, resulting in difficulties with flexion and extension. Severe pain may occur with squatting or pivoting.

Chronic meniscus tears generally occur in older patients and are the result of degenerative changes in the meniscus that are typical of aging. Patients with such tears will have insidious onset of knee pain and effusion. There is often no discrete history of trauma. The pain is exacerbated by activity and improved with rest. The knee effusion may be variable in size based on the patient's recent activity level.

Physical Findings

Patients with acute traumatic meniscus tears will have tenderness to palpation along the joint line in the area of the tear. Thus, those with medial meniscus tears will have medial joint line tenderness, and those with lateral tears will have lateral joint line tenderness. A knee effusion is also likely to be present. The McMurray test, which is performed by extending a flexed knee while exerting an internal or external rotation force on the tibia may elicit pain and a pop or click; this pop/click is the result of the torn edge of the meniscus being caught between the tibia and femoral condyle as the knee comes from flexion to extension.

PATIENT ASSESSMENT

1. Acute tears associated with identified significant twisting injury
2. Chronic tears associated with age and degenerative joint disease (DJD)
3. Acute tears associated with young adults
4. Occasional locking, catching, and giving way
5. Localized tenderness over the joint line
6. Rule out avascular necrosis in older adults

NOT TO BE MISSED

- Cruciate ligament tear
- Collateral ligament sprain
- Pes anserine bursitis
- Avascular necrosis of medial femoral condyle
- Fracture

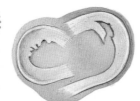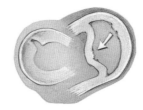

Figure 22.1 Schematic of torn medial meniscus. **Left:** Small flap tear. **Right:** Large, "bucket-handle" tear.

The Apley grind test can also be performed to assess for meniscal pathology. This test is performed by having the patient lie prone on the examination table with the knee flexed to 90 degrees. The test is performed by pushing the foot and leg downward and rotating them while flexing and extending the knee. A positive test will elicit pain and popping along the joint line.

Patients with chronic, degenerative meniscus tears may have fewer positive physical findings. Anatomically, degenerative tears involve more meniscal fraying and fissuring; such tears do not often have large pieces of torn meniscus in the knee joint space that can produce mechanical symptoms. Therefore, tests such as the McMurray and Apley may not be positive. The absence of such positive provocative tests does not rule our chronic meniscus tear. Patients will consistently demonstrate medial joint line tenderness. Patients with chronic tears will also often some degree of coexisting DJD.

Studies

Initial studies for any patient with an acute knee injury, pain, and an effusion include AP and lateral plain x-rays of the knee to look for fractures. If these studies are negative and the diagnosis of meniscus tear is suspected based on history and physical, MRI is warranted, as this modality is highly sensitive and specific; MRI has been demonstrated to be 80% to 90% accurate in diagnosing such tears[1] (Figs. 22.1–22.3).

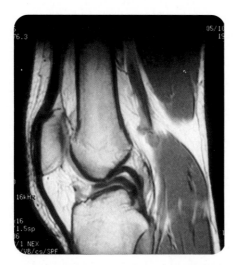

Figure 22.2 Locked bucket-handle medial meniscus producing the double posterior cruciate ligament sign on MRI. A tear of this size would most likely produce mechanical symptoms of catching or locking in the knee.

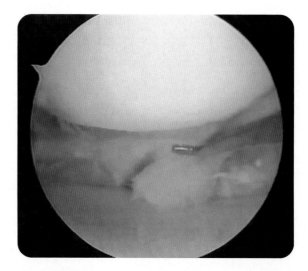

Figure 22.3 Diagnostic arthroscopy of the knee. Visualization of the posterior horn of the medial meniscus demonstrating a degenerative tear. (From Koval KJ, Zuckerman JD. *Atlas of Orthopaedic Surgery: A Multimedial Reference.* Philadelphia: Lippincott Williams & Wilkins; 2004.)

For patients with a suspected degenerative meniscus tear, initial imaging studies should include AP and lateral weight-bearing knee x-rays. Patients with chronic meniscus tears will often have some degree of DJD with medial or lateral compartment arthritis. If on plain x-ray patients are determined to have DJD and the clinical exam and history indicate meniscus tear, such patients should be referred to an orthopaedic surgeon for further management and determination of the need for MRI.

Treatment

1. Acute tears with large segments can be repaired arthroscopically.

2. Small acute tears can be excised.

3. Degenerative tears may not be symptomatic unless associated with mechanical symptoms.

4. For chronic tears, arthroscopic debridement can offer some benefit only if mechanical symptoms are present.

Treatment of meniscal tears is predicated on the size of the tear and the severity of symptoms in the patient as well as patient age and activity level. Patients with isolated small meniscus tears that do not produce pain or mechanical symptoms can be treated successfully with nonoperative measures such as rest, ice, physical therapy, and activity modifications. Physical therapy including knee range of motion and quadriceps and hamstring stretching and strengthening should also be initiated. Older patients with degenerative tears that are minimally symptomatic can also be managed with such strategies. Intra-articular corticosteroid preparations may also be utilized to reduce inflammation and pain.

Patients with large tears that produce mechanical symptoms require arthroscopic surgery. Young patients with large tears may occasionally undergo arthroscopic repair of the meniscus (depending on its location), while older patients with degenerative tears will often undergo partial meniscectomy.

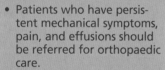 **Refer to Physical Therapy**

WHEN TO REFER

• Patients who have persistent mechanical symptoms, pain, and effusions should be referred for orthopaedic care.

• Patients with meniscus tear and combined cruciate or collateral ligament injury by MRI scan should be referred.

• Patients with small, asymptomatic tears do not need to be referred to an orthopaedist unless new complaints or problems arise.

Clinical Course

Most patients with large, acute meniscus tears will continue to be symptomatic with mechanical locking, pain, and recurrent effusion if no surgical treatment is performed.

However, patients with small, stable tears that do not produce symptoms can often be treated successfully without surgery. Such patients will respond well to physical therapy, NSAIDs, and activity modifications.

ICD9
836.0 Tear of medial cartilage or meniscus of knee, current
836.1 Tear of lateral cartilage or meniscus of knee, current
836.2 Other tear of cartilage or meniscus of knee, current
717.0 Old bucket handle tear of medial meniscus
717.1 Derangement of anterior horn of medial meniscus
717.2 Derangement of posterior horn of medial meniscus
717.3 Other and unspecified derangement of medial meniscus
717.40 Derangement of lateral meniscus, unspecified
717.41 Bucket handle tear of lateral meniscus
717.42 Derangement of anterior horn of lateral meniscus
717.43 Derangement of posterior horn of lateral meniscus
717.49 Other derangement of lateral meniscus
717.5 Derangement of meniscus, not elsewhere classified

Reference

1. Ma CB, Rodeo SA. Meniscal injuries. In: Garrick JG, ed. *Orthopaedic Knowledge Update, Sports 3.* Rosemont, IL: American Academy of Orthopaedic Surgeons; 2004.

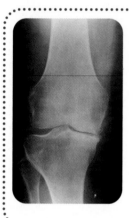

A 70-year-old woman reports a several-year history of right knee pain, intermittent swelling, and stiffness. There is no history of trauma to the right knee. The pain has had a waxing and waning character over the last few years, with intervals of decreased pain followed by periods of more severe pain. The pain is worse with activity and better with rest.

Clinical Presentation

When evaluating an elderly patient with knee pain, it is important to remember that degenerative joint disease (DJD)/OA of the knee is the most common cause of knee pain in such patients; additionally, the knee is the most common joint in the body affected by OA.[1]

The clinical presentation of knee DJD is variable. The most common presentation will be an individual in the seventh or eighth decade of life with insidious knee pain, swelling, and stiffness that has gradually become more severe. There is rarely a history of discrete trauma. Patients may also describe a weather-related variation of their symptoms, with pain worse on cold, humid days. The pain is most often exacerbated by activity and relieved by rest. Patients will often relate a gradual decrease in their ambulation tolerance. Patients with DJD can have night pain, but unrelenting severe night pain should raise concern for diagnoses other than DJD, such as malignancy.

Younger patients with previous knee trauma such as chronic anterior cruciate ligament rupture, tibial plateau fracture, osteochondritis dissecans, meniscus tear, femur fracture, and other injuries are at increased risk for DJD of the knee at an early age.

Physical Findings

Physical exam findings of patients with suspected diagnosis of OA should begin with gross observation of gait. Patients with OA will often have an antalgic gait. Bow legs or varus malalignment is most common in patients with OA. In such patients, the medial compartment is the most affected by DJD. Alternatively, patients may present with OA and knock-kneed or valgus posture (Fig. 23.1). Such patients will often have more severe lateral compartment OA, with attenuation of medial structures.

CLINICAL POINTS

- The condition is the most common cause of knee pain in older adults.

- The knee is joint most frequently affected by osteoarthritis (OA).

- Pain may be worse in cold, humid weather.

- Patients may report gradual decrease in ambulation tolerance.

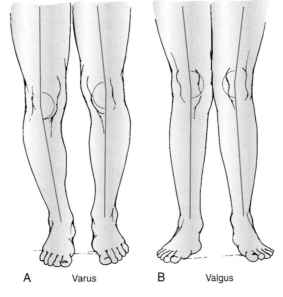

Figure 23.1 Varus and valgus alignment of the knee. **A:** In varus alignment of the knee, the angle formed by lines through the femur and tibia opens medially. **B:** In valgus alignment of the knee, the angle formed by lines through the femur and tibia opens laterally. (From Oatis CA. *Kinesiology: The Mechanics and Pathomechanics of Human Movement*. Baltimore: Lippincott Williams & Wilkins; 2004.)

Tenderness to palpation around the knee is common; osteophytes may be palpable. Crepitus (crackling) with knee flexion and extension is typical.

Studies

The most useful radiologic studies for the diagnosis of knee OA include weight-bearing AP and lateral x-rays of the knee (Fig. 23.2). These x-rays can reveal joint space narrowing, osteophytes, subchondral sclerosis, and cyst formation, all of which are indicative of DJD. Additional x-ray views that may reveal DJD in the posterior condyles of the femur include PA weight-bearing views with the knees in 30 degrees of flexion. Finally, Merchant/sunrise views are also helpful in assessing the degree of patellofemoral arthritis.

MRI of the arthritic knee is almost universally unnecessary and adds very little to the diagnostic picture. However, in patients with mild OA who present with acute knee pain, an MRI should be obtained to rule out osteonecrosis or a meniscus tear.

Treatment

1. Early OA should be treated with NSAIDs and activity modification.
2. Later treatments require NSAIDs and occasional intra-articular steroid injection.
3. Mid stage may benefit from distal supplementation.
4. End stage requires total knee replacement.

Initial treatment of patients with knee DJD includes weight loss, activity modifications, and analgesics

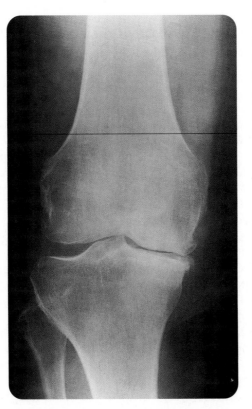

Figure 23.2 Preoperative weight-bearing radiographs demonstrate varus OA: AP view.

such as acetaminophen and/or NSAIDs. High-impact activities such as running should be avoided. Nonimpact exercises such as swimming are beneficial.

Other treatment options include intra-articular steroid injections, although they should not be given more than three or four times per year and may be best avoided in patients with diabetes mellitus because it may increase endogenous glucose levels. Viscosupplementation therapy with hyaluronic acid preparations is being used with increasing frequency. Literature reports have demonstrated mixed results of viscosupplementation. One recent double-blind, placebo-controlled investigation indicated that patients aged 60 years and older with moderate to severe DJD would derive the greatest benefit from viscosupplementation therapy.[2] Valgus bracing for medial compartment arthritis may offer some relief. However, patients with very advanced DJD and knees in >20 degrees of varus are unlikely to benefit.[3]

Finally, assistive devices such as a walking cane can also provide some pain relief and increase walking tolerance. Total joint replacement is appropriate when nonoperative treatments fail to adequately relieve the patient's pain.

 Refer to Patient Education

 Refer to Physical Therapy

Clinical Course

The natural history of OA of the knee varies in terms of the rate of progression of disease, deformity, loss of motion, and severity of symptoms.

WHEN TO REFER

- When patients have failed all conservative modalities described previously, referral to an orthopaedic surgeon for possible surgical treatment is warranted. Surgical options include high tibial osteotomy, uni-compartmental knee arthroplasty, and total knee arthroplasty.

ICD9

715.00 Osteoarthrosis, generalized, involving unspecified site
715.04 Osteoarthrosis, generalized, involving hand
715.09 Osteoarthrosis, generalized, involving multiple sites
715.80 Osteoarthrosis involving or with mention of more than one site, but not specified as generalized, and involving unspecified site
715.89 Osteoarthrosis involving or with mention of multiple sites, but not specified as generalized
715.90 Osteoarthrosis, unspecified whether generalized or localized, involving unspecified site
715.91 Osteoarthrosis, unspecified whether generalized or localized, involving shoulder region
715.92 Osteoarthrosis, unspecified whether generalized or localized, involving upper arm
715.93 Osteoarthrosis, unspecified whether generalized or localized, involving forearm
715.94 Osteoarthrosis, unspecified whether generalized or localized, involving hand
715.95 Osteoarthrosis, unspecified whether generalized or localized, involving pelvic region and thigh

715.96 Osteoarthrosis, unspecified whether generalized or localized, involving lower leg

715.97 Osteoarthrosis, unspecified whether generalized or localized, involving ankle and foot

715.98 Osteoarthrosis, unspecified whether generalized or localized, involving other specified sites

References

1. Shaffer B. The knee and the leg. In: Wiesel SA, Delahay JN, eds. *Principles of Orthopaedic Medicine and Surgery*. Philadelphia: WB Saunders; 2001:711–766.
2. Bellamy N, Campbell J, Robinson V, et al. Viscosupplementation for the treatment of osteoarthritis of the knee. *Cochrane Database Syst Rev* 2006;(2):CD005321.
3. Lindenfeld TN, Hewett TE, Andriacchi TP. Joint loading with valgus bracing in patients with varus gonarthrosis. *Clin Orthop Relat Res* 1997;(344):290–297.

CHAPTER 24 Baker Cyst

Sharat Kusuma and Jess H. Lonner

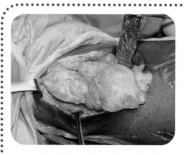

A 50-year-old man with mild, chronic medial knee pain after a twisting injury several months ago has noted a fullness in the medial aspect of his thigh. An MRI scan performed to evaluate the knee pain reveals a medial meniscus tear and also a posteromedial cystic mass between the semimembranosus and medial head of the gastroc muscle.

CLINICAL POINTS

- Cysts may increase in size in the presence of meniscus tears or degenerative arthritis.

- There are generally no symptoms except for fullness and mild pain.

- Ruptured cysts may cause pain and swelling in the calf resulting from fluid leakage.

Clinical Presentation

Baker cysts are normal anatomic structures that represent a bursal sac that is located most often on the medial side of the knee between the semimembranosus and medial head of the gastroc. These cysts have intra-articular communication and often increase in size in response to some type of intra-articular pathology, most often a meniscus tear or degenerative arthritis. Patients may complain of a fullness and mild pain in the posteromedial aspect of the knee, but otherwise the cysts are usually asymptomatic. Rarely, cysts may grow large enough in size to produce a large amount of swelling in the popliteal area. Occasionally, a ruptured Baker cyst will leak fluid into the calf, causing calf pain and swelling.

Physical Findings

Patients will demonstrate a palpable mass or fullness in the posteromedial aspect of the knee. Patients with meniscal pathology will have joint line tenderness and other physical exam findings consistent with a meniscus tear.

Studies

Baker cyst is typically found on MRI or ultrasound (Fig. 24.1).

Treatment

1. Asymptomatic, no treatment required
2. Can aspirate and inject with cortisone

SECTION 5 Knee

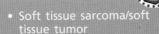

PATIENT ASSESSMENT

1. Pain and swelling in the posterior aspect of the knee

2. Usually associated with some intra-articular pathology

3. Diffuse complaint of fullness and pain and minor achiness in posterior aspect of the knee

4. Occasionally, rupture that causes acute symptoms resembling thrombophlebitis

NOT TO BE MISSED

- Soft tissue sarcoma/soft tissue tumor
- Meniscal cyst
- Deep venous thrombosis
- Popliteal artery aneurysm
- Thrombophlebitis
- Septic arthritis

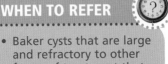

WHEN TO REFER

- Baker cysts that are large and refractory to other forms of treatment that are symptomatic may need surgical excision. This scenario is rare, but if it does arise, referral for orthopaedic specialty care is warranted.

- Patients with MRI evidence of a soft tissue mass or tumor that is not a Baker cyst should be referred to a musculoskeletal oncologist.

- Patients who have thrombophlebitis or deep venous thrombosis should undergo appropriate anticoagulation.

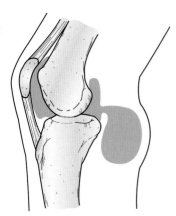

Popliteal cyst

Figure 24.1 Popliteal cysts are fluid-filled herniations of the synovial membrane of the knee joint. This schematic depicts the formation of a popliteal cyst.

3. May recur

4. Generally resolves spontaneously if intra-articular pathology addressed

5. Rarely requires surgical excision

Baker cysts that are asymptomatic do not need to be treated. Conservative treatment of a symptomatic Baker cyst involves NSAIDs and a compressive knee wrap. Often, if the intra-articular pathology is addressed (i.e., meniscus tear), the cyst will decrease in size and disappear or become asymptomatic. Baker cysts are rarely aspirated or surgically excised. In cases where cysts recur despite these measures, surgical resection is an option.

 Refer to Physical Therapy

Clinical Course

Most Baker cysts will resolve spontaneously once the intra-articular pathology has been addressed. Many cysts may wax and wane in size and may be minimally symptomatic and therefore not require treatment.

ICD9
727.51 Synovial cyst of popliteal space

Ankle

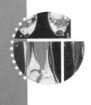
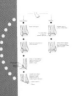
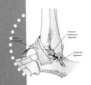

25 Achilles Tendon

David Pedowitz and Enyi Okereke

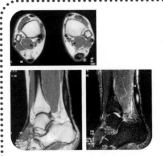

A 28-year-old female tennis player presents with posterior calf/heel pain that is worse with activity and has been gradually worsening over the past 3 months. She reports that she started training for a triathlon 4 months ago with an intense running program. (Figure from Thordarson DB. Foot and Ankle. *Philadelphia: Lippincott Williams & Wilkins; 2004.*)

CLINICAL POINTS

- Inflammatory injuries may lead to discomfort and swelling.
- Degenerative injuries may cause no symptoms.
- Tendon rupture may be either acute or chronic.

Clinical Presentation

Achilles tendon injuries comprise a large spectrum of pathology from peritendinitis to frank rupture. For the purposes of this chapter, they have been separated into paratenonitis, tendinosis, insertional tendinitis, and rupture. While these may seem somewhat arbitrary divisions in similar disease processes, clinical practice among foot and ankle surgeons has necessitated this separation, since the aforementioned diagnoses require unique diagnostic and treatment algorithms to achieve resolution.

Paratenonitis of the Achilles tendon refers to inflammation of the paratenon or fascial sheath that covers the tendon.[1] Tendinosis is when there is actual intratendinous degeneration. Unlike tendinosis, which is not characterized by an inflammatory process, insertional tendinitis is an inflammatory condition that occurs at and around the Achilles tendon insertion into the calcaneus. Achilles tendon rupture can either be acute or chronic, and while these entities present their own challenges, they both require surgical repair and will be discussed below.[2]

Paratenonitis (peritendinitis) is most often seen in athletes, especially long- and middle-distance runners. Due to its vascularity, the paratenon is susceptible to inflammation and presents as diffuse discomfort and swelling of the tendon. Acutely, the Achilles can appear sausagelike secondary to inflammatory edema. Tender nodules can occur within the paratenon, reflecting localized hypertrophy of connective tissue.[3]

The etiology of this irritation to the paratenon seems to be from external pressure from poor-fitting shoes that cause friction between the Achilles and the overlying paratenon. Additionally, fluid may accumulate adjacent to the tendon, and adhesions can develop. Grossly, the tendon becomes thick and adheres to the normal surrounding tissue or to the tendon itself.[3] Histologically, capillary proliferation and inflammatory infiltrate confined to the paratenal tissue is seen.

While paratenonitis is predominantly an inflammatory process, tendinosis is a degenerative process in which there is little inflammation. This is likely due to the fact that the tendon itself has sparse cellularity and vascularity, both of which impair the inflammatory process. The tendon becomes thicker, softer, and yellowish, owing to an accumulation of mucinoid material within the tendon. Degeneration within the tendon itself is often insidious and asymptomatic. It is thought to occur as a result of repetitive microtrauma, aging, or a combination of both. Due to its asymptomatic nature, tendinosis progresses unnoticed and often presents in the office at its end stage; as full-thickness or partial rupture of the tendon. These ruptures typically occur in middle-aged men who have suddenly increased their levels of physical activity.[2,3]

Insertional tendinitis is a true inflammatory process within the tendinous insertion of the Achilles. It is often associated with a Haglund deformity (bone spur anterior to the insertion site) and as well with hill running and interval workouts. Training errors such as improper stretching prior to exertion or excessive increases in exercise intensity can quickly exacerbate this condition. Insertional tendinitis presents with posterior heel pain thought to be due to bony impingement from the calcaneus, local bursitis, or both.[3]

Achilles tendon rupture is classically described by middle-aged athletes (weekend warriors) who have experienced a sudden pain with an audible "pop" in the back of their heels. Many report the sensation of being hit in the posterior calf. Most authorities suggest that the pathogenesis of these ruptures is secondary to a degenerative process within the tendon itself and that it eventually leads to rupture. Interestingly, >15% of patients with an acute rupture report a history of prior symptoms.

Physical Findings

Pain is the cardinal symptom of Achilles tendinopathy. In the early phase of paratenonitis, patients may complain primarily of pain following strenuous exercise and, if progressive, can develop pain that accompanies routine activities. For athletes, the pain can be disabling enough to curtail training regimens.

On physical examination, findings can vary depending on the degree of inflammation present within the paratenon. Decreased ankle dorsiflexion and hamstring tightness are commonly found in patients with Achilles pathology. It is important to note that in patients with paratenonitis, a tenderness and thickness that remains fixed with active range of motion of the ankle will be exhibited. Nodularity within the paratenon can be detected on palpation. There is often palpable tenderness on both sides of the tendon, with the medial side being more tender than the lateral.[3]

Clinically, it is important to note the contour of the tendon, any areas of widening, and the presence or absence of nodules. Most runners present with a gradual evolution of symptoms, including pain and swelling approximately 2 to 3 cm proximal to the calcaneal insertion. A distinguishing

PATIENT ASSESSMENT

1. Patients who experience rupture typically describe a "popping" sensation in their leg.

2. On physical exam, assess the contour of the tendon.

3. The Thompson test can help to evaluate the integrity of the tendon.

4. MRI is helpful in assessing tendon degeneration and rupture.

feature of tendinosis from paratenonitis is the mobility of the intratendinous nodule or thickening with the point of maximal tenderness during active range of motion (painful arc sign).[3] Differentiating between the conditions that cause posterior heel pain can be difficult and can perhaps be thought of as a spectrum of a single disease process. However, insertional tendinitis requires that patients have tenderness at the bone–tendon interface, and examination will reveal point-specific pain at the insertional interface, often posterolaterally. There is also limited dorsiflexion. If the tendinitis becomes chronic in nature, the tendon can also become palpably thickened.

Rupture is perhaps the easiest diagnosis to make regarding the Achilles tendon. Patients are often unable to bear weight secondary to pain. Of note, those patients with partial tears will complain of more pain than those with complete ruptures. Current thinking is that a partially torn tendon is still experiencing loads that put tension across the rupture site causing pain, while the tendon ends in those patients with complete ruptures are not tethered to the surrounding soft tissues. The patient with an Achilles rupture will be unable to plantarflex the ankle. The Thompson test is quite sensitive in picking up a rupture. This test is classically performed in the prone position with the knee flexed at 90 degrees. Keeping the patient in this position allows the foot to passively assume a plantigrade position from which to reference. An active squeeze of the gastrocnemius-soleus complex with the examiner's hand should produce ankle plantarflexion if there is continuity of fibers in the tendon. Lastly, a palpable gap is often felt 2 to 6 cm proximal to the tendon insertion.[3] This specific location is a watershed area for the Achilles blood supply and is a frequent site of tendon rupture.

Chronic rupture or neglected rupture of the Achilles tendon is more difficult to appreciate on physical examination. Any diagnosis made later than 4 weeks following rupture should be considered chronic, because after 2 weeks, any gap in the tendon ends has filled with a disorganized scar and has likely undergone some retraction into the more proximal calf. Most patients are able to ambulate, although with a markedly decreased push-off strength and difficulty with stairs (also, driving a car if the right side is involved). The most reliable clinical parameter is a hyperdorsiflexion sign where the patient's ankle can be brought into much more dorsiflexion than the unaffected side due to the tendon being in a lengthened position.[4]

Studies

Imaging of the Achilles is primarily dependent on two modalities: ultrasonography and MR. Ultrasound of a patient with paratenonitis will frequently reveal fluid surrounding the tendon acutely and more chronically can reveal peritendinous adhesions that can be visualized as thickening of the hypoechoic paratenon. On MRI, T1 imaging will show a thickened paratenon, with a high signal seen within the paratenon on T2 imaging (halo sign).[5]

On ultrasound, tendinosis can appear as a hypoechoic lesion with or without intratendinous calcification.[5,6] MRI would also reveal tendon

SECTION 6 Ankle

NOT TO BE MISSED

- Achilles tendon rupture
- Achilles tendinosis
- Insertional Achilles tendinitis
- Achilles paratenonitis
- Retrocalcaneal bursitis
- Calcaneal stress fracture

abnormalities such as tendon thickening on sagittal imaging and altered signal appearance within the tendon tissue.

In most clinical scenarios, radiographs are helpful and should be obtained. They can reveal a prominence of the posterior calcaneal tuberosity, avulsions, fractures, possible calcification, or intratendinous spurs. MRI can be used to rule out abnormalities within the tendon and can demonstrate high signal intensity within the retrocalcaneal bursa and is often best seen on T2 imaging. It can also reveal degenerative or inflammatory changes within the tendon insertion.

Overall, the imaging study of choice is MR, which can define intratendinous, paratendinous, and insertional problems as well as chronic or acute ruptures. This modality, when compared with ultrasound, is both easily available and less reliant on a skillful technician, which in most practices makes it the most useful imaging study.[6]

Treatment and Clinical Course

1. Ruptured tendon should be evaluated by a surgeon in an expeditious manner.
2. Tendinitis should be treated with activity modification, cross training, consideration of orthosis, and NSAIDs.

As with all overuse injuries of the Achilles tendon in general, initial conservative treatment should be directed toward relieving symptoms, correcting training errors, limb malalignment with orthoses, and improving flexibility. This typically consists of modification of training regimens (such as a staged cross-training regimen), rest, ice massage, and NSAIDs. A small heel lift or a shock-absorbing orthotic can also help to reduce acute symptoms. Physical therapy, concentrating on enhancing dorsiflexion, is beneficial given that most patients with chronic tendinopathy possess limited passive dorsiflexion. To treat the excess pronation that is often found in these patients, a full-length, flexible, or semirigid orthotic device has been found to work well, and a shock-absorbing insole can also be helpful. For patients with severe symptoms without rupture, a temporary short leg cast or removable walker may be used. Once symptomatic resolution has been achieved, patients should be counseled regarding activity modification and appropriate shoe-wear changes.

It is critical to note that the use of corticosteroids in chronic tendinopathy is contraindicated due to the risk of creating a frank rupture. If a patient fails to respond adequately to conservative treatment within a 3- to 6-month period, attention should be directed toward managing the pathology operatively.

While rupture has historically been treated conservatively with acceptable results, recent advances in surgical technique have yielded superior results in most studies comparing operative versus nonoperative management. Surgical intervention, in the case of an acute rupture, involves a primary repair of the tendon while in the chronic setting demands a more complicated surgical reconstruction, often with tendon transfers. In general, surgical treatment results in excellent outcomes, and conservative management of these entities should be reserved for poor surgical candidates or those with limited physical demands and functional expectations.

WHEN TO REFER

- Evidence of a rupture (palpable gap, positive calf-squeeze Thompson test)
- Recalcitrant to short course of physical therapy
- Severe pain with inability to bear weight

⟨⊶⟩ Refer to Physical Therapy

ICD9

726.71 Achilles bursitis or tendinitis
727.06 Tenosynovitis of foot and ankle
727.67 Nontraumatic rupture of Achilles tendon
845.09 Other ankle sprain

References

1. Allenmark C. Partial Achilles tendon tears. *Clin Sports Med* 1992;11(4):759–769.
2. Saltzman CL, Tearse DS. Achilles tendon injuries. *J Am Acad Orthop Surg* 1998;6(5):316–325.
3. Coughlin M. Disorders of tendons. In: Coughlin MJ, ed. *Surgery of the Foot and Ankle,* 7th ed. Philadelphia: Mosby; 1999.
4. Gabel S, Manoli A 2nd. Neglected rupture of the Achilles tendon. *Foot Ankle Int* 1994;15(9):512–517.
5. Fornage BD. Achilles tendon: US examination. *Radiology* 1986;159(3):759–764.
6. Pope CF. Radiologic evaluation of tendon injuries. *Clin Sports Med* 1992;11(3):579–599.

SECTION 6 Ankle

CHAPTER 26 Ankle Sprains

David Pedowitz and Enyi Okereke

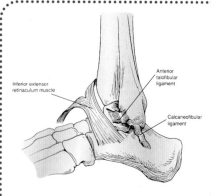

A 19-year-old male basketball player landed awkwardly during a game and felt a "pop" on the lateral aspect of his ankle, with the onset of pain and swelling. (Figure from Kitaoka HB. Masters Techniques in Orthopaedic Surgery: Foot and Ankle, *2nd ed. Philadelphia: Lippincott Williams & Wilkins; 2002.)*

CLINICAL POINTS

- Ankle sprains are common injuries, especially in athletes.
- Many patients suffer long-term effects.
- An overwhelming majority of injuries involve the lateral structures of the ankle.
- Medial ankle sprains and high ankle sprains are less common.

Clinical Presentation

Ankle sprains are some of the most common injuries seen by physicians, comprising nearly one in every ten emergency room visits. Additionally, nearly half of all athletic injuries consist of ankle sprains. With the overwhelming prevalence of these injuries, it behooves the astute clinician to be well acquainted with the presentation, diagnosis, and treatment of acute episodes of ankle instability.[1] Underscoring the importance of recognizing these injury patterns is the knowledge that long-term sequelae from lateral ankle sprains have been estimated to occur in up to 50% of patients. For the purposes of this chapter, ankle sprains will be separated into three distinct entities: lateral sprains, medial sprains, and high ankle sprains.

The vast majority of ankle sprains consist of injury to the lateral structures of the ankle. Typically, this involves injury to either of two specific ligaments, the anterior talofibular ligament (ATFL) and/or the calcaneofibular ligament (CFL) (Fig. 26.1). The ATFL functions mainly to restrict internal rotation of the talus underneath the bony mortise (the arch of bone formed by the lateral malleolus, distal tibial plafond, and medial malleolus, in which the talus sits) of the ankle. The CFL primarily resists adduction. Most lateral ligament injuries occur with inversion, plantar flexion, or internal rotation. Given this mechanism and the fact that the ATFL is the weaker of these two ligaments, the ATFL is most frequently torn in lateral ligamentous injuries.

Medial ankle sprains involve injury to the deltoid ligament alone and are, by themselves, unusual. The deltoid ligament is divided into both a superficial and deep ligament, each with its own particular constituents (Fig. 26.2). Typically, medial sprains and tears occur in combination with an injury to the lateral ligamentous structures or a fracture.

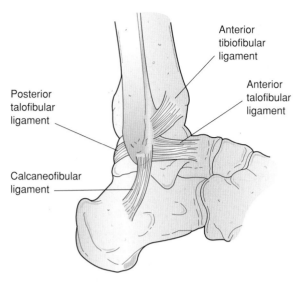

Figure 26.1 Lateral collateral ligaments of the ankle and the anterior syndesmotic ligament. (From Bucholz RW, Heckman JD. *Rockwood and Green's Fractures in Adults*, 5th ed., Vol. 2. Philadelphia: Lippincott Williams & Wilkins; 2001.)

SECTION 6 Ankle

The term *high ankle sprain*, refers to a sprain of the syndesmotic ligaments. The syndesmosis is the complex of ligaments responsible for stability at the inferior tibiofibular joint (Fig. 26.3). Diastasis, or gross separation of these two bones, is not necessary to define a sprain in this area. High ankle sprains therefore encompass the wide spectrum of injury from the minor sprain to the complete disruption of these structures, leading to diastasis. While they mostly exist in the setting of medial/lateral or bony injury, they can present in isolation and are generally thought to result from an external rotation injury.[2]

Physical Findings

Ankle sprains are traditionally classified according to grades I to III. A grade I sprain is an intraligamentous tear with pain but no instability. Grade II sprains are incomplete tears with pain and mild to moderate instability. Grade III sprains are complete ligamentous ruptures with gross instability, pain, and often the inability to bear weight. Patients sustaining these injuries usually describe an inversion or eversion injury with an audible "pop." Whether or not a tearing sensation and audible noise can be appreciated at the time of injury, most patients present with pain, loss of support, and difficulty with weight bearing. While palpating the area of tenderness can usually determine the anatomic site of the injury, the clinician must be cognizant of the tendency for the accuracy of physical exam findings to depreciate significantly as the time between injury and presentation increases.[1,2]

Most patients with ankle sprains will report an inversion or internal rotation injury often occurring during cutting or landing from a jump. They will be particularly tender laterally and, depending on which ligament has been injured, be more tender anteriorly or inferiorly to the tip of the lateral malleolus. Medial tenderness indicates a concomitant deltoid ligament injury. When the ATFL has been torn, an anterior drawer test (with knee flexed over the end of the examination table and the foot dangling, the examiner stabilizes the tibia with one hand and attempts to anteriorly translate the foot forward with the other hand grasping the heel) will produce pain and demonstrate instability. The foot

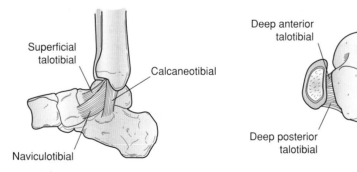

Superficial deltoid ligament   Deep deltoid ligament

Figure 26.2 Medial collateral ligaments of the ankle. Sagittal plane **(A)** and transverse plane **(B)** views. The deltoid contains a superficial component and a deep component. Superficial fibers mostly arise from the anterior colliculus and attach broadly from the navicular across the talus and into the medial border of the sustentaculum tali and the posterior medial talar tubercle. The deep layer of the deltoid ligament originates from the anterior and posterior colliculi and inserts on the medial surface of the talus. (From Bucholz RW, Heckman JD. *Rockwood and Green's Fractures in Adults*, 5th ed., Vol. 2. Philadelphia: Lippincott Williams & Wilkins; 2001.)

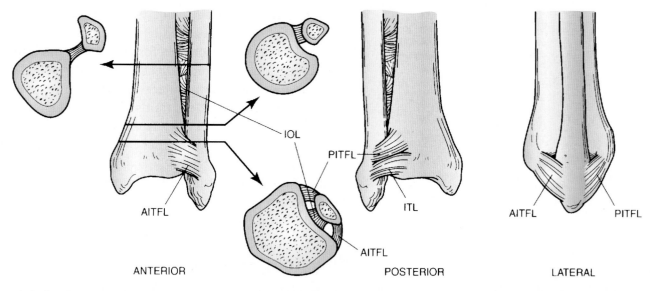

Figure 26.3 Three views of the tibiofibular syndesmotic ligaments. Anteriorly, the anterior inferior tibiofibular ligament (*AITFL*) spans from the anterior tubercle and anterolateral surface of the tibia to the anterior fibula. Posteriorly, the tibiofibular ligament has two components: the superficial posterior inferior tibiofibular ligament (*PITFL*), which constitutes the posterior labrum of the ankle, and the stout interosseous ligament (*IOL*), which resides between the anterior and posterior tibiofibular ligaments. (From Bucholz RW, Heckman JD. *Rockwood and Green's Fractures in Adults*, 5th ed. Vol. 2. Philadelphia: Lippincott Williams & Wilkins; 2001.)

should be plantar flexed when this test is performed so that the ATFL is in a tightened position and its integrity can be fully appreciated. It is important to note that patients with partial ligamentous tears often have more pain with provocative tests than those with complete tears.

When the CFL has been injured, inversion of the ankle and subtalar joints will yield instability and pain. Additionally, the anterior drawer test with the foot dorsiflexed can also produce a positive test result (since the ligament becomes taut in this position). For syndesmotic injury, if the examination is performed soon after injury, patients will be tender specifically over the anterolateral ankle joint, with little to no tenderness over the lateral malleolus, ATFL, or CFL. Medial malleolar tenderness is not uncommon in the setting of a syndesmotic sprain. The "squeeze test" should be performed. This test involves squeezing the midcalf, which, if an injury is present, will cause separation at the origin of the syndesmotic ligaments.[2,3]

Studies

Despite history and physical examination being the most useful tools in evaluating injuries to the ankle, imaging studies can be invaluable in specific circumstances. While a meticulous examiner can easily appreciate gross instability with complete rupture of the ligaments, recent studies suggest that with physical examination alone, more subtle injuries will often be missed. The Ottawa Ankle Rules are commonly recognized criteria for obtaining radiographs in the presence of an ankle injury and should be referred to when encountering a patient with a history of ankle instability. Based on the Ottawa criteria, radiographs are only required for patients with tenderness at the posterior edge or the tip of the medial or lateral malleolus, inability to bear weight initially or at presentation (four

NOT TO BE MISSED

- Ankle fracture (medial malleolus, lateral malleolus)
- Systemic disorders such as rheumatoid arthritis or Lyme disease (Ehlers-Danlos syndrome)
- Tarsal coalition
- Osteochondral lesion of the talus

steps in the emergency room), or pain at the base of the fifth metatarsal. When indicated, the standard three views (AP, lateral, and mortise) should be obtained. Stress views of the ankle, including but not limited to talar tilt, anterior drawer, external rotation, inversion, and eversion, can be obtained if there is suspicion of a tear. Arthrography is also a modality that has shown great accuracy. Although these views provide the clinician with valuable information, they are not easily performed without the aid of appropriate intra-articular anesthesia or sedation.

When the diagnosis is in doubt or when objective documentation is necessitated, MRI is the study of choice. In addition to defining the anatomic lesion, MRI can also help to grade the degree of injury.

Treatment and Clinical Course

1. Rest, ice, compression, and evaluation (RICE)
2. NSAIDs
3. A period of immobilization for severe sprains
4. Possibly, surgical stabilization for recurrent sprains

While conservative management is the mainstay of treatment for the vast majority of ankle sprains, it is imperative to recognize that prevention is preferable. Taping, bracing, proper shoe wear, and muscle and proprioceptive training regimens should all be advocated for those active patients at particular risk for ankle trauma. Short of prevention, most ankle sprains of any grade will show great improvement with the classic RICE protocol. NSAIDs should also be added to this regimen and used liberally in patients who can tolerate them. Additionally, a short period of immobilization (4–6 weeks) with protected weight bearing should be prescribed for those in which there is suspicion for a grade III sprain. For most patients, immobilization in a removable walker with crutches will suffice. While there is no consensus among experts on the method or length of time of immobilization or whether or not to allow weight bearing as tolerated, any combination of these modalities is likely to be met with clinical satisfaction.

When patients can bear all of their weight on the injured ankle, they should be converted to a lace-up or stirrup brace for stability. Initially, this should be worn at all times and then weaned to only during at-risk activities such as sports.[2,3]

Predicated on any treatment protocol is also the recognition that in addition to ligamentous laxity, injury to the neuromuscular sleeve of the ankle also occurs during a severe sprain. Neuromuscular deficits can persist as deficiencies in proprioception, impaired balance, and slower firing of the peroneal musculature, which can lead to chronic or recurrent instability. The author therefore recommends a supervised proprioceptive and strengthening physical therapy regimen following a return to full weight bearing and no tenderness to palpation.[1,2,4]

The author does not advocate corticosteroid injections into the ligamentous areas or ankle joint following a sprain, as there is further risk of complete rupture with intraligamentous injection.

SECTION 6 Ankle

WHEN TO REFER

- Chronic instability
- Recalcitrant to short course of immobilization and physical therapy
- When associated with a fracture or cartilaginous lesions in the talus or tibia
- Child or adolescent with recurrent or chronic ankle sprains

Surgical management of the acute sprain is a controversial topic, and operative intervention is generally reserved for recalcitrant instability regardless of its anatomic location. Referral for surgical care should be contemplated in those cases where subjective instability persists following resolution of the initial symptoms and conservative care—including a supervised therapy program. When a concomitant fracture exists, surgical indications may exist independent of the ligamentous injury and should be evaluated by an orthopaedic surgeon.

 Refer to Patient Education

 Refer to Physical Therapy

ICD9

845.00 Unspecified site of ankle sprain
845.01 Deltoid (ligament), ankle sprain
845.02 Calcaneofibular (ligament) ankle sprain
845.03 Tibiofibular (ligament) sprain, distal
845.09 Other ankle sprain

References

1. Clanton TO, McGarvey W. Athletic injuries to the soft tissues of the foot and ankle. In: Coughlin MJ, Mann RA, and Saltzman CL, eds. *Surgery of the Foot and Ankle*, 8th ed. Philadelphia: Mosby; 2007:1425.
2. Scoli M. Injuries about the ankle: instability of the ankle and subtalar joint. In: *Myerson's Foot and Ankle Disorders*. Philadelphia: WB Saunders; 2000:1399.
3. Guyton GP. Chronic ankle instability. In: E. Greer Richardson, ed. *Orthopaedic Knowledge Update Foot and Ankle 3*. Rosemont, IL: American Academy of Orthopaedic Surgeons; 2003:103.
4. Penner MJ. Instability of the ankle. In: Johnson DH and Pedowitz RA, eds. *Johnson and Pedowitz's Practical Orthopaedic Sports Medicine and Arthroscopy*. Philadelphia: Lippincott Williams & Wilkins; 2007:861.

27 Fractured Fibula: Nondisplaced/Avulsion Fracture

Sudheer Reddy and Enyi Okereke

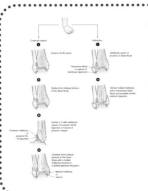

A 45-year-old woman slipped on ice and fell. She immediately noticed swelling and a sharp pain along the lateral aspect of her ankle and was unable to ambulate.

Clinical Presentation

Ankle fractures are common entities encountered by both the primary care physician and the orthopaedic surgeon. These fractures are the most common fracture treated by orthopaedic surgeons.[1] A fractured fibula is one variant of an ankle fracture that generally occurs after sustaining a rotational injury to the ankle. Avulsion injuries are due to a rupture of the ligamentous insertion to bone, in which the attachment fails and pulls a small fragment of bone off the fibula. Patients will typically give a history of a low-energy injury such as twisting and falling on an ankle.[2] They will complain of pain and swelling in the area of injury. Furthermore, the patient can have varying levels of discomfort when trying to ambulate.

Ankle fractures generally manifest in older populations, and their incidence and severity are increasing in patients over the age of 65.[3] This may be a consequence of the improved longevity and increased activity observed in older individuals.[1] Additionally, obesity and a history of smoking have been correlated with an increased incidence of ankle fractures.[4]

Treating physicians should also be aware of other entities that could potentially present acutely with swelling and pain, such as a Charcot arthropathy in a patient with diabetic neuropathy.[2] As a result, it is important for the clinician to inquire about comorbid conditions such as diabetes, peripheral vascular disease, malnutrition, and tobacco use, as they can adversely affect fracture healing.

CLINICAL POINTS

- Ankle fractures are often seen by physicians.
- Common symptoms include pain and swelling.
- Patients may have fallen awkwardly on an ankle.
- Injuries typically occur in older individuals.

Physical Findings

Physical examination will reveal swelling and tenderness to palpation at the area of injury. There may be a limitation in range of motion depending

SECTION 6 Ankle

on the degree of swelling and pain. The clinician should also evaluate the circulatory and neurologic status of the extremity to detect if there is underlying vascular disease or neuropathy. Compromise of the neurologic status of the extremity can occur in the presence of a dislocation of the ankle. Furthermore, the clinician should also look for any lacerations or abrasions indicating that the injury (fracture) communicates with the outside environment (open fracture). Both of these situations are emergent conditions and require evaluation and treatment by an orthopaedic surgeon.[2] Proximal leg tenderness with no clearly visible swelling at the level of the ankle is also a cause for concern. This could potentially indicate a high fibular fracture (Maisonneuve injury).[4]

Studies

Radiographs are necessary when evaluating a suspected fibular fracture. Standard radiographs include the AP, mortise, and lateral nonweight-bearing views.[4] However, not all injured ankles require radiographs. The Ottawa Ankle Rules were designed to aid health care professionals in deciding for whom to order radiographs to diagnose a suspected ankle fracture.[4] The Ottawa Ankle Rules state that radiographs are required to diagnose an ankle fracture if the patient has tenderness near one or both malleoli and has at least one of the following present:[4]

- Age 55 or older
- Inability to bear weight
- Bone tenderness at the posterior edge or tip of either malleolus

The use of these rules has been shown to have nearly 100% sensitivity in evaluating ankle fractures and has allowed treating physicians to reduce the number of radiographs obtained in an emergency setting.[4]

There are two general classification systems that are used to both evaluate and communicate the pertinent details of the injury. These include the Dennis-Weber system (Table 27.1) and the Lauge-Hansen system

Table 27.1   Dennis-Weber Classification System for Rotational Ankle Fractures

TYPE	DESCRIPTION
A	Fracture below the syndesmosis. Probable avulsion injuries associated frequently with oblique or vertical medial malleolar fractures (correlates with supination-adduction injury).
B	Fracture begins at joint level and extends proximally in an oblique fashion. May be accompanied with transverse medial malleolus fracture or with deltoid ligament rupture (correlates with supination–external rotation injury).
C	Fractures above the joint line, generally with syndesmotic injury. Can be associated with transverse avulsion medial malleolus fracture or deltoid ligament rupture (similar to pronation-eversion fracture).

From Thordarson DB. Foot and ankle trauma. In: Thordarson DB, ed. *Orthopaedic Surgery Essentials.* Philadelphia: Lippincott Williams & Wilkins; 2004:289.

Table 27.2 Lauge-Hansen Classification System for Rotational Ankle Fractures	
TYPE	**DESCRIPTION**
Supination–external rotation	Correlates to Weber B
Pronation–external rotation	Correlates to Weber C
Supination adduction	Correlates to Weber A
Pronation abduction	Oblique fracture of fibula above ankle mortise with medial malleolar fracture or deltoid ligament tear

(Table 27.2, Fig. 27.1). Within the Lauge-Hansen system, the names of the individual injuries pertain to the position of the foot at the time of injury and the actual deforming force creating the injury.[2] As well, the specific rotational injury patterns are categorized into stages I to IV. The greater the degree of injury, the greater the stage number ascribed to the particular type of injury. Supination-external rotation is the most common injury pattern observed, and it occurs in approximately 85% of all ankle fractures.[3]

Treatment and Clinical Course

1. Nondisplaced fractures are generally treated nonoperatively.
2. Displaced fractures generally require operative treatment.

For nondisplaced fractures, such as nondisplaced fibular fractures or avulsions, in which the ankle joint is anatomically reduced, nonoperative treatment is pursued. Patients can be placed in a splint in the emergency room setting to allow for acute swelling to subside. Once the swelling has subsided, the patient can then be placed in a short, nonweight-bearing cast for approximately 4 to 6 weeks. It is important to closely follow these patients to ensure that the fracture does not displace following initial treatment.

Isolated lateral malleolar fractures are injuries that can be managed by a primary care physician without the need for referral to a specialist. Specifically, isolated lateral malleolar injuries are defined as those with clear evidence of a nondisplaced fibular fracture, without a medial malleolar fracture, medial ankle tenderness (indicating potential injury to the deltoid ligament), or disruption of the ankle mortise. Injuries that do not fit these criteria need to be referred to an orthopaedic surgeon promptly. Additional scenarios that require referral include ankle dislocations, additional fractures, syndesmotic injuries, and fractures that are not healing appropriately. Ankle fractures occurring in patients with neuropathy or vascular insufficiency need to be referred, as healing is frequently delayed in these patients, and they are prone to ulcer formation if not treated and followed carefully.[5,6]

SECTION 6 Ankle

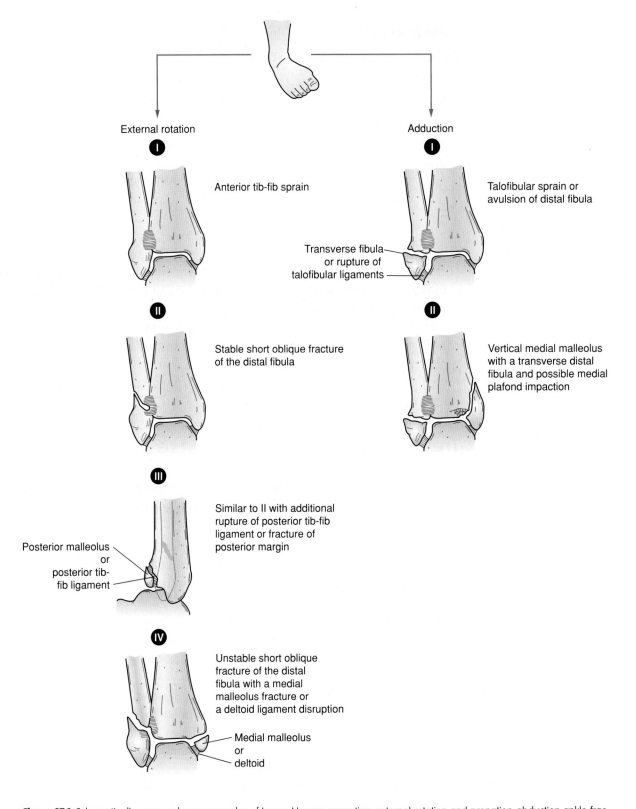

External rotation

Ⅰ

Anterior tib-fib sprain

Adduction

Ⅰ

Talofibular sprain or avulsion of distal fibula

Transverse fibula or rupture of talofibular ligaments

Ⅱ

Stable short oblique fracture of the distal fibula

Ⅱ

Vertical medial malleolus with a transverse distal fibula and possible medial plafond impaction

Ⅲ

Similar to II with additional rupture of posterior tib-fib ligament or fracture of posterior margin

Posterior malleolus or posterior tib-fib ligament

Ⅳ

Unstable short oblique fracture of the distal fibula with a medial malleolus fracture or a deltoid ligament disruption

Medial malleolus or deltoid

Figure 27.1 Schematic diagram and case examples of Lauge-Hansen pronation–external rotation and pronation-abduction ankle fractures. (From Bucholz RW, Heckman JD. *Rockwood and Green's Fractures in Adults*, 6th ed., Vol. 2. Philadelphia: Lippincott Williams & Wilkins; 2005.)

WHEN TO REFER (?)

- Displaced fibular fracture/ Disruption of ankle mortise

- Ankle dislocation

- Presence of comorbid conditions (diabetes, vascular disease)

- Syndesmotic injury

- Associated orthopaedic injuries (tibia fracture, fracture of tarsal bones, etc.)

- Delayed healing/ nonhealing fracture (nonunion)

ICD9

823.01 Closed fracture of upper end of fibula
823.21 Closed fracture of shaft of fibula
823.41 Torus fracture, fibula alone
823.81 Closed fracture of unspecified part of fibula
823.11 Open fracture of upper end of fibula
823.31 Open fracture of shaft of fibula
823.91 Open fracture of unspecified part of fibula

References

1. Michelson JD. Fractures about the ankle. *J Bone Joint Surg Am* 1995;77(1):142–152.
2. Thordarson DB. Foot and ankle trauma. In: Thordarson DB, ed. *Orthopaedic Surgery Essentials*. Philadelphia: Lippincott Williams & Wilkins; 2004:288–292.
3. Michelson JD. Ankle fractures resulting from rotational injuries. *J Am Acad Orthop Surg* 2003;11:403–412.
4. Marsh JL, Saltzman CL. Ankle fractures. In: Bucholz RW, Heckman JD, Court-Brown C., eds. *Rockwood and Green's Fractures in Adults*. Philadelphia: Lippincott Williams & Wilkins; 2006:2147–2247.
5. Flynn JM, Rodriguez-del Rio F, Piza PA. Closed ankle fractures in the diabetic patient. *Foot Ankle Int* 2000;21:311–319.
6. Wuest T. Injuries to the distal lower extremity syndesmosis. *J Am Acad Orthop Surg* 1997;5(3):172–181.

SECTION 6 Ankle

28 Retrocalcaneal Bursitis

Sudheer Reddy and Enyi Okereke

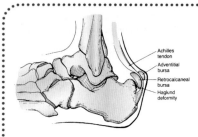

Achilles tendon
Adventitial bursa
Retrocalcaneal bursa
Haglund deformity

A 35-year-old man complains of dull, aching posterior heel pain that is aggravated by activity and shoe wear. He notices that the pain is most pronounced when arising from a seated position or when arising from bed in the morning. (Figure from Thordarson DB. Foot and Ankle. Philadelphia: Lippincott Williams & Wilkins; 2004.)

CLINICAL POINTS

- Pain anterior to the Achilles tendon is typical.
- Pathology involves inflammation of the retrocalcaneal bursa, which may injure the Achilles tendon.
- Younger adults, such as those in their 30s, are most likely to be affected.

PATIENT ASSESSMENT

1. Dull, aching pain in the retrocalcaneal area
2. Be mindful and perform thorough Achilles tendon exam during evaluation

Clinical Presentation

Retrocalcaneal bursitis is a distinct entity that is characterized by pain anterior to the Achilles tendon and involves inflammation of the retrocalcaneal bursa[1] (Fig. 28.1). This type of bursitis generally manifests in younger populations (those in their 30s) and is often seen in athletes who train uphill due to the extreme dorsiflexion that their ankles experience.[2] The bursa is horseshoe shaped and is 4 mm in width and 8 mm in depth[3,4] (Fig. 28.2). The anterior surface of the bursa is composed of fibrocartilage and is adjacent to the posterior aspect of the calcaneus, while the posterior aspect of the bursa merges with the paratenon of the Achilles. The bursa can become inflamed, hypertrophied, and adherent to the underlying Achilles that can, in turn, lead to degenerative changes within the Achilles, typically at the insertion of the Achilles (insertional tendinosis or tendinopathy). Haglund deformity is an enlarged, prominent portion of the posterosuperior angle of the calcaneus, which causes mechanical irritation of the retrocalcaneal bursa. The entity of Haglund syndrome is that of insertional Achilles tendinosis, retrocalcaneal bursitis, and adventitial bursitis, with the adventitial bursa being located between the Achilles tendon and the skin.[1] Each of these three components of Haglund syndrome can also occur separately. Anatomically, the bursa is important in maintaining a constant distance between the axis of the ankle joint and the Achilles, allowing the tension within the gastrocnemius-soleus group to remain constant during dorsiflexion and plantar flexion.[5]

Physical Findings

Patients with a Haglund deformity and retrocalcaneal bursitis will complain of dull, aching pain in the retrocalcaneal area that is aggravated during

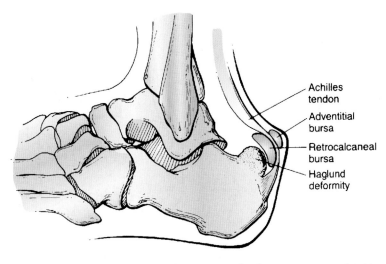

Figure 28.1 Illustration of Haglund deformity. (From Thordarson DB. *Foot and Ankle*. Philadelphia: Lippincott Williams & Wilkins; 2004.)

start-up activity. It is not typically associated with an acute onset of pain. If pain is acutely present, the clinician should be concerned with an Achilles rupture. The two-finger squeeze test is perhaps the best diagnostic sign due to the location of the bursa. Pain is elicited by applying pressure medially and laterally anterior to the Achilles insertion.[6] Of note, it is important to distinguish Haglund deformity/retrocalcaneal bursitis from what is commonly known as a "pump bump." Pump bump is an inflammation of the adventitial bursa that lies between the skin and Achilles tendon due to an abrasive heel counter.[2]

The clinician should also be mindful to carefully palpate the Achilles down to its insertion in order to identify insertional tendinosis, which may be tender to palpation and swollen. Dorsiflexion of the foot will tend to aggravate the pain due to compression of the bursa between the calcaneus and Achilles. The presence of a Haglund deformity can also be palpated in the superior portion of the heel directly anterior to the Achilles and may be associated with an overlying callus due to the prominence of the Haglund deformity (Fig. 28.3). An adventitial bursitis will lead to pain on palpation directly over the Achilles rather than anterior to it, as seen in retrocalcaneal bursitis. The presence or absence of an Achilles tendon contracture that could lead to increased tension at the Achilles insertion should also be assessed.[1]

Studies

IMAGING

Routine radiographs should be obtained that include a standing lateral view of the foot. If present, the Haglund deformity will be readily observed. The posterior calcaneal angle can be measured (Fig. 28.4), with greater angles being observed in those with Haglund disease.[1]

Other radiographic features to be observed include loss of the lucent retrocalcaneal recess anterior to the Achilles that is indicative of retrocalcaneal bursitis as well as a convexity of soft tissues posterior to Achilles

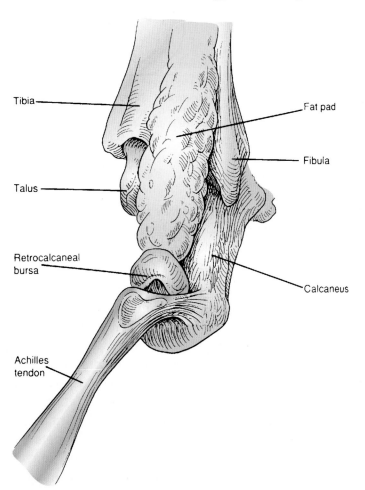

Figure 28.2 Anatomy of retrocalcaneal bursa. (From Kitaoka HB. *Masters Techniques in Orthopaedic Surgery: Foot and Ankle*, 2nd ed. Philadelphia: Lippincott Williams & Wilkins; 2002.)

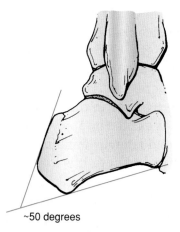
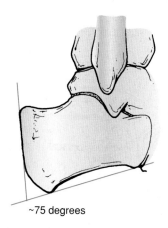
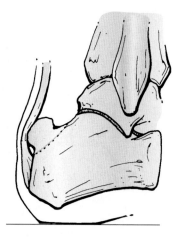

~50 degrees

~75 degrees

Figure 28.3 Measurement of the posterior calcaneal angle. The normal angle is shown on the left and the abnormal on the right. Upper level of normal is considered to be 69°. (From Thordarson DB. *Foot and Ankle*. Philadelphia: Lippincott Williams & Wilkins; 2004.)

tendon insertion that is indicative of superficial Achilles bursitis. MRI scans, while not necessary for reaching the diagnosis of a Haglund deformity or retrocalcaneal bursitis, is useful in visualizing abnormalities in the Achilles tendon, retrocalcaneal bursa, or the posterosuperior aspect of the calcaneus (Fig. 28.5).

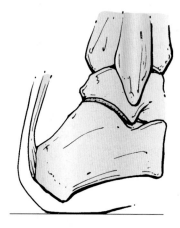

Figure 28.4 Diagram of Haglund deformity before and after resection. (From Thordarson DB. *Foot and Ankle*. Philadelphia: Lippincott Williams & Wilkins; 2004.)

Treatment and Clinical Course

1. Stretching exercises, activity modification, and NSAIDs are helpful.
2. Severe cases may require immobilization.

Nonsurgical management should be employed, consisting of rest, orthoses, and physical therapy (stretching of the gastrocnemius complex). An example of stretching of the Achilles tendon complex would be placing only the forefoot on a stair and allowing the individual's weight to depress the hindfoot and stretch the Achilles. Modification of training regimens and NSAIDs can also be helpful. Abnormal external pressure, such as from a hard athletic shoe heel counter, should be alleviated. If these methods are unsuccessful, then a short period of immobilization in a short leg walking cast with the ankle in 10 to 15 degrees of plantarflexion and a heel post for 4 to 8 weeks can be used to reduce symptoms. Night splints can also be utilized to improve dorsiflexion and reduce morning start-up pain. If Achilles tendinosis is present, a molded ankle–foot orthosis may help to reduce symptoms over a 6- to 9-month period.[1] Injection of steroids into the bursa should be avoided due to the risk of precipitating an Achilles rupture. Occasionally, however, a patient

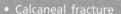

NOT TO BE MISSED

- Calcaneal fracture
- Tendinitis: Achilles, posterior tibial, flexor hallucis longus, flexor digitorum longus
- Neurologic: tarsal tunnel syndrome, entrapment of medial calcaneal nerve
- Tendon rupture: posterior tibial tendon, plantaris, Achilles
- Bony disorders: calcaneal periostitis, Sever disease (calcaneal epiphysitis—children), Haglund deformity
- Systemic disorders: rheumatoid arthritis, seronegative spondyloarthropathies (ankylosing spondylitis, Reiter syndrome), connective tissue disease, infection

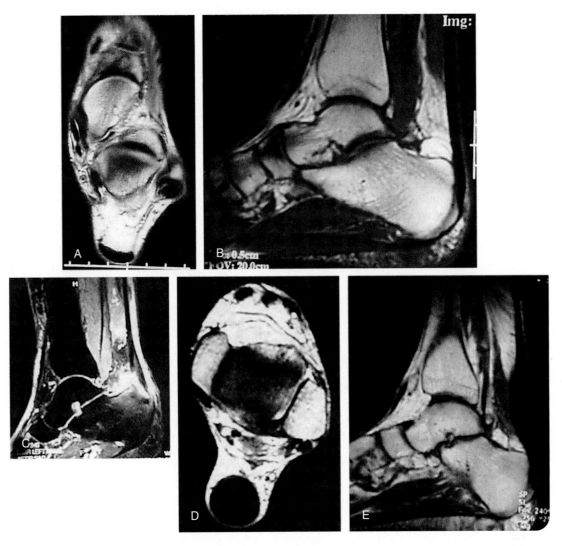

Figure 28.5 MRI of Achilles tendon. **A:** Axial MRI scan of normal Achilles tendon showing normal shape of the Achilles. **B:** Sagittal MRI scan of normal Achilles tendon showing normal shape of Achilles. **C:** Sagittal MRI scan showing increased signal in the insertion of the Achilles tendon consistent with tendinosis. There is increased fluid demonstrating an inflamed bursa surrounding the Haglund deformity. **D, E:** Axial and sagittal MRI scans demonstrating chronic tendinosis of the Achilles with marked fusiform swelling of the tendon. (From Thordarson DB. *Foot and Ankle*. Philadelphia: Lippincott Williams & Wilkins; 2004.)

may fail these conservative measures and require surgical intervention. Surgical management for the spectrum of retrocalcaneal pathology is dependent on the specific condition that is present.

WHEN TO REFER ?

- Unresponsive to conservative measures
- Achilles tendon rupture
- Concomitant hindfoot/forefoot deformity

ICD9

726.79 Other enthesopathy of ankle and tarsus

References

1. Wapner KL, Puri RD. Heel and subcalcaneal pain. In: Thordarson DB, ed. *Orthopaedic Surgery Essentials: Foot and Ankle*. Philadelphia: Lippincott Williams & Wilkins; 2004:182–194.
2. Coughlin M. Disorders of tendons. In: Mann RA, Coughlin MJ, eds. *Surgery of the Foot and Ankle*. Philadelphia: Mosby; 1999:786–861.
3. Frey C. Calcaneal prominence resection. In: Kitaoka H, ed. *Masters Techniques in Orthopaedic Surgery: The Foot and Ankle*. Philadelphia: Lippincott Williams & Wilkins; 2002:357–367.
4. Schepsis AA, Jones H, Haas HL. Achilles tendon disorders in athletes. *Am J Sports Med* 2002;30(2):287–303.
5. Paavola M, Kannus P, Jarvinen TAH, et al. Achilles tendinopathy. *J Bone Joint Surg Am* 2002;84(11): 2062–2076.
6. Schepsis AA, Wagner C, Leach RE. Surgical management of Achilles tendon overuse injuries. *Am J Sports Med* 1994;22(5):611–619.

SECTION 6 Ankle

Foot

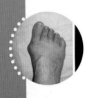

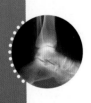
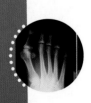
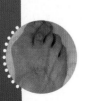

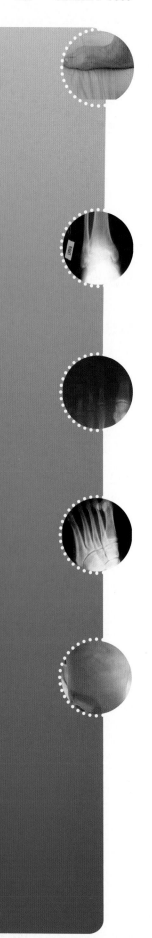

29 Bunion/Hallux Valgus

Keith Wapner

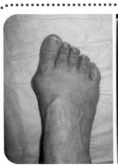 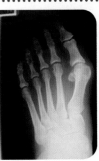

A 41-year-old woman presents with a history of pain, discomfort, and deformity over the first metatarsophalangeal (MTP) joints bilaterally, greater on the right than the left.

Clinical Presentation

Patients often have a history of pain and an increasing deformity at the first MTP joint and often note an increasingly large "bump" over the medial aspect of the first MTP joint. They complain of their shoes no longer fitting and being unable to wear high heels or pointed-toe shoes.

CLINICAL POINTS

- Pain and deformity of the first MTP joint are typical.
- Reports of an increasingly large "bump" over the first MTP joint are frequent.
- Patients may complain of problems with the way their shoes fit.

Physical Findings

On presentation, bilateral feet often reveal obvious hallux valgus deformities. Dorsalis pedis pulse and posterior tibialis pulses are typically palpable bilaterally.

Musculoskeletal exam should reveal a normal gait pattern. On inspection of both lower extremities, there should be no other misalignment, asymmetry, crepitation, defect, or effusions. The patient typically has bilateral hallux valgus deformities, with pain over the medial eminence. The first MTP joints bilaterally are reducible. Muscle strength of both lower extremities should reveal no atrophy or abnormal movements. Muscle strength for the anterior tibial muscles, posterior tibial muscles, peroneal muscles, and gastroc-soleus muscles should be normal. Neurologic examination should demonstrate normal coordination, reflexes, and sensation of both lower extremities.

PATIENT ASSESSMENT

1. Normal gait pattern
2. Typically a bilateral finding
3. Weight-bearing x-rays of the forefoot can be helpful

Studies

Weight-bearing x-rays of the affected foot should be obtained in AP, lateral, and oblique planes (Fig. 29.1). The 1-2 intermetatarsal angle (normal <9 degrees) and hallux valgus angle (normal <15 degrees) are measured to evaluate the severity of the deformity.

NOT TO BE MISSED

- Hallux rigidus
- Rheumatoid arthritis

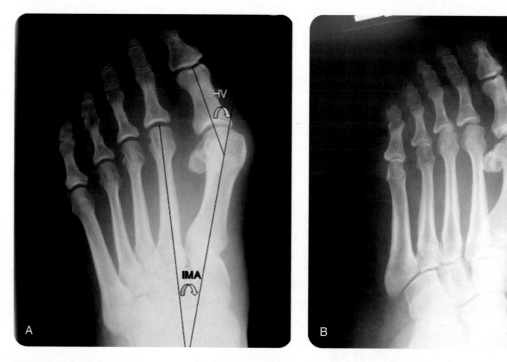

Figure 29.1 Weight-bearing anterior–posterior (AP) **(A)** and oblique **(B)** views of a patient with hallux valgus deformity. IMA, intermetatarsal angle.

Treatment and Clinical Course

1. Conservative treatment usually helps, consisting of wearing a wide-toe box shoe.
2. Increasing deformity should be evaluated by an orthopaedist.

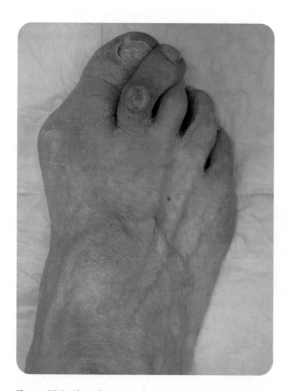

Figure 29.2 Clinical picture of a patient with a bunion who has progressively also developed a hammer toe in response to the first MTP deformity.

WHEN TO REFER (?)

- Progressive deformity
- Increasing pain in the first MTP joint
- Subluxation of the second MTP joint

The vast majority of patients with bunions realize significant benefit from conservative management. On first examination, the patient should be advised to forgo pointed-toe shoes. Shoes with wider toe boxes or a straight medial last will be more comfortable. Bunion splints, toe spacers, and injections are not recommended, as they have not been proven to be clinically effective. Conservatively, there is no other treatment for patients until they become more symptomatic.

Over time, many patients will continue to have the development of progressive deformity. This may be associated with increasingly restrictive shoe wear, pain, and discomfort. When the first toe abuts the second, the patient may develop second MTP synovitis, subluxation, hammer toe (Fig. 29.2), or crossover toe. Eventually, these patients may seek surgical interventions to treat the hallux valgus deformity.

ICD9
727.1 Bunion
735.0 Hallux valgus (acquired)

SECTION 7 Foot

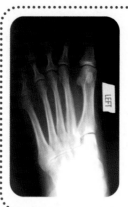

A 65-year-old woman presents with a history of bilateral forefoot pain and discomfort in the area of the second and third metatarsals. She describes aching and burning pain of moderate severity. The pain is intermittent in duration and stable in context. She states that she feels like she is walking on pebbles.

Clinical Presentation

The primary symptom of metatarsalgia is pain at one or more of the metatarsal heads. Diffuse forefoot pain and midfoot pain are often present. The pain typically is aggravated during the midstance and propulsion phases of walking or running. A history of gradual chronic onset is more common than acute presentation.

Physical Findings

Musculoskeletal exam typically reveals a normal gait pattern. On inspection of both lower extremities, there is no misalignment, asymmetry, crepitation, defect, or effusions. There is often tenderness to palpation at the affected MTP joints. The physician may be able to appreciate some fat pad atrophy over the plantar surface of the forefoot bilaterally.

Examination for range of motion reveals symmetric motion of the ankles in dorsiflexion and plantar flexion, subtalar joints in inversion and eversion, transverse tarsal joints in abduction and adduction, and MTP joints in dorsiflexion and plantar flexion, without any evidence of contracture or crepitation. A drawer test for stability of the MTP joint may reveal instability of the joint.

Studies

Weight-bearing views of the left and right foot are obtained in AP, lateral, and oblique planes (Fig. 30.1). Careful attention is paid to the symptomatic MTP joints to look for medial or lateral deviation of the joint, subluxations, joint space narrowing, or arthritic changes. Additionally, the cascade of the MTP joints, from medial to lateral, should be noted. This cascade should resemble an inverted parabola.

CLINICAL POINTS

- Metatarsal pain is typical.
- Pain is often worse when the patient walks or runs.
- Onset tends to be gradual.

PATIENT ASSESSMENT

1. Typically, forefoot pain in the region of the metatarsals
2. Tenderness to palpation over the metatarsophalangeal (MTP) joint
3. May notice fat atrophy in the forefoot
4. Normal gait pattern

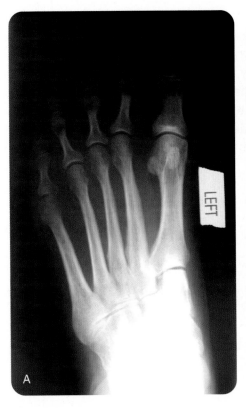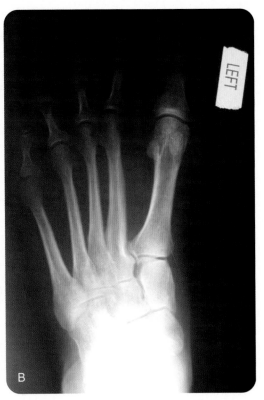

Figure 30.1 Weight-bearing AP **(A)** and oblique **(B)** views of the left foot. Both x-rays demonstrate a medial deviation of the second MTP joint.

NOT TO BE MISSED

- Morton neuroma
- MTP subluxation or dislocation
- Hammer toe/Claw toe
- Psoriatic arthritis
- Gout
- Osteoarthritis/Rheumatoid arthritis
- Stress fracture

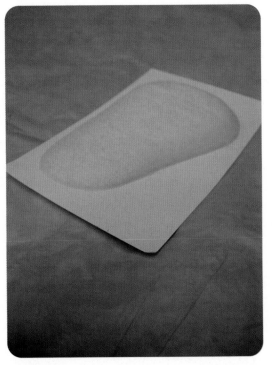

Figure 30.2 Clinical picture of a metatarsal pad (Hapad) used for dissipating pressure more proximally on the metatarsal.

Treatment and Clinical Course

1. Recommend use of a metatarsal pad (Hapad)

The goal of treatment is to decrease the amount of stress placed on the MTP joint with gait. On first examination, the patient should be advised to forgo high heels or pointed-toe shoes. A metatarsal pad (such as a Hapad) (Fig. 30.2) should be utilized to distribute pressure more proximally throughout the metatarsal shaft. This can be accompanied with an insole to help cushion the plantar surface of the foot. Finally, the MTP joint can be taped in neutral dorsiflexion and plantar flexion. Corticosteroid injections

WHEN TO REFER

- Progressive deformity
- Intractable pain

into the MTP joint are not recommended, as they have been associated with ruptures of the plantar plate and collateral ligaments.

For many patents, conservative treatments are effective. Some patients may require larger metatarsal pads. In those patients where pain continues, the MTP joint may sublux laterally or medially and develop into a crossover toe. Additionally, some patients may develop a hammer toe or claw toe deformity. For patients who experience progressive deformity or recalcitrant pain, surgical intervention is required.

 Refer to Patient Education

ICD9
726.70 Enthesopathy of ankle and tarsus, unspecified

31 Plantar Fasciitis

Keith Wapner

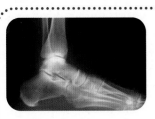

A 61-year-old woman with a history of fibromyalgia presents for evaluation of right heel pain. The pain has been ongoing for approximately 6 months. The patient states that the pain is most severe in the morning with her first few steps. Additionally, she states that she experiences severe pain in the right heel after sitting for prolonged periods of time.

CLINICAL POINTS

- Patients are often runners.
- Repetitive microtrauma may trigger symptoms.
- Etiology may be multifactorial.

PATIENT ASSESSMENT

1. Heel pain is the primary complaint.
2. Medial plantar fascia tenderness is elicited on exam.
3. Consider calcaneal stress fracture in the differential diagnosis.

Clinical Presentation

The cause of plantar fasciitis is unclear and may be multifactorial. Because of the high incidence in runners, it is best postulated to be caused by repetitive microtrauma. Possible risk factors include obesity, occupations requiring prolonged standing, heel spurs, pes planus (excessive pronation of the foot), and reduced dorsiflexion of the ankle.

Physical Findings

Musculoskeletal exam typically reveals a normal gait pattern. There is often tenderness to palpation of the heel at the insertion of the medial band of the plantar fascia. There is also pain with mediolateral compression test of the calcaneus. When the patient has more tenderness with mediolateral compression of the posterior body of the calcaneus than at the insertion of the plantar fascia, a diagnosis of a calcaneal stress fracture must be entertained.

Oftentimes, examination of the ankle for range of motion reveals decreased ankle dorsiflexion on the affected side as compared with that found on the normal contralateral side, suggesting a tight gastroc-soleus complex. There is typically symmetric motion of the ankles in plantar flexion.

Studies

Weight-bearing views of the foot are obtained in AP, lateral, and oblique planes (Fig. 31.1). Clinically, when the mediolateral compression test is positive, a bone scan or MRI is recommended to evaluate for the presence of a calcaneal stress fracture. On the bone scan, the insertion site of the plantar fascia and the calcaneus will demonstrate increased signal intensity.

On the MRI, the T2 images will be bright in the area of the insertion of the plantar fascia as well as the calcaneal marrow proximal to the insertion site of the plantar fascia (Fig. 31.2).

Treatment and Clinical Course

1. Conservative modalities are the mainstay of treatment, including immobilization, stretching exercises, night splints, and NSAIDs.
2. Cortisone injections should be avoided.
3. Resistant cases should be evaluated by an orthopaedist.

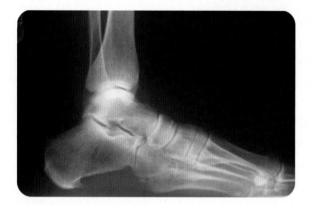

Figure 31.1 A weight-bearing lateral view of the left foot demonstrates the presence of a plantar calcaneal osteophyte.

Initially, if the patient has a positive mediolateral calcaneal compression test, the foot should be immobilized in either a CAM Walker or a short leg-walking cast. Patients are re-examined at a 3- to 4-week interval. Once the mediolateral calcaneal compression test is negative, the patient can be advanced out of the cast or boot and into a well-padded, regular shoe. A silastic heel cup (Fig. 31.3) may be beneficial at this time. Furthermore, a program of night splints, stretching of the gastroc-soleus complex and plantar fascia, and well-padded shoes (such as running shoes) should be implemented.

Patients who present with a negative mediolateral calcaneal compression test can be treated initially with a CAM Walker if their pain is severe; otherwise, a program of night splints, stretching of the gastroc-soleus complex and plantar fascia, well-padded shoes (such as running shoes), and a silastic heel cup should be implemented. These patients should be re-examined at 4- to 6-week intervals.

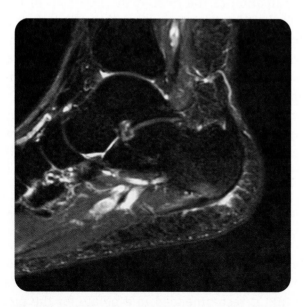

Figure 31.2 T2 MRI of a patient with a positive mediolateral compression test. The bright signal in the plantar fascia insertion as well as the calcaneus are indicative for plantar fasciitis with a calcaneal stress fracture.

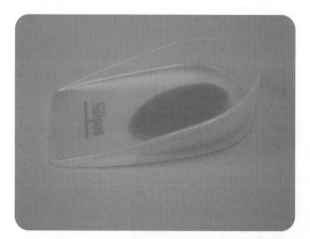

Figure 31.3 Silastic heel cup insert used for cushioning the heel and helping to prevent progression/recurrence of plantar fasciitis.

Plantar fascial corticosteroid injections are not recommended, as these have been shown to be associated with a higher rate of plantar fascial rupture.[1,2] High-energy extracorporeal shockwave therapy has been shown to be effective for the patient with recalcitrant plantar fasciitis.[3] At this time, clinical data does not support the efficacy of low-energy extracorporeal shockwave therapy.

The majority of patients will get better over time; however, this can be a long, frustrating process for the patient, as treatment length is usually correlated with length of pretreatment symptoms. It is critical for the physician to constantly reassure the patient with recalcitrant plantar fasciitis, because these patients will make the slowest progress. Finally, continued stretching should be emphasized, even after symptoms resolve, as this may help to prevent recurrences of plantar fasciitis.

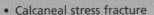

WHEN TO REFER

- Calcaneal stress fracture
- Recalcitrant plantar fasciitis

Refer to Patient Education

Refer to Physical Therapy

ICD9
728.71 Plantar fascial fibromatosis

SECTION 7 Foot

References

1. Acevedo JI, Beskin JL. Complications of plantar fascia rupture associated with corticosteroid injection. *Foot Ankle Int* 1998;19:91–97.
2. Sellman JR. Plantar fascia rupture associated with corticosteroid injection. *Foot Ankle Int* 1994;15: 376–381.
3. Wang CJ, Wang FS, Yang KD, et al. Long-term results of extracorporeal shockwave treatment for plantar fasciitis. *Am J Sports Med* 2006;34:592–596.

32 Morton Neuroma

Keith Wapner

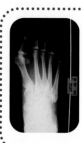

A 68-year-old woman presents complaining of aching and burning pain of moderate to severe intensity in the third web space of the right foot. It is constant in duration and worsening in context.

CLINICAL POINTS

- Pathology involves tissue thickening, not tumor formation.
- Precipitating factors include irritation and trauma.
- Women are more likely to be affected.

PATIENT ASSESSMENT

1. Most frequently develops between the third and fourth toe
2. Is eight to ten times more frequent in women than in men
3. Mulder sign

Clinical Presentation

Morton neuroma is not actually a tumor but a thickening of the tissue that surrounds the digital nerve leading to the toes. It occurs as the nerve passes under the ligament connecting the metatarsals in the forefoot. Morton neuroma most frequently develops between the third and fourth toes, usually in response to irritation, trauma, or excessive pressure. The incidence of Morton neuroma is eight to ten times greater in women than in men.

Physical Findings

Musculoskeletal exam typically reveals a normal gait pattern. On inspection of both lower extremities, there is no other misalignment, asymmetry, crepitation, defect, or effusions. There is usually tenderness in the third web spaces of the affected foot.

To diagnose Morton neuroma, the physician should palpate the web space to elicit pain, squeezing the toes from the side. Next, an attempt should be made to feel the neuroma by pressing a thumb into the toe web space. The physician should try to elicit the Mulder sign by holding the patient's first, second, and third metatarsal heads with one hand and the fourth and fifth metatarsal heads in the other and pushing half the foot up and half the foot down slightly. In many cases of Morton neuroma, this causes an audible click, known as the *Mulder sign*. Range-of-motion tests will rule out arthritis or joint inflammations. X-rays may be required to rule out a stress fracture or arthritis of the joints.

Studies

Weight-bearing x-ray views of the foot are obtained in AP, lateral, and oblique planes (Fig. 32.1).

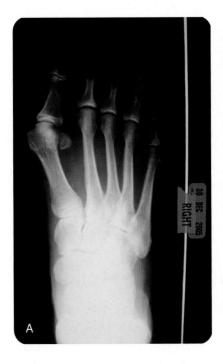

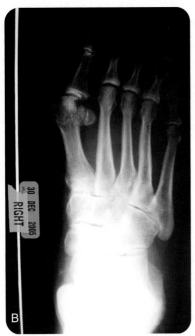

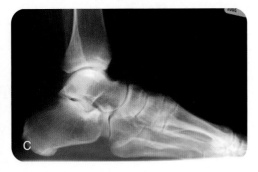

Figure 32.1 Weight-bearing AP **(A)**, oblique **(B)**, and lateral **(C)** views of the right foot.

SECTION 7 Foot

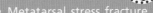

NOT TO BE MISSED

• Metatarsal stress fracture

WHEN TO REFER

• Intractable pain

• Associated pathologies, such as hammer toes

Treatment and Clinical Course

1. May benefit from use of a metatarsal pad
2. Corticosteroid injections used sparingly

If an interdigital neuroma is suspected, the patient can be treated initially with a metatarsal Hapad support (refer to Fig. 30.2). This support minimizes the force over the interdigital areas and helps to distribute force throughout the midarch and metatarsals. It is recommended that patients begin with a small Hapad. Patients should be re-evaluated every 4 to 6 weeks. If the patient is experiencing minimal relief, the Hapad should continually be increased in size, from small to medium to large.

Interdigital injections with short-term anesthetics can be diagnostic. Corticosteroid interdigital injections should be used sparingly, as the steroid can lead to fat atrophy and skin discolorations.

Patients can be treated successfully with conservative methods. These patients should continue to wear Hapads of the appropriate size, even after symptoms have resolved. Patients who continue to have pain that is debilitating should seek surgical intervention.

ICD9
355.6 Lesion of plantar nerve

CHAPTER 33 Hammer Toes

Keith Wapner

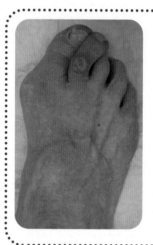

A 58-year-old woman presents complaining of her second right toe becoming more crooked. She states that it is bending more often and that she has a callus developing over the second toe. She no longer wears pointed-toe shoes, as they are unable to accommodate for her toe deformity. Even with a deeper toe box, the patient continues to have a worsening deformity of the second toe.

Clinical Presentation

People with hammer toe may have corns or calluses on the top of the middle joint of the toe or on the tip of the toe. They may also feel pain in their toes or feet and have difficulty finding comfortable shoes. As a group, these deformities can be secondary to overcrowding in closed-toe shoes that are too small for the foot, a muscle imbalance, or a combination of one or more other factors.

CLINICAL POINTS

- Corns or calluses may be present.
- Pain in the toes or feet may occur.
- Finding comfortable shoes may be a problem.

Physical Findings

A hammer toe exists when there is a flexion deformity of the PIP joint. A mallet toe exists when there is a flexion deformity of the distal interphalangeal joint (DIP). When either the DIP or PIP joint is involved with the MTP joint, the diagnosis is claw toe.

Studies

Weight-bearing views of the foot are obtained in AP, lateral, and oblique planes (Fig. 33.1). Careful attention is paid to the affected digit, looking for dorsal subluxation of the MTP joint or arthritic changes.

Treatment and Clinical Course

1. Treat initially with wider and deeper toe box shoes.
2. Taping of the MTP joint in neutral can be helpful.
3. When the deformity becomes fixed and painful, surgical options may be considered.

PATIENT ASSESSMENT

1. Hammer toe exists when there is a flexion deformity of the proximal interphalangeal (PIP) joint.

2. When the metatarsophalangeal (MTP) joint is involved along with a flexion deformity of the interphalangeal joint, the diagnosis is claw toe.

3. X-rays can be helpful to evaluate associated degenerative joint disease.

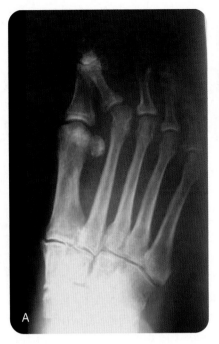

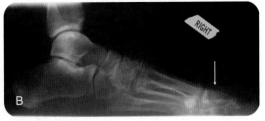

Figure 33.1 Weight-bearing AP **(A)** and lateral **(B)** views of the right foot.

NOT TO BE MISSED

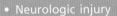

- Neurologic injury

WHEN TO REFER

- Intractable pain
- Continued or worsening deformity

Initially, hammer toes are flexible and can be corrected with simple measures, but if left untreated, they can become fixed and require surgery.

If the deformity is flexible, patients can initially attempt to wear shoes with wider and deeper toe boxes. Simultaneously, patients can tape the MTP joint in neutral or try a metatarsal pad. These modalities can help to reposition the toe and minimize pressure over the flexed joint.

If the toe has become inflexible, the conservative management options are few other than utilizing a higher toe box shoe. The options mentioned previously can be attempted; however, for patients with continued symptoms, surgical intervention must be considered.

ICD9

735.4 Other hammer toe (acquired)
735.2 Hallux rigidus

CHAPTER 34

Pronation/Adult Flatfoot/Posterior Tibial Tendon Dysfunction

Keith Wapner

A 60-year-old woman presents with a chief complaint of increasing pain and discomfort affecting the left hindfoot over the past year.

Clinical Presentation

Posterior tibial tendon dysfunction (PTTD) is an inflammation and/or overstretching of the posterior tibial tendon in the foot. An important function of the posterior tibial tendon is to help support the arch. But in PTTD, the tendon's ability to perform that job is impaired, often resulting in a flattening of the foot. The posterior tibial tendon is a fibrous cord that extends from a muscle in the leg. It descends the leg and runs along the inside of the ankle, down the side of the foot, and into the arch. This tendon serves as one of the major supporting structures of the foot and helps the foot to function while walking. PTTD is often called *adult-acquired flatfoot* because it is the most common type of flatfoot developed during adulthood. Although this condition typically occurs in only one foot, some people may develop it in both feet.

The natural history of PTTD is not clearly understood; however, there are four stages of dysfunction, and treatment is undertaken based on the stage. Patients with higher stages are more likely to require surgery. In stage 1 PTTD, patients have no changes in posture of the foot. There is tenderness along the course of the posterior tibial tendon. Patients are able to perform a single heel raise. In stage 2 PTTD, patients have a flexible pes planus deformity. The deformity is not present when the patient is nonweight bearing; however, once weight is placed on the foot, the pes planus deformity becomes evident. Stage 3 patients have fixed pes planus deformity. Associated with this are a hindfoot valgus alignment, possible subfibular impingement, and the inability to perform a single heel raise. Stage 4 PTTD has associated arthritis of the tibiotalar/ankle joint.

Physical Findings

On examination, there typically is tenderness to palpation along the course of the posterior tibialis tendon as well as pain in the subfibular area of the ankle. When the patient stands, a pes planus posture is observed.

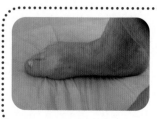

CLINICAL POINTS

- Inflammation and/or overstretching of the posterior tibial tendon may lead to flatfoot.

- Usually, only one foot is affected.

- Not all conditions are equally severe; not all patients have a deformity.

Examination for range of motion commonly reveals symmetric motion of the ankles in dorsiflexion and plantar flexion, subtalar joints in inversion and eversion, transverse tarsal joints in abduction and adduction, and metatarsophalangeal joints in dorsiflexion and plantar flexion, without any evidence of contracture or crepitation.

Muscle strength of both lower extremities reveals no atrophy or abnormal movements but typically reveals weakness of the posterior tibialis muscle. The patient often has difficulty in attempting to perform a single heel rise on the affected foot. The affected hindfoot is aligned in valgus with weight bearing, and the patient has a positive "too many toes" sign (when the feet are viewed from the back, more of the lateral toes are seen on the affected foot rather than on the unaffected foot) (Fig. 34.1).

Studies

Weight-bearing views of the left foot are obtained in AP, lateral, and oblique planes. The talo–first metatarsal axis (normal is aligned) on the lateral view is noted to evaluate the extent of talonavicular sag. The talonavicular–first metatarsal angle (normal is 0 degrees) on the AP view is measured to assess the amount of talonavicular subluxation. MRI is very helpful in making the diagnosis. On MRI, a posterior tibial tendon that is twice the size of the flexor digitorum longus tendon, >8 mm in size, has fluid in the posterior tendon sheath, has a gross tear, or is absent may signify PTTD (Fig. 34.2).

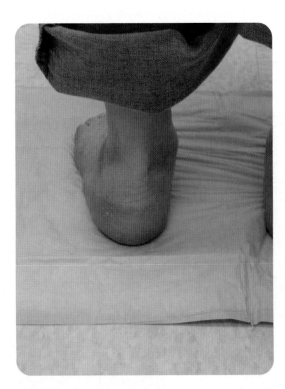

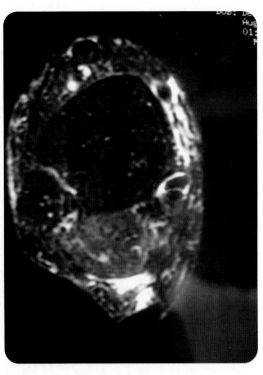

Figure 34.1 The affected hindfoot is aligned in valgus with weight bearing, and the patient has a positive "too many toes" sign.

Figure 34.2 T2 MRI of the left foot demonstrates a high signal around the posterior tibial tendon. This coupled with the clinical exam is suggestive of a PTTD.

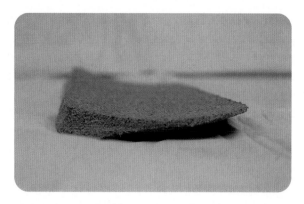

Figure 34.3 Typical medial heel wedge used in the early stages of posterior tibial dysfunction.

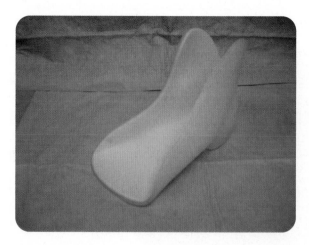

Figure 34.4 UCBL orthotics.

Treatment and Clinical Course

1. Early on, NSAIDs and the use of various bracing options can be considered.

2. If pain and deformity persist, then consideration for surgical treatment should be given.

Treatment is based on the stage of the dysfunction. Patients with higher stages are more likely to require surgery. In stage 1 or 2, a medial heel wedge (Fig. 34.3), a University of California Berkley Laboratories (UCBL) orthotic (Fig. 34.4), an Arizona brace (Fig. 34.5), a molded ankle foot orthosis (MAFO) (Fig. 35.6), or a short leg-walking cast can be prescribed to treat

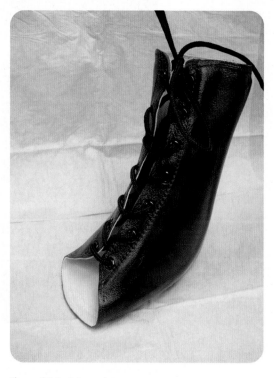

Figure 34.5 Arizona brace.

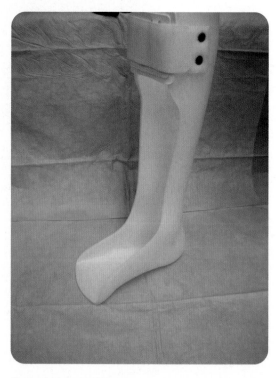

Figure 34.6 Typical MAFO.

- Intractable pain
- Continued functional loss

the patient. In stage 2 PTTD, patients are initially treated conservatively, like stage 1 patients. Following diminution of pain, patients are enrolled in a physical therapy program that focuses on enhancing range of motion and strength of the posterior tibial tendon. When such a program is successful, patients may have resolution of their symptoms. Stage 3 patients have fixed pes planus deformity. The patients can also be treated conservatively with the methods described in stage 1 and 2; however, the UCBL and medial heel wedge are not recommended for stage 3 PTTD, as the deformity is fixed. Patients who fail conservative care may elect to have surgical intervention. The surgical procedure utilized is dictated by the stage.

ICD9

734.00 Flatfoot
736.79 Other acquired deformities of ankle and foot

SECTION 7 Foot

CHAPTER 35 Osteoarthritis: Foot/Ankle Joints

Keith Wapner

Ankle Arthritis

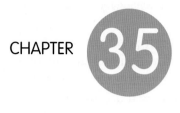

A 74-year-old man started having increasing pain in the right ankle following a fall. He had immediate onset of pain and swelling. His pain has persisted since that time.

CLINICAL POINTS

- Any joint in the foot or ankle may be involved.
- Symptoms may vary, depending on which joint is affected.
- Pain and swelling are common.

Clinical Presentation

Osteoarthritis can practically affect any joint in the foot and ankle and in any combination of joints. The more common locations of osteoarthritis include the following:

- Ankle (tibiotalar joint)
- Three joints of the hindfoot: the subtalar or talocalcaneal joint, the talonavicular joint, the calcaneocuboid joint
- Midfoot (metatarsocuneiform joint)
- Great toe (first metatarsophalangeal [MTP] joint)

Signs and symptoms of arthritis of the foot vary, depending on which joint is affected. Common symptoms include pain or tenderness, stiffness or reduced motion, and swelling. Walking is often difficult.

Physical Findings

Musculoskeletal exam commonly reveals a mild antalgic gait pattern. On inspection, there is usually asymmetry with swelling of the affected ankle. There is tenderness to palpation of the ankle and pain with ankle motion. Range of motion is typically reduced as compared with that found in the contralateral ankle, with particular reduction in dorsiflexion and plantar flexion on the ankle. Muscle strength of both lower extremities reveals no atrophy or abnormal movements.

Studies

Weight-bearing x-ray views of the ankle are obtained (AP, lateral, and mortise views) (Fig. 35.1). On the x-rays, the clinician should look for alignment, joint space narrowing, subchondral sclerosis, osteophyte formation, and degenerative cyst formation.

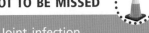

PATIENT ASSESSMENT

1. Patients commonly present with pain, stiffness, and swelling of the ankle joint.

2. Walking can be painful.

3. With physical examination, compare the affected joint with the contralateral foot.

4. On exam, patients typically have decreased range of motion.

5. X-rays are helpful in making a diagnosis.

NOT TO BE MISSED

- Joint infection
- Tendon rupture

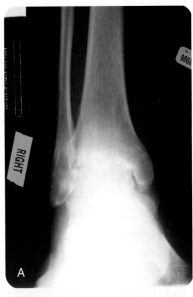

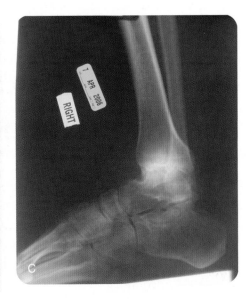

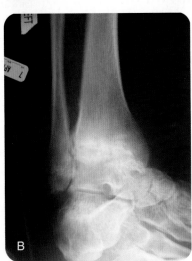

Figure 35.1 Weight-bearing AP **(A)**, mortise **(B)**, and lateral **(C)** views of the right ankle demonstrate severe ankle joint (tibiotalar) arthritis. There is joint space obliteration, subchondral sclerosis, and osteophyte formation.

Treatment and Clinical Course

1. Treatment depends on the nature and severity of the arthritis.

2. Clearly, the early use of nonoperative treatment consisting of weight reduction, activity modification, and NSAIDs can be helpful.

Patients with ankle arthritis can be managed conservatively with NSAIDs. Immobilization to restrict range of motion of the ankle can be attempted as well. Immobilization can be successfully achieved with an Arizona brace or molded ankle foot orthosis (MAFO). Intra-articular corticosteroid-anesthetic injections can be attempted, but no more frequently than once every 4 months. Hyaluronic acid substitutes, such as Synvisc or Hyalgan, have not been FDA approved for use in the ankle, as the clinical data has not shown the efficacy of this treatment. Glucosamine and chondroitin sulfate has been studied in the knee, yielding conflicting results in the treatment of osteoarthritis.[1–4] Once patients have end-stage osteoarthritis of the ankle, an ankle fusion or total ankle arthroplasty may be entertained.

WHEN TO REFER

- Ankle deformity
- Intractable pain
- Loss of quality of life
- Unable to perform activities of daily living

Although patients may wax and wane in their response to different conservative measures for ankle arthritis, over an extended period of time, patients will continue to worsen. It is important for the patient to realize that the arthritis is not curable.

Subtalar Arthritis

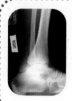

A 28-year-old man presents with a history of increasing pain and discomfort of the right ankle. He has a history of a prior ankle sprains to that ankle, after which he states that he did have discomfort.

Physical Findings

Musculoskeletal exam typically reveals an antalgic gait pattern. On inspection of both lower extremities, there is usually no other misalignment, asymmetry, crepitation, defect, or effusions. Patient will typically have significant pain to palpation over the anterior aspect of the ankle and with all attempted subtalar ranges of motion.

Examination for range of motion reveals symmetric motion of the ankles in dorsiflexion and plantar flexion. Subtalar motion of the affected lower extremity is limited, with only minimal inversion and eversion. There is pain with passive range of motion of the subtalar joint. Muscle strength of both lower extremities reveals no weakness.

Studies

Weight-bearing views of the right foot are obtained in AP, lateral, and oblique planes (Fig. 35.2). Particular attention is paid to the subtalar joints to look for evidence of osteoarthritis, such as subchondral sclerosis, joint space narrowing, cyst formation, and osteophytes.

CT scans or MRIs of the ankle are more sensitive in showing the amount of osteoarthritis present, joint space narrowing, subchondral cyst formation, and bony anatomy (Fig. 35.3).

Treatment and Clinical Course

1. Treatment depends on the nature and severity of the arthritis.
2. Clearly, the early use of nonoperative treatment consisting of weight reduction, activity modification, and NSAIDs can be helpful.
3. In severe cases, surgical treatment may be necessary.

Depending on the severity of symptoms, the patient can be initially treated with a variety of conservative modalities such as NSAIDs and immobilization. Immobilization to restrict range of motion of the ankle can be attempted with an Arizona brace, MAFO, or University of California Berkley Laboratories (UCBL) orthotic. Intra-articular corticosteroid-anesthetic injections can be attempted, but it can be difficult to inject in

PATIENT ASSESSMENT

1. Patients usually report pain in the region of the heel.
2. There may be difficulty when walking on uneven surfaces.
3. On physical examination, decreased ability to pronate/supinate the subtalar joint is noted.
4. On x-ray, the talocalcaneal joint should be assessed.

NOT TO BE MISSED

- Talar fracture
- Tendon rupture

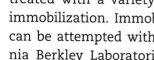

SECTION 7 Foot

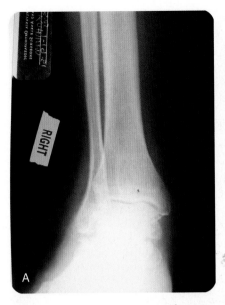 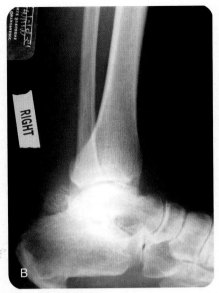 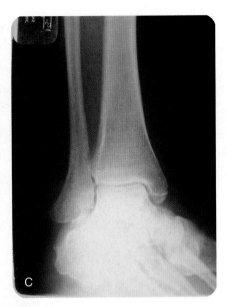

Figure 35.2 Weight-bearing AP **(A)**, oblique **(B)**, and lateral **(C)** views of the right ankle demonstrate joint space narrowing and subchondral sclerosis of the subtalar joint.

WHEN TO REFER

- Intractable pain
- Inability to perform activities of daily living
- Loss of quality of life

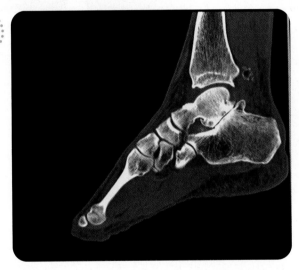

Figure 35.3 CT scan of the right ankle reveals osteophytes, joint space narrowing, and articular surface irregularities of the subtalar joint, consistent with subtalar arthritis.

an arthritic subtalar joint. This should definitely be reserved for an orthopaedist. Once patients have end-stage osteoarthritis of the subtalar joint, a subtalar fusion may be entertained. Many patients, over time, will continue to have the development of progressive pain. Eventually, these patients will seek surgical interventions to treat the subtalar fusion.

SECTION 7 Foot

Midfoot Arthritis

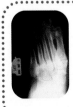 *A 62-year-old woman presents with complaints of right foot pain. She had a right foot fracture after a motor vehicle accident in 1971. She was treated with casting. She describes aching pain of moderate to severe intensity.*

Physical Findings

Musculoskeletal exam commonly reveals a normal gait pattern. There is asymmetry of the feet, with a dorsal exostosis being present at the midfoot on the affected foot.

PATIENT ASSESSMENT

1. Patients usually report pain in the midportion of the foot.

2. Typically, patients will have a normal gait.

3. Weight-bearing x-rays of the foot are needed.

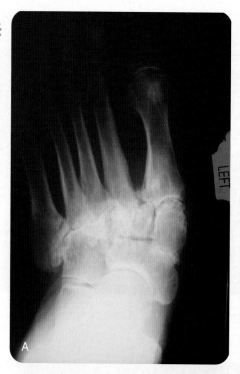
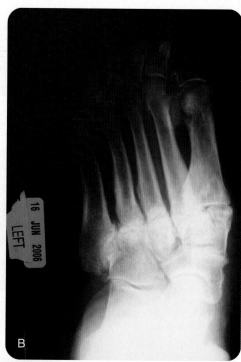
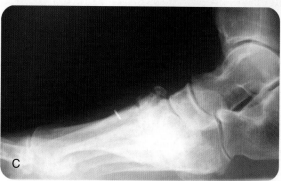

Figure 35.4 Weight-bearing AP **(A)**, oblique **(B)**, and lateral **(C)** views of the left foot demonstrate joint space narrowing and subchondral sclerosis of the second, third, and fourth tarsometatarsal joints.

NOT TO BE MISSED

• Tendon rupture

• Midfoot instability (Lis-Franc injury)

Studies

Weight-bearing x-rays of the foot and ankle are obtained in AP, lateral, and oblique planes. The ankle, subtalar, and midfoot joints are evaluated for pathology (Fig. 35.4).

A CT scan can be used to supplement the x-ray findings. On CT scan, the alignment of the bones and the degree of degenerative changes can be seen more readily and accurately.

Treatment and Clinical Course

1. Treatment depends on the nature and severity of the arthritis.

2. Clearly, the early use of nonoperative treatment consisting of weight reduction, activity modification, and NSAIDs can be helpful.

3. In severe cases, surgical treatment may be necessary.

WHEN TO REFER

- Intractable pain
- Inability to perform activities of daily living
- Subtalar deformity
- Loss of quality of life

Conservative options such as a CAM Walker or short leg-walking cast can be initially tried to decrease the joint inflammation. This can be followed by the use of a stiff, steel shank shoe, a UCBL orthotic, Arizona brace, or MAFO. Medications, such as NSAIDs, can supplement immobilization. Intra-articular corticosteroid-anesthetic injections can be attempted, but it can be difficult to enter an arthritic midfoot joint. Once patients have end-stage osteoarthritis of the midfoot joints, a fusion of the appropriate joint must be entertained. Again, many patients, over time, will continue to have the development of progressive pain. Eventually, these patients will seek surgical interventions to treat the midfoot condition. Selective fusion of the involved joint as determined by a preoperative CT scan is generally successful.

Hallux Rigidus

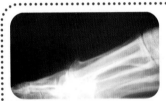

A 65-year-old woman presents with a chief complaint of pain and discomfort at the level of the first MTP joint. She has a history of increasing pain and dorsal spurring of the first MTP joint.

PATIENT ASSESSMENT

1. Pain is noted in the region of first MTP joint, particularly on the dorsum of the foot.

2. On physical examination, there is markedly decreased range of motion of the first MTP as compared with that found in the contralateral foot.

3. Weight-bearing views of the forefoot looking specifically at the first MTP are necessary.

Physical Findings

Most patients present with complaints of loss of mobility of the first toe MTP joint and may even complain of impingement of the dorsal spur against a closed-toe shoe.

Musculoskeletal exam reveals a normal gait pattern. On inspection of both lower extremities, there is no other misalignment, asymmetry, crepitation, defect, or effusions. There is typically tenderness at the level of the symptomatic first MTP joint and an associated large dorsal spur formation.

Examination for range of motion reveals symmetric range of motion of the ankles in dorsiflexion and plantar flexion and subtalar joints in inversion and eversion. Patients typically have negligible motion at the symptomatic first MTP joint with 0 degrees of dorsiflexion and 20 degrees of plantar flexion, as opposed to approximately 15 and 30 degrees on the normal side.

Studies

Weight-bearing views of the right foot are obtained (Fig. 35.5). There are three radiographic stages of hallux rigidus: stage I, with maintenance of joint space and minimal spurring; stage II, with joint space narrowing, subchondral cysts and sclerosis, and some spurring; and stage III, with no joint space, loose bodies, and prominent spurring.

Treatment and Clinical Course

1. Treatment depends on the nature and severity of the arthritis.
2. Use of a wide-toe box shoe can help to improve symptoms.
3. Surgery may be necessary in severe cases.

NOT TO BE MISSED

- Gout
- Early diabetic ulcer
- Turf toe

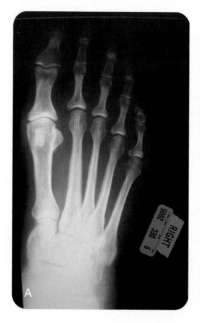

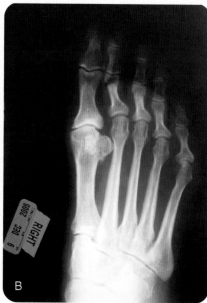

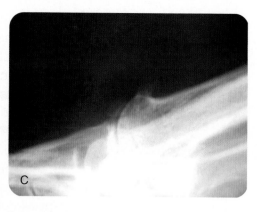

Figure 35.5 Weight-bearing AP **(A)**, oblique **(B)**, and lateral **(C)** views of the right foot demonstrate joint space narrowing, subchondral sclerosis, and dorsal metatarsal osteophyte formation of the first MTP joint.

Conservative considerations for this type of patient include a stiffer-soled shoe. Also, the patient can attempt to wear shoes with wider and larger toe boxes. NSAIDs, intra-articular corticosteroid-anesthetic injections, and glucosamine and chondroitin sulfate are all fairly ineffective in treating this condition. Once patients have end-stage osteoarthritis of the first MTP or debilitating stage I or II hallux rigidus, a fusion of the joint may be considered. For stage I or II hallux rigidus, a cheilectomy (excision of the dorsal spurs and dorsal portion of the metatarsal head) may be utilized. Joint replacement remains controversial, and long-term results have not been favorable.

ICD9

715.17 Osteoarthrosis, localized, primary, involving ankle and foot
715.27 Osteoarthrosis, localized, secondary, involving ankle and foot
715.37 Osteoarthrosis, localized, not specified whether primary or secondary, involving ankle and foot
715.97 Osteoarthrosis, unspecified whether generalized or localized, involving ankle and foot

WHEN TO REFER

- Intractable pain
- Inability to perform activities of daily living
- Loss of quality of life
- Consideration for surgery

References

1. McAlindon TE, LaValley MP, Gulin JP, et al. Glucosamine and chondroitin for treatment of osteoarthritis: a systematic quality assessment and meta-analysis. *JAMA* 2000;283:1469–1475.
2. Reginster JY, Deroisy R, Rovati LC, et al. Long-term effects of glucosamine sulfate on osteoarthritis progression: a randomized, placebo-controlled trial. *Lancet* 2001;357:251–256.
3. Michel BA, Stucki G, Frey D, et al. Chondroitins 4 and 6 sulfate in osteoarthritis of the knee: a randomized, controlled trial. *Arthritis Rheum* 2005;52(3):779–786.
4. Richy F, Bruyere O, Ethgen O, et al. Structural and symptomatic efficacy of glucosamine and chondroitin in knee osteoarthritis: a comprehensive meta-analysis. *Arch Intern Med* 2003;163(13):1514–1522.

36 Third Metatarsal Stress Fracture

Keith Wapner

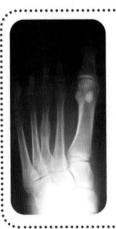

A 41-year-old male overnight package delivery worker presents with a history of pain in his left forefoot. The pain occurs after being on the job for 2 to 3 hours. The patient visited the emergency room approximately 2 weeks ago, where x-rays of the left foot were obtained. The patient states that these x-rays were negative. The patient has been self-medicating with Motrin but has not had any relief with it.

Clinical Presentation

The second and third metatarsals are relatively fixed in position within the foot; the first, fourth, and fifth are relatively mobile. More stress is placed on the second and third metatarsals when ambulating, so these are at increased risk for stress fracture. Patients usually report increased intensity or duration of an exercise regimen. Dull pain occurs initially only with exercise, progressing to pain at rest. Pain is initially diffuse and then localizes to the site of the fracture. Menstrual irregularities should be explored in female patients, due to a high association between female athletics, amenorrhea, and osteoporosis (the "female athletic triad").

Physical Findings

On physical exam, the physician should inspect the foot for swelling, bruising, or warmth. The unaffected foot should always be inspected for a side-by-side comparison. Palpate to find the point of maximal tenderness. Specifically seek to determine if the point of maximal tenderness is related to bony or soft tissue problems.

Studies

Weight-bearing views of the foot are obtained in AP, lateral, and oblique planes (Fig. 36.1). The third metatarsal is carefully examined to see if there are any lesions, cortical breaks, or malalignments. It may take up to 3 to 4 weeks for the x-rays to have any evidence of the stress fractures. For this reason, other modalities, such as MRI or bone scan, can be helpful in making the diagnosis.

CLINICAL POINTS

- The second and third metatarsals are at increased risk.
- Patients usually report increased intensity or duration of an exercise regimen.
- In female patients, menstrual irregularities may be present.

PATIENT ASSESSMENT

1. Dull pain occurs initially with exercise, progressing to pain at rest.
2. Pain is initially diffuse and then localizes to the site of the fracture.
3. On physical examination, seek to determine if the point of maximal tenderness is related to the bone or surrounding soft tissue.
4. X-rays and MRI, in some cases, are indicated.

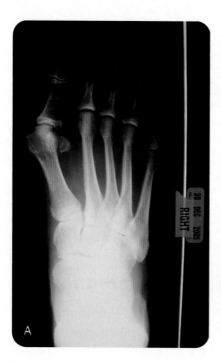

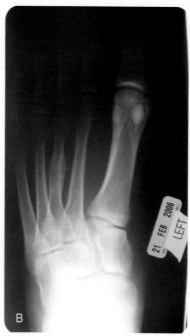

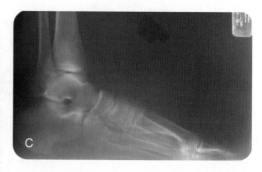

Figure 36.1 Weight-bearing AP **(A)**, oblique **(B)**, and lateral **(C)** views of the left foot demonstrate cortical thickening in the area of the third metatarsal diaphysis.

MRI of the foot is helpful in identifying suspected cases of stress fracture that are not apparent on the radiographs. Cortical defects and bone marrow edema, suggestive of stress fractures, are readily visualized on T2 MRIs (Fig. 36.2).

Bones scans can be used to identify an area of increased metabolic activity in the foot and ankle. This can be suggestive for the stress fracture diagnosis (Fig. 36.3).

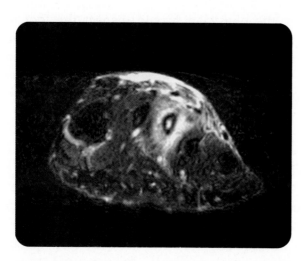

Figure 36.2 T2 coronal MRI demonstrates bone marrow edema in the third metatarsal of this patient. This is indicative of a stress fracture of the third metatarsal.

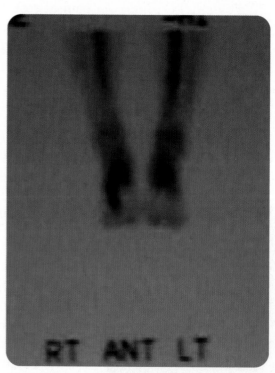

Figure 36.3 A bone scan in this patient demonstrates increased uptake in the area of the third metatarsal. This is consistent with a stress fracture of the third metatarsal.

Treatment and Clinical Course

1. Most stress fractures respond well to activity modification and a short period of immobilization.

2. In severe cases, consideration should be given to the use of a bone stimulator and a workup for osteoporosis.

Suspected stress fractures can be successfully treated with conservative methods. Metatarsal taping, CAM Walkers, and short leg nonweight-bearing casts all aid in stress shielding the metatarsal, allowing time for healing to occur. If weight-bearing activities are restricted, it can take 4 to 6 weeks for the stress fracture to heal. If patients continue to weight bear, however, it may take more than 8 weeks to heal. The majority of patients are treated successfully with conservative methods. At times, stress fractures can be recalcitrant and symptomatic for months. In these cases, a bone stimulator, either ultrasound or pulsed electromagnetic field units, can be attempted to heal the lesion.

ICD9
733.94 Stress fracture of the metatarsals

CHAPTER 37 Fractures of the Fifth Metatarsal

Keith Wapner

There are a variety of fifth metatarsal fractures that have been described. Some of the more common fracture patterns include the "dancer's" fracture (a fracture of the diaphysis), a "Jones" fracture (at the level of the metaphysis–diaphysis), and an avulsion fracture.

Clinical Presentation

The patient with an avulsion fracture experiences the sudden onset of pain at the base of the fifth metatarsal. These fractures occur after forced inversion with the foot and ankle in plantar flexion.

Jones Fracture

A 35-year-old man presents with left foot pain after turning his foot over playing basketball. The pain is localized to the base of the fifth metatarsal.

CLINICAL POINTS

- Sudden pain at the base of the fifth metatarsal is characteristic of an avulsion fracture.

- Forced inversion with the foot and ankle in plantar flexion results in avulsion fractures.

Physical Findings

In a fracture of fifth metatarsal, pain and tenderness are present at the base of fifth metatarsal, along with swelling, ecchymosis, and difficulty in weight bearing. This fracture is sometimes hard to differentiate from an ankle injury because the swelling can be near the region of the lateral malleolus.

Studies

Weight-bearing x-rays of the foot are obtained in AP, lateral, and oblique planes (Fig. 37.1). Fractures that are at the fifth metatarsal, metaphyseal–diaphyseal junction, entering the fourth and fifth metatarsal articulation medially are true Jones fractures.

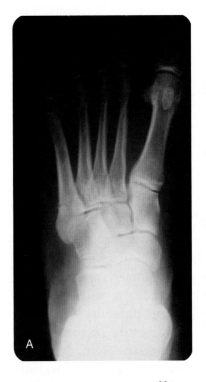
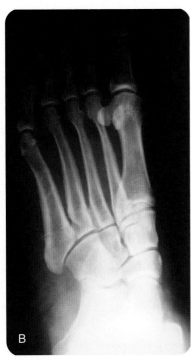
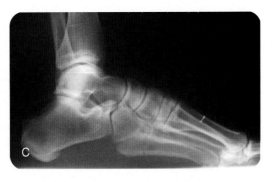

Figure 37.1 Weight-bearing AP **(A)**, oblique **(B)**, and lateral **(C)** views of the left foot demonstrate a Jones fracture, with the fracture exiting laterally in the fourth and fifth metatarsal articulation.

PATIENT ASSESSMENT

1. Patients present with lateral-sided hindfoot pain, typically after an inversion injury.
2. Walking is painful.
3. Weight-bearing x-rays of the foot are necessary.

NOT TO BE MISSED

- Charcot foot
- Tendon rupture

WHEN TO REFER

- At the time of injury

Treatment and Clinical Course

1. Treatment generally consists of a nonweight-bearing cast.
2. Elite athletes and dancers may need operative fixation of this fracture.

The recommended treatment for a Jones fracture depends on patient demographics.

Because of low vascularization and high stresses at this site, Jones fractures are associated with a poor outcome. Nonunions and delayed unions are common, particularly in patients who have received less than optimal treatment. Elite athletes and dancers should be treated surgically with an open reduction and internal fixation to minimize recovery time and lessen the risk of a nonunion. All other patients should be treated conservatively in a nonweight-bearing short leg cast.

Patients treated conservatively can expect to be in a nonweight-bearing short leg cast for approximately 10 to 12 weeks. Nonunion rates are up to 44% in patients treated nonsurgically.[1] Nonunions can be treated with a bone stimulator, either ultrasound or pulsed electromagnetic field units. When this fails, surgical intervention should be considered.

Avulsion Fractures of the Fifth Metatarsal (Pseudo-Jones Fracture)

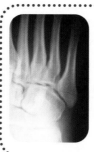

A 24-year-old male dancer presents complaining of a right foot injury. The patient sustained an inversion injury to his right foot a day ago, when he landed on another dancer's foot during rehearsal. The pain is localized to the base of the fifth metatarsal.

Physical Findings

Similar to a Jones fracture, with a pseudo-Jones fracture, there is pain and tenderness present at the base of fifth metatarsal, along with swelling, ecchymosis, and difficulty in weight bearing. This fracture is sometimes hard to differentiate from an ankle injury because the swelling can be near the region of the lateral malleolus.

Studies

Weight-bearing x-rays of the foot are obtained in AP, lateral, and oblique planes (Fig. 37.2). In a pseudo-Jones fracture, there will be a nondisplaced fracture of the fifth metatarsal tuberosity.

Treatment and Clinical Course

1. Treatment generally consists of a weight-bearing cast or orthopaedic boot (CAM Walker).

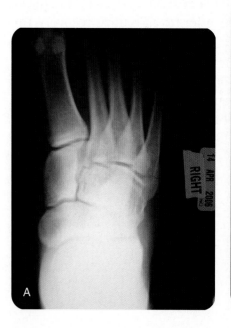

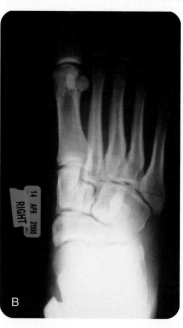

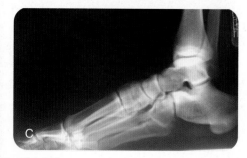

Figure 37.2 Weight-bearing AP **(A)**, oblique **(B)**, and lateral **(C)** views of the right foot demonstrate an avulsion fracture of the base of the fifth metatarsal.

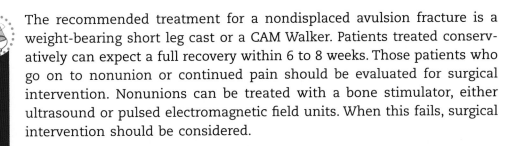

1. Patients present with lateral-sided hindfoot pain, typically after an inversion injury.
2. Walking is painful.
3. Weight-bearing x-rays of the foot are necessary.

NOT TO BE MISSED

- Jones fracture
- Charcot foot

WHEN TO REFER

- Failure to respond to conservative treatment
- Jones fracture

The recommended treatment for a nondisplaced avulsion fracture is a weight-bearing short leg cast or a CAM Walker. Patients treated conservatively can expect a full recovery within 6 to 8 weeks. Those patients who go on to nonunion or continued pain should be evaluated for surgical intervention. Nonunions can be treated with a bone stimulator, either ultrasound or pulsed electromagnetic field units. When this fails, surgical intervention should be considered.

ICD9

825.25 Fracture of metatarsal bone(s), closed
825.35 Fracture of metatarsal bone(s), open

Reference

1. Rubino RL, Miller MD. What's new in sports medicine. *J Bone Joint Surg Am* 2006;88:457–468.

38 Diabetic Foot

Keith Wapner

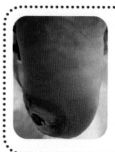

A 58-year-old diabetic male hospital employee presents complaining of pain and swelling of the right foot. His pain has been increased over the past month. He has had unrelenting edema and warmth in the right foot.

CLINICAL POINTS

- Foot ulcers occur in 15% of people with diabetes during their lifetimes.

- The risk of lower extremity amputation (LEA) increases substantially once an ulcer develops.

- Peripheral neuropathy, particularly sensory neuropathy, causes the problem.

Clinical Presentation

Diabetic foot ulcers (DFUs) precede 85% of nontraumatic LEAs. Approximately 3% to 4% of individuals with diabetes currently have foot ulcers or deep infections. During their lifetimes, 15% of diabetics develop foot ulcers. Their risk of LEA increases by a factor of 8 once an ulcer develops.

The etiology of this problem is peripheral neuropathy, which affects sensory, motor, and autonomic pathways. Sensory neuropathy deprives the patient of early warning signs of pain or pressure from footwear, from inadequate soft tissue padding, or from infection. This neuropathy appears in a stocking-glove distribution, with many of these individuals complaining of burning or searing pain. The primary risk factor for the development of DFUs is loss of protective sensation, best measured by insensitivity to the Semmes-Weinstein 5.07 (10 g) monofilament. Abnormal WBC function and the presence of peripheral vascular disease allow wounds to become contaminated and infected by normally nonpathogenic organisms. This explains the identification of unusual bacteria from the wounds of patients with diabetes.

It has been estimated that 2% of people with diabetes develop Charcot joint. This is a condition in which certain joints, most commonly the midfoot, collapse and degenerate. This occurs only in people who have peripheral neuropathy. The earliest stage consists of a red, hot, swollen foot. This is often mistaken for an infection. X-rays will often show severe destruction and erosions of the involved joints. Later stages are without the inflammation but may show either a completely flattened arch or the classical "rocker-bottom" foot.

Physical Findings

How does the clinician determine if there is an active infection? This is usually done by clinical evaluation. For example, redness, swelling, pain, and pus all point to infection. Keep in mind that all ulcers will have some drainage. Since the skin (which is ordinarily a barrier to prevent dehydration) is disrupted, drainage (which is usually watery or blood tinged) will be present. This is in distinction to drainage that is thick, white and creamy, which usually indicates pus and an infection. Also, culture swabs should not be used alone as an indication of infection, because most diabetic ulcers will have bacterial colonization on the surface of the ulcer but do not represent a true infection. Culture swabs are most useful as a means of determining which bacterial organisms are causing an infection once a diagnosis of infection has been made from clinical findings.

Studies

Weight-bearing views of the foot are obtained in AP, lateral, and oblique planes (Fig. 38.1). X-rays are helpful in assessing for associated joint destruction or Charcot joint.

MRI of a Charcot foot may show joint subluxations, marrow edema due to stress reactions, fractures, and soft tissue edema (Fig. 38.2). It is important to differentiate these changes from osteomyelitis. If the bone marrow edema is not associated with an ulcer, it is unlikely that the edema is secondary to osteomyelitis.[1]

CT scans aid in the understanding of the changed bony anatomy of a Charcot lower extremity (Fig. 38.3). The bony structures and relationships can be evaluated and understood more readily with a CT scan.

A three-phase bone scan is helpful is differentiating Charcot foot from osteomyelitis and cellulitis (Fig. 38.4). A negative bone scan rules out bony pathology. If phases 1 and 2 (arteriogram and blood pool phases, respectively) are positive but the third phase is negative, the symptoms are secondary to cellulitis and soft tissue inflammation. If all three phases are bright, bony pathology should be considered. An indium WBC tagged scan can differentiate infection from Charcot changes.

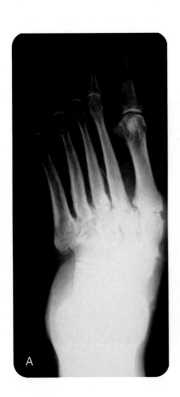

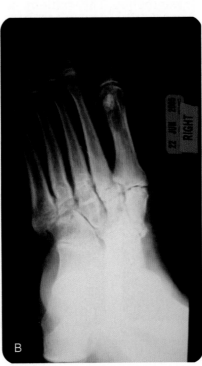

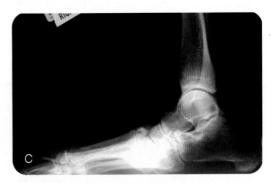

Figure 38.1 Weight-bearing AP **(A)**, oblique **(B)**, and lateral **(C)** views of a typical Charcot joint demonstrates collapse and fragmentation of the midfoot and subluxation of the midtarsal joints.

WHEN TO REFER

- Progressive deformity
- Infection
- Fracture
- Intractable pain

Treatment and Clinical Course

1. Patients with DFUs should be referred to an orthopaedist for consideration of total contact casting, debridement, and/or vascular evaluation.

Treatment for the Charcot patient varies depending on the clinical stage of the patient. In general, when patients present with edema and rubor but no ulcer, a total contact cast can be used to maintain structure and anatomy. This cast should be applied by an orthopaedic surgeon who is experienced in the application of these casts. The cast should be changed at 7- to 10-day intervals, as the edema subsides and the cast loosens. The cast is continued until the edema and warmth resolve. At this point, patients are placed in the appropriate orthotic.

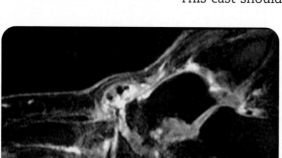

Figure 38.2 T2 sagittal MRI shows areas of bone marrow edema, subluxations, and soft tissue edema.

For patients with ulcers, appropriate wound care is applied routinely. A variety of advanced wound care products are now available, including enzymatic products to aid in debridement, growth factor products to enhance epithelialization and vascularization, antimicrobials, and the vacuum-assisted wound closure system. Occasionally, patients may require admission for surgical debridements.

The Eichenholtz classification system is used to classify the Charcot foot. Stage 1 is the fragmentation stage (acute Charcot). It is characterized by periarticular fracture and joint dislocation, which leads to an unstable, deformed foot. Stage 2 is the coalescence stage (subacute Charcot). Here, patients present with resorption of bone fragments. The consolidation stage (chronic Charcot) is associated with restabilization of the foot with fusion of the involved fragments. The patient will now have a stable but deformed foot.

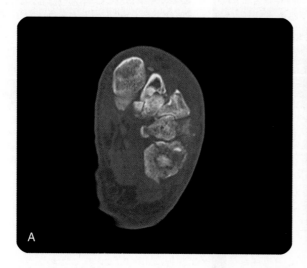
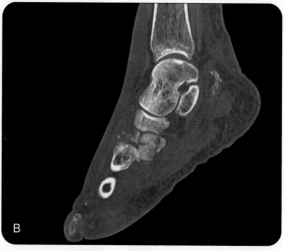

Figure 38.3 Axial **(A)** and sagittal **(B)** CT images clearly demonstrate the subluxation of joints and fragmentation of bone.

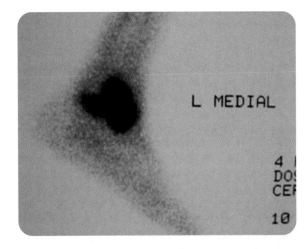

Figure 38.4 A three-phase bone scan in a Charcot ankle.

ICD9

Code Type of Diabetes First:

250.61 Diabetes mellitus with neurological manifestations, type I (juvenile type) not stated as uncontrolled
250.62 Diabetes mellitus with neurological manifestations, type II or unspecified type, uncontrolled
250.81 Diabetes mellitus with other specified manifestations, type I (juvenile type) not stated as uncontrolled
250.82 Diabetes mellitus with other specified manifestations, type II or unspecified type, uncontrolled

Code Type of Diabetic Problem Second:

707.14 Ulcer of heel and midfoot
707.15 Ulcer of other part of foot
357.2 Polyneuropathy in diabetes
713.5 Arthropathy associated with neurological disorders

SECTION 7 Foot

Reference

1. Craig JG, Amin MB, Wu K, et al. Osteomyelitis of the diabetic foot: MR imaging—pathologic correlation. *Radiology* 1997;203(3):849–855.

Shoulder

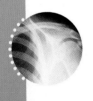
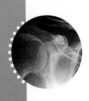

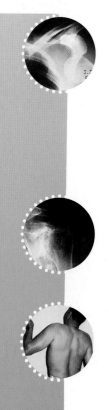

39 Tendinitis/Bursitis/ Subacromial Impingement

Joseph A. Abboud

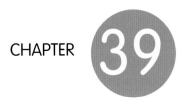

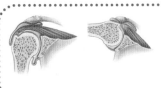

A 43-year-old female tennis player presents with right shoulder pain. She states that she has had the pain for the past 2 months.

CLINICAL POINTS

- Pathology involves inflammation of the bursa between the rotator cuff and the acromion.
- The most common symptom is pain.
- The condition is more common in adults who are >40 years of age.

Clinical Presentation

Subacromial impingement, also known as *rotator cuff tendinitis* or *bursitis*, occurs when the rotator cuff becomes irritated underneath the acromion. The reason why this happens is unclear. Some people are thought to be born with a "hooked" acromion that will predispose them to impingement. Other patients develop impingement due to intrinsic rotator cuff weakness. Because the rotator cuff is a humeral head centralizer, weakness of the cuff will allow it to ride up and impinge on the acromion. The result is inflammation of the bursa between the rotator cuff and the acromion.

The typical patient presents with a recent history of overactivity and onset of moderate to occasionally severe pain with active range of motion of the shoulder.[1] A complete history of the patient is critical in the diagnosis of subacromial impingement syndrome, and it is important to identify predisposing factors, such as participation in sports- or work-related activities, that involve overhead motion. Patients often complain of pain on the top and front of the shoulder. Either way, pain is the most common symptom. Symptoms also include localized tenderness, inflammation, edema, and loss of function. Weakness and stiffness of the shoulder also may occur, but this is usually secondary to pain and not muscle weakness. When the pain is eliminated, the weakness and stiffness generally resolve. If the weakness persists, the patient should be evaluated for a tear of the rotator cuff or a neurologic etiology (i.e., cervical radiculopathy or suprascapular nerve entrapment). If the stiffness persists, the patient may have a frozen shoulder, inflammatory arthritis, or calcific tendinitis.

It is important to establish the position of maximum pain, quality of the pain (dull or severe), timing of the pain (during the day or at night), and association between pain and activity (i.e., the presence or absence of pain during sleep and during movement). Most symptoms of impingement begin gradually and have a chronic component that progresses over several months.[2] Sometimes, the bursitis that occurs with rotator cuff tendinitis can cause a mild popping or cracking sensation in the shoulder that can be annoying to the patient. Finally, it is important to document all treatment modalities attempted, including changes in lifestyle, physical therapy regimens, use of NSAIDs, subacromial injections, and operative procedures on the shoulder.

Impingement syndrome is more common in patients who are >40 years of age. However, in patients who are <40 years, the diagnosis of impingement syndrome must be approached cautiously, as these patients may have subtle glenohumeral instability as the underlying problem.[3] Unfortunately, these two processes cannot be differentiated on the basis of an accurate history alone. However, it is rare that someone <40 years presents with isolated impingement syndrome.

Physical Findings

The physical examination should help in confirming or refuting the initial diagnosis that is made on the basis of the history. A careful examination of the cervical spine should be performed to rule out any abnormalities, including radiculopathy and degenerative joint disease that may cause referred pain in the shoulder. It is important to remember that patients can have problems with their neck and shoulder, and this needs to be further substantiated or refuted on exam. Next, the shoulder is inspected and palpated, and the muscle strength as well as the range of motion is assessed. Range of motion of the shoulder is performed actively and passively and compared with that of the asymptomatic side.[4]

Several tests are helpful in diagnosing impingement syndrome. The impingement sign, as described by Neer (Fig. 39.1), is elicited by standing behind the patient and passively elevating the arm in the scapular plane while stabilizing the scapula.[5]

Pain usually is elicited in the arc between 50 and 130 degrees of forward elevation (Fig. 39.2). The acromiohumeral distance is decreased substantially in this range of motion as the greater tuberosity passes under the acromion. This distance is decreased further by internally rotating the humerus, spur formation, or the presence of an acromial spur (Fig. 39.3). Hawkins and Kennedy modified the maneuver by passively internally rotating the arm after passively elevating the arm to 90 degrees[2] (Fig. 39.4). Remember, it may be difficult to elicit the impingement or Hawkins sign in a patient who has a stiff shoulder that is unable to pass through this range of motion.

The *impingement test* can be a useful adjunct in diagnosing impingement. After sterile injection of 10 mL of lidocaine (Xylocaine) into the subacromial space, the test for the impingement sign is repeated. When the abnormality

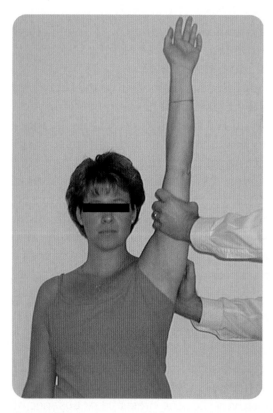

Figure 39.1 Impingement sign is elicited by standing behind the patient and passively elevating the arm in the scapular plane while stabilizing the scapula.

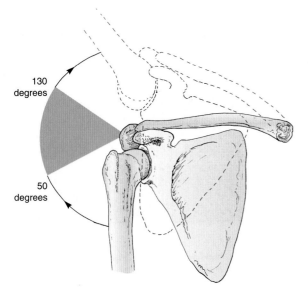

Figure 39.2 With impingement, the painful arc of motion is generally between 50 and 130 degrees of forward elevation. The mid arc range of motion.

is confined to the subacromial space, the injection eliminates the pain in most patients.[4]

Abnormalities of the acromioclavicular joint should be ruled out by direct palpation of the joint, internal rotation of the extended arm, and adduction of the arm across the chest (Fig. 39.5). However, these maneuvers also may cause impingement in the subacromial space and therefore may not be specific for the identification of abnormalities of the acromioclavicular joint. Selective injections into both the acromioclavicular joint and the subacromial bursa can be helpful in identifying the source of symptoms. However, accurate injection into the acromioclavicular joint can be challenging.

It is also important to evaluate the patient for a rupture of the long head of the biceps tendon, which can occur secondary to impingement (Fig. 39.6). This tendon may rupture at the superior aspect of the bicipital groove, just adjacent to the insertion of the supraspinatus tendon. If a patient presents with a rupture of the long head of the biceps tendon and pain in the proximal part of the shoulder, an evaluation should be made for impingement and a possible rotator cuff tear.[2]

So what if the clinician is concerned about impingement with an associated partial-thickness rotator cuff tear or full-thickness rotator cuff tear? With a partial-thickness tear, strength is generally preserved on clinical examination. However, pain inhibition may result in both apparent loss of strength and a decrease in active range of motion in patients with a partially intact cuff. Partial-thickness tears are often associated with pain on testing for the classic Jobe sign (active resistance to shoulder abduction with the shoulder positioned in 90 degrees of abduction) (Fig. 39.7).

Weakness to resisted external rotation with the arm at the side can also be indicative of a rotator cuff tear affecting the posterior cuff (infraspinatus and teres minor) (Fig. 39.8). Discernible weakness (unrelated to

SECTION 8 Shoulder

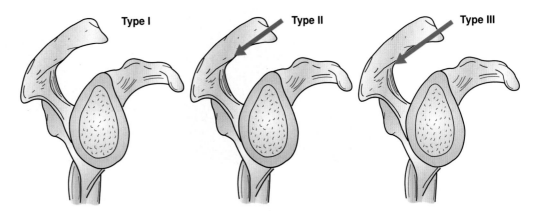

Figure 39.3 Three types of acromion: type I, flat; type II, curved; and type III, hooked. (From Baker CL, Whaley AL, Baker M. Subacromial impingement and full thickness rotator cuff tears in overhead athletes. In: Krishnan SG, Hawkins RJ, Warren RF, eds. *The Shoulder and the Overhead Athlete.* Philadelphia: Lippincott Williams & Wilkins; 2004:150.)

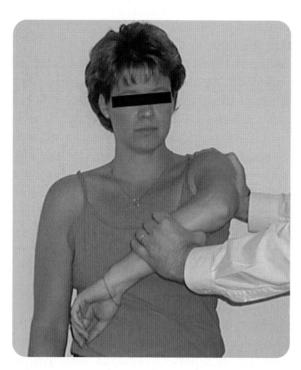

Figure 39.4 Hawkins sign—modification of the Neer sign. This test is performed by placing the arm in 90 degrees of forward flexion, with the elbow flexed 90 degrees. The examiner then passively internally rotates the arm maximally. A positive test is signified by production of pain.

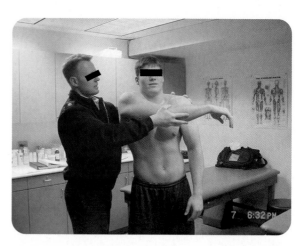

Figure 39.5 This is a cross body adduction maneuver that compresses the acromioclavicular joint. A positive test produces pain on top of the shoulder. (From Tokish JM. Clinical examination of the overhead athlete: the differential directed approach. In: Krishnan SG, Hawkins RJ, Warren RF, eds. *The Shoulder and the Overhead Athlete.* Philadelphia: Lippincott Williams & Wilkins; 2004:33.)

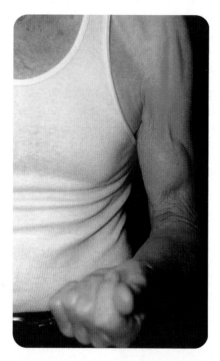

Figure 39.6 Patient with a long history of pain in the shoulder. Rupture of the long head of the biceps is noted as a lump on the anterior lateral aspect of the arm. (From Iannotti JP, Williams GR. *Disorders of the Shoulder: Diagnosis and Management.* Philadelphia: Lippincott Williams & Wilkins; 1999:173.)

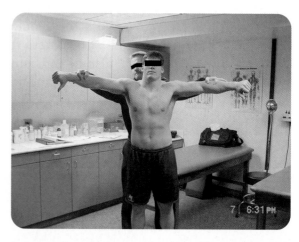

Figure 39.7 Jobe test. This test is performed by placing the patient in 90 degrees of elevation in the scapular plane, classically with the thumb pointed down. The position is held against downward resistance. This test isolates the supraspinatus and is positive when there is asymmetric weakness. Caution should be used in the patient with pain, because pain can simulate weakness in patients with painful subacromial impingement. (From Tokish JM. Clinical examination of the overhead athlete: the differential directed approach. In: Krishnan SG, Hawkins RJ, Warren RF, eds. *The Shoulder and the Overhead Athlete.* Philadelphia: Lippincott Williams & Wilkins; 2004:31.)

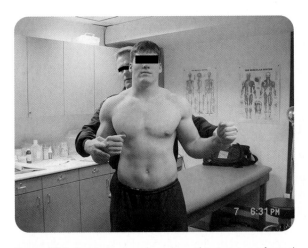

Figure 39.8 Resisted external rotation. This test is performed with the patient's elbows at his or her side and flexed 90 degrees. A positive test is signified by asymmetric weakness. (From Tokish JM. Clinical examination of the overhead athlete: the differential directed approach. In: Krishnan SG, Hawkins RJ, Warren RF, eds. *The Shoulder and the Overhead Athlete.* Philadelphia: Lippincott Williams & Wilkins; 2004:31.)

NOT TO BE MISSED

- Full-thickness rotator cuff tears
- Septic shoulder
- Brachial plexus injury
- Peripheral nerve injury
- Spinoglenoid notch cyst
- Radiculopathy
- Axillary-subclavian venous thrombosis
- Referred pain of cardiac, pulmonary, or visceral origin
- Soft tissue or bone tumor

discomfort) and atrophy of cuff musculature indicate a high likelihood of full-thickness involvement.

As mentioned previously, the diagnosis of impingement in young patients (<40 years of age) should be approached with skepticism. Younger patients who have signs and symptoms of impingement syndrome have been reported extensively in the literature.[2,3,6–8] These patients may have secondary impingement due to subtle glenohumeral instability. Therefore, the apprehension and relocation tests described by Jobe should be performed when examining these patients (Fig. 39.9). The apprehension test is performed first. With the patient in the supine position and the affected shoulder in 90 degrees of abduction, the arm is externally rotated beyond 90 degrees. The test is positive when the patient is apprehensive as the humeral head begins to subluxate anteriorly. Next, the relocation test is performed by directing a posterior force on the proximal humerus, thereby relieving the apprehension by the patient. The examiner must exercise caution in avoiding overaggressive examination, which can result in dislocation in the office.

Studies

LABORATORY

Laboratory studies are generally not helpful in the diagnosis of bursitis/impingement unless there is concern about a septic shoulder.

RADIOGRAPHIC EVALUATION

Routine radiographs are helpful in making the diagnosis of subacromial impingement. AP radiographs may show subchondral cysts or sclerosis of the greater tuberosity with corresponding areas of sclerosis or spur formation on the anterior edge of the acromion (Fig. 39.10). In addition, AP radiographs may help in identifying other abnormalities such as osteoarthritis of the acromioclavicular joint, calcific tendinitis, evidence of glenohumeral instability (an osseous Bankart lesion or a Hill-Sachs lesion), and osteoarthritis of the glenohumeral joint. An axillary radiograph may be needed to diagnose an unfused acromial epiphysis. The subacromial space, however, is best visualized on a supraspinatus outlet view because the clinician is able to avoid the superimposition of the scapular spine and body (Fig. 39.11).

OTHER IMAGING MODALITIES

If the history, physical examination, and radiographs are consistent with subacromial impingement syndrome and an intact rotator cuff, additional imaging studies are not needed. However, if a tear of the rotator cuff is suspected or the patient fails to respond to conservative treatment after 3 months, additional imaging studies may be indicated. The use of MRI

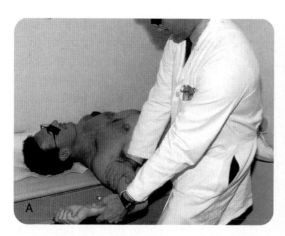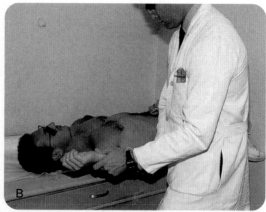

Figure 39.9 A: The apprehension test is performed with the patient supine by stressing the shoulder in maximum abduction and external rotation. The patient may exhibit guarding or other actions that may make the patient or the examiner apprehensive, resulting in a positive test. This is the most reliable clinical test for anterior instability, because it is easy to perform and is very sensitive for producing symptoms in the anteriorly unstable patient. **B:** Relocation test for instability. This test is performed the same way as the apprehension test, except that a positive sign is signified by apprehension or a feeling that the shoulder will come out if further external rotation is applied. Such apprehension should disappear with a posteriorly directed force while holding the arm in external rotation. With this posteriorly directed force, the arm can be moved into further external rotation without discomfort. (From Iannotti JP, Williams GR. *Disorders of the Shoulder: Diagnosis and Management.* Philadelphia: Lippincott Williams & Wilkins; 1999:259.)

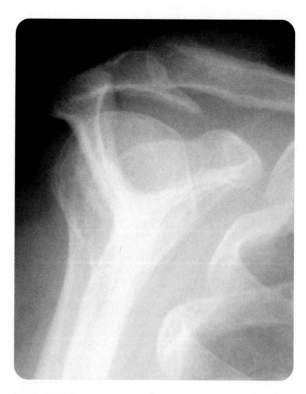

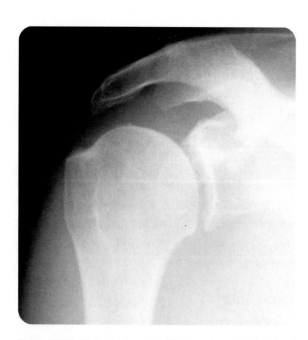

Figure 39.10 AP view shows osteophytes on the lateral border of the acromion. (From Tokish JM. Clinical examination of the overhead athlete: the differential directed approach. In: Krishnan SG, Hawkins RJ, Warren RF, eds. *The Shoulder and the Overhead Athlete.* Philadelphia: Lippincott Williams & Wilkins; 2004:149.)

Figure 39.11 Supraspinatus outlet view shows the shape of the acromion. This patient has a type III acromion because of the osteophyte formation that impinges on the rotator cuff. (From Tokish JM. Clinical examination of the overhead athlete: the differential directed approach. In: Krishnan SG, Hawkins RJ, Warren RF, eds. *The Shoulder and the Overhead Athlete.* Philadelphia: Lippincott Williams & Wilkins; 2004:148.)

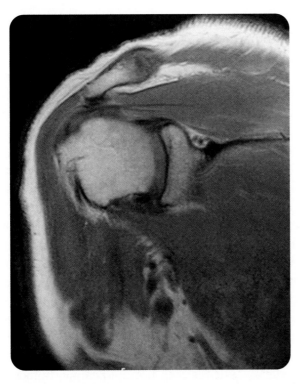

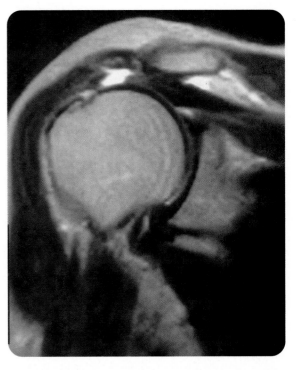

Figure 39.12 T1-weighted MRI showing evidence of an acromial spur and partial-thickness rotator cuff tear involving the supraspinatus tendon.

Figure 39.13 MRI with contrast shows a full-thickness tear of the supraspinatus tendon. (From Tokish JM. Clinical examination of the overhead athlete: the differential directed approach. In: Krishnan SG, Hawkins RJ, Warren RF, eds. *The Shoulder and the Overhead Athlete.* Philadelphia: Lippincott Williams & Wilkins; 2004:150.)

SECTION 8 Shoulder

has increased the ability to diagnose partial tears (Fig. 39.12) and small full-thickness tears (Fig. 39.13).

MRI is also helpful in evaluating the acromioclavicular joint, unfused acromial epiphysis (os acromiale), and lateral acromial morphology. In patients who are unable to undergo MRI, ultrasound is a viable option for further evaluating the rotator cuff. However, this technique is operator dependent, and referral should be made to centers with extensive experience in the use of ultrasound to evaluate the shoulder.

Treatment

1. NSAIDs
2. Subacromial injections with cortisone and/or bupivacaine (Marcaine)
3. Arthroscopy for failure of conservative therapy and impingement

Most patients who have impingement syndrome eventually recover with conservative treatment. The best initial interventional modalities include modification of activity, the use of NSAIDs, consideration of subacromial injections (Fig. 39.14) of steroids, and physical therapy programs. The use of newer arthroscopic procedures to decompress the subacromial space has decreased the morbidity associated with operative treatment. Therefore, a shorter period of nonoperative treatment may be appropriate

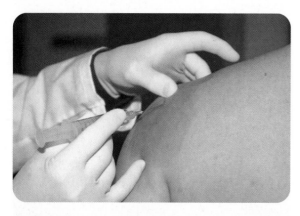

Figure 39.14 Subacromial injection. This injection is performed from the back by using the posterolateral border of the acromion as a landmark. The injection is placed into the subacromial space by advancing the needle directly under the acromion anteriorly and slightly medially. In exceptionally large individuals, the needle must be long enough to reach the anterior one third of the subacromial area, because the pathology exists anteriorly. Alternatively, lateral and anterior injection techniques can be used in injecting the subacromial space. (From Tokish JM. Clinical examination of the overhead athlete: the differential directed approach. In: Krishnan SG, Hawkins RJ, Warren RF, eds. *The Shoulder and the Overhead Athlete*. Philadelphia: Lippincott Williams & Wilkins; 2004:39.)

before operative intervention is attempted. However, a minimum 6-month trial of nonoperative intervention is recommended.

Individuals with suspected partial-thickness rotator cuff tears are treated in the same manner as patients with impingement syndrome. Subacromial bursal inflammation is controlled with activity modification, NSAIDs, and the occasional use of injectable corticosteroids. Physical therapy is advanced as inflammation and pain decrease. Therapy should first be directed at eliminating capsular contractures and regaining full motion. Posterior capsular contracture is addressed by progressive stretching in adduction and internal rotation. As the pain subsides and the stiffness resolves, attention is focused on strengthening the periscapular musculature and rotator cuff.[2] The function of the rotator cuff as a dynamic stabilizer of the humeral head is improved by using a program emphasizing progressive resistive exercises involving the use of elastic bands. Rehabilitation of the periscapular musculature is crucial, as it restores normal scapulothoracic mechanics, which should minimize dynamic impingement secondary to scapulothoracic dyskinesis.[2]

Patients with impingement believed to be secondary to instability are also treated initially with the control of inflammation and pain. Again, attention is focused on rehabilitating the rotator cuff and periscapular muscle groups. Restoration of proper shoulder mechanics is crucial in overhead athletes.

 Refer to Patient Education

 Refer to Physical Therapy

Clinical Course

Most patient with impingement syndrome or small rotator cuff tearing will recover and return to normal function within 6 months. Supervised physical therapy and NSAIDs and/or analgesia are valuable. In time, the symptoms gradually subside. The minority of patients who have persistent or increasing symptoms should be evaluated for possible surgical interventions. However, surgery should be avoided for at least 6 months.

In summary, regardless of the etiology of shoulder impingement, most patients will improve with conservative measures over 6 months, and some continue to improve up to 18 months from initiation of treatment.

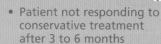

WHEN TO REFER

- Patient not responding to conservative treatment after 3 to 6 months
- Traumatic glenohumeral instability
- Full-thickness rotator cuff tears
- Symptomatic os acromiale
- Spinoglenoid notch cyst (Ganglion cyst of the shoulder)
- Recalcitrant adhesive capsulitis

ICD9

726.2 Other affections of shoulder region, not elsewhere classified
726.10 Disorders of bursae and tendons in shoulder region, unspecified
726.0 Adhesive capsulitis of shoulder

References

1. Bigliani LU, Levine WN. Subacromial impingement syndrome. *J Bone Joint Surg Am* 1997;79:1854–1868.
2. McConville OR, Iannotti JP. Partial-thickness tears of the rotator cuff: evaluation and management. *J Am Acad Orthop Surg* 1999;7:32–43.
3. Baker CL, Whaley AL, Baker M. Subacromial impingement and full thickness rotator cuff tears in overhead athletes. In: Krishnan SG, Hawkins RJ, Warren RF, eds. *The Shoulder and the Overhead Athlete.* Philadelphia: Lippincott Williams & Wilkins; 2004:146–162.
4. Arroyo JS, Flatow EL. Management of rotator cuff disease: intact and repairable cuff. In: Iannotti JP, Williams GR, eds. *Disorders of the Shoulder: Diagnosis and Management.* Philadelphia: Lippincott Williams & Wilkins; 1999:31–56.
5. Tokish JM. Clinical examination of the overhead athlete: the differential directed approach. In: Krishnan SG, Hawkins RJ, Warren RF, eds. *The Shoulder and the Overhead Athlete.* Philadelphia: Lippincott Williams & Wilkins; 2004:23–49.
6. Ellman H. Diagnosis and treatment of incomplete rotator cuff tears. *Clin Orthop Relat Res* 1990;254:64–74.
7. Hawkins RJ, Hobeika PE. Impingement syndrome in the athletic shoulder. *Clin Sports Med* 1983;2:391–405.
8. Post M, Silver R, Singh M. Rotator cuff tear. Diagnosis and treatment. *Clin Orthop Relat Res* 1983;173:78–91.

CHAPTER 40 Calcific Tendinitis

Joseph A. Abboud

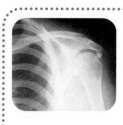

A 52-year-old woman presents with severe shoulder pain without history of trauma or repetitive use. (Figure from Craig EV. Master Techniques in Orthopaedic Surgery: The Shoulder. Philadelphia: Lippincott Williams & Wilkins; 2003.)

Clinical Presentation

Calcifying tendinitis, or calcific tendinopathy of the rotator cuff, is a common disorder of unclear etiology in which multifocal, cell-mediated calcification of a tendon is usually followed by spontaneous resorption (Fig. 40.1). The clinical presentation of calcific tendinitis is variable. Patients may have minimal or no symptoms during the formative phase, while some may have acute symptoms during the resorptive phase.[1,2] The resorptive phase, which occurs later in the cycle of calcifying tendinitis, is commonly characterized by acute symptoms such as pain. However, some patients have deposits that are found incidentally as part of a workup for impingement syndrome.

The pain seen in the resorptive stage is related to the increase in intratendinous pressure from vascular proliferation, influx in inflammatory cells, edema, and swelling. As tendon volume increases, the restrictive dimensions of the subacromial space may lead to additional pressure on the involved tendon and even to secondary impingement. During the acute phase, pain can be intense; patients can also have a sensation of painful catching caused by a localized impingement of the calcified mass on the coracoacromial arch.

Physical Findings

The physical examination should help to confirm or refute the initial diagnosis. A careful examination of the cervical spine should first be performed to rule out any abnormalities; next, the shoulder is inspected and palpated, and the muscle strength as well as the range of motion is assessed. Range of motion of the shoulder is performed actively and passively and compared that of the asymptomatic side.[3] Again, the physical examination characteristics are dependent on the phase of presentation of calcific tendinitis. With the subacute or chronic phase, examination findings often mimic subacromial impingement, with mild decreases in range of motion and a positive impingement sign.

CLINICAL POINTS

- Clinical presentation is variable; the condition may be discovered incidentally.
- An increase in intratendinous pressure leads to pain.
- Pain may be intense during the acute phase.

PATIENT ASSESSMENT

1. Acute onset of pain
2. Pain on motion
3. Well-localized tenderness
4. X-rays may show calcific deposits

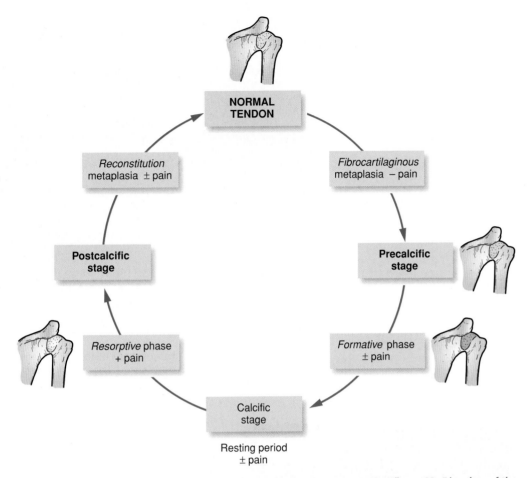

Figure 40.1 Summary of the natural cycle of calcifying tendinitis. (From Iannotti JP, Williams GR. *Disorders of the Shoulder: Diagnosis and Management.* Philadelphia: Lippincott Williams & Wilkins; 1999;132.)

In the chronic phase of calcifying tendinitis, the patient may also present with supraspinatus and infraspinatus atrophy.[1] In this phase, the severe pain leads to guarding against any motion. Even if the patient allows motion, the glenohumeral motion and even the scapulothoracic motion may be severely limited secondary to muscle spasm. Strength testing is prohibited by the pain and can be misleading to the novice examiner. During this phase, provocative tests such as the impingement sign can be nearly impossible to perform due to the significant loss of motion.[1]

Studies (Labs, X-rays)

Laboratory studies are generally not helpful in the diagnosis of calcific tendinitis unless there is concern about a septic shoulder, which should always be part of the differential diagnosis.

RADIOGRAPHIC EVALUATION

Radiographs should be obtained whenever calcification of the cuff is suspected. Radiographic evaluation is also important during follow-up examinations, because it allows the physician to monitor changes in the density and extent of calcification. Initial radiographs should include AP views with

NOT TO BE MISSED

- Septic shoulder
- Acute brachial plexitis (Parsonage-Turner syndrome)
- Full-thickness rotator cuff tears

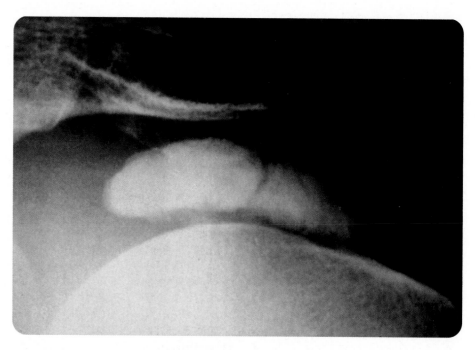

Figure 40.2 A magnified AP radiograph of the shoulder demonstrating calcific tendinitis in the subacromial space involving the supraspinatus tendon. (From Iannotti JP, Williams GR. *Disorders of the Shoulder: Diagnosis and Management.* Philadelphia: Lippincott Williams & Wilkins; 1999:138.)

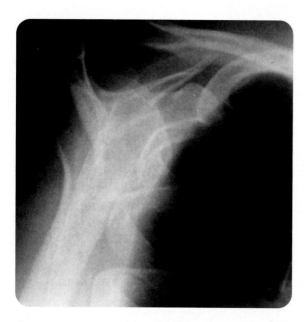

Figure 40.3 A supraspinatus outlet view demonstrating calcium deposition in the supraspinatus tendon (From Iannotti JP, Williams GR. *Disorders of the Shoulder: Diagnosis and Management.* Philadelphia: Lippincott Williams & Wilkins; 1999:137.)

the shoulder in neutral position, internal rotation, and external rotation. Deposits in the supraspinatus are usually visible on films obtained in neutral rotation (Fig. 40.2), whereas deposits in the infraspinatus and teres minor are best visualized on internal rotation films. Although calcifications in the subscapularis rarely occur, a radiograph obtained in external rotation can be obtained to rule them out. The author also recommends an axillary radiograph as part of the radiologic workup. Finally, the supraspinatus outlet view (Fig. 40.3) can help to determine whether a calcification is causing impingement.[1,2]

Calcium deposits are often barely visible on radiographs; MRI may be necessary in rare circumstances. Plain films are usually adequate to make the diagnosis of calcific tendinitis when the rotator cuff is intact; however, MRI is recommended if a tear of the rotator cuff is suspected. On T1-weighted images, calcifications appear as areas of decreased signal intensity; T2-weighted images frequently show a focal band of increased signal intensity compatible with edema.[4]

Treatment

1. NSAIDs
2. Intrabursal injection of cortisone
3. Surgical removal of calcium if patient fails to respond to conservative care

There have been a variety of treatment methods proposed for calcific tendinitis, all of which have had some success. Nonoperative treatment is nearly always the first line of treatment; the treatment protocol is similar to that for rotator cuff tendinitis and generally includes physical therapy, NSAIDs, and steroid injections. Although these modalities individually have not been shown to be critical in resolving the symptoms of calcific tendinitis, combination therapy appears to provide good treatment success rates. Although the calcific deposit will often remain, the symptoms usually resolve nicely.

The patient with calcific tendinitis should be started on a daily exercise program to avoid loss of mobility of the glenohumeral joint and should keep the arm in abduction as much as possible. This can be done by putting a pillow or small beach ball in between the patient's side and the elbow. The application of heat and the use of ultrasound can be beneficial, although there is no evidence that these methods accelerate the disappearance of calcium deposits. Intrabursal injection of corticosteroids can be beneficial during the formative phase of calcific tendinitis; needling of the dense deposits, while described in the literature, has never been attempted by the author's group.

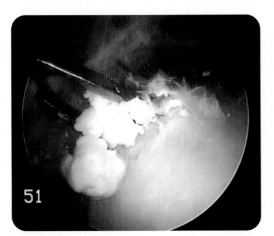

Figure 40.4 A small arthroscopic grabber is used to remove calcium deposition in the rotator cuff. (From Craig EV. *Master Techniques in Orthopaedic Surgery: The Shoulder.* Philadelphia: Lippincott Williams & Wilkins; 2003:187.)

Extracorporeal shock wave therapy has recently been used to treat calcific deposits. However, this technique is still under investigation, and longer follow-up studies and reports from other centers are needed before it can be recommended.

Surgery is recommended in the following situations: when symptoms continue to progress despite treatment, the pain interferes with activities of daily living, and when symptoms do not respond to conservative care over a period of 3 to 6 months.

SECTION 8 Shoulder

Refer to Physical Therapy

WHEN TO REFER

- Patient not responding to conservative treatment after 3 to 6 months
- Patient developing recalcitrant adhesive capsulitis

Clinical Course

Nonoperative treatment is successful in approximately 80% of patients. When surgery is indicated, good results are achieved in 85% to 90% of patients after arthroscopic excision (Fig. 40.4).

> **ICD9**
> *726.11 Calcifying tendinitis of shoulder*

References

1. Hennigan SP, Romeo AA. Calcifying tendonitis. In: Iannotti JP, Williams GR, eds. *Disorders of the Shoulder: Diagnosis and Management.* Philadelphia: Lippincott Williams & Wilkins; 1999:129–157.

2. Uhthoff HK, Loehr JW. Calcific tendinopathy of the rotator cuff: pathogenesis, diagnosis, and management. *J Am Acad Orthop Surg* 1997;5:183–191.

3. Arroyo JS, Flatow EL. Management of rotator cuff disease: intact and repairable cuff. In: Iannotti JP, Williams GR, eds. *Disorders of the Shoulder: Diagnosis and Management*. Philadelphia: Lippincott Williams & Wilkins; 1999:31–56.

4. Kneeland JB. Magnetic resonance imaging: general principles and techniques. In: Iannotti JP, Williams GR, eds. *Disorders of the Shoulder: Diagnosis and Management*. Philadelphia: Lippincott Williams & Wilkins; 1999:911–925.

41 Acromioclavicular Joint Arthritis

Joseph A. Abboud

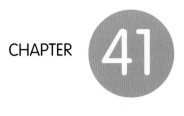

A 47-year-old male laborer presents with gradually worsening activity-related shoulder pain. (Figure from Shaffer BS. Painful conditions of the acromioclavicular joint. J Am Acad Orthop Surg 1998;7:179.)

CLINICAL POINTS

- Shoulder pain is a common symptom.
- Shoulder movement, especially in a horizontal direction, aggravates the pain.
- Typical complaints include inability to sleep on the affected side.

PATIENT ASSESSMENT

1. Localized pain and swelling over the AC joint
2. Pain on cross body adduction
3. Pain on vigorous physical activity, like push ups
4. X-rays show degenerative changes on AC joint

Clinical Presentation

Osteoarthritis of the acromioclavicular (AC) joint is a common source of shoulder pain that is often neglected by physicians. Patients typically present with shoulder pain that unfortunately is not well localized to the AC joint; there is usually a dull ache involving the deltoid area that is exacerbated by motion.[1] Although most planes of motion will cause the patient pain, horizontal cross body adduction (such as occurs when reaching over the front of the body) will tend to be the most symptom provoking. Patients will also often complain of an inability to sleep on the affected side; this vague description of pain is likely due to irritation of the underlying subacromial bursa by inferior-projecting osteophytes from the AC joint.[2]

Physical Findings

The clinical presentation of AC osteoarthritis can be deceiving even to experienced physicians. A careful examination of the cervical spine should be performed to rule out any abnormalities, including radiculopathy and degenerative joint disease that may cause referred pain in the shoulder. The shoulder is inspected and palpated, and the muscle strength as well as the range of motion is assessed. Range of motion of the shoulder is performed actively and passively and compared with that of the asymptomatic side.[3] This may reveal joint prominence or asymmetry.

Range of motion tends to vary greatly, as there may be coexisting rotator cuff or capsule pathology. In addition, when AC osteoarthritis has been symptomatic for a prolonged period of time, adhesive capsulitis may set in. Overall, most patients should have nearly full but painful passive range of motion. It is common for a painful arc in a range greater than that associated with rotator cuff impingement to be present (i.e., pain in the 120- to 180-degree vs. 60- to 120-degree range).[1]

Pain is usually reliably reproduced with passive horizontal cross body adduction at 90 degrees of forward flexion. While the patient is in a sitting

SECTION 8 Shoulder

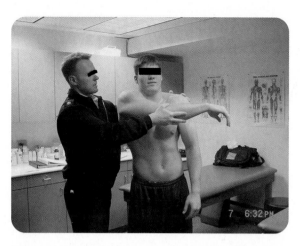

Figure 41.1 AC compression test. This is a cross body adduction maneuver that compresses the AC joint. A positive test produces pain on the top of the shoulder. (From Tokish JM. Clinical examination of the overhead athlete: the differential directed approach. In: Krishnan SG, Hawkins RJ, Warren RF, eds. *The Shoulder and the Overhead Athlete*. Philadelphia: Lippincott Williams & Wilkins; 2004:33.)

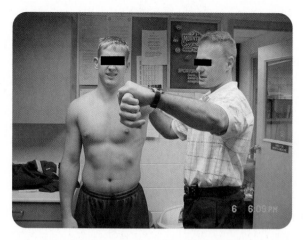

Figure 41.2 Active compression test (O'Brien test). This test is performed by having the patient place his or her arm forward flexed to 90 degrees with 10 degrees of horizontal adduction and internal rotation (thumb down). A positive test is signified by pain on top of the shoulder when the arm is pushed in a downward direction, which is lessened when the test is repeated with the arm in external rotation (thumb up). (From Tokish JM. Clinical examination of the overhead athlete: the differential directed approach. In: Krishnan SG, Hawkins RJ, Warren RF, eds. *The Shoulder and the Overhead Athlete*. Philadelphia: Lippincott Williams & Wilkins; 2004:33.)

position, the examiner passively forward flexes the arm to 90 degrees and then horizontally adducts the arm as far as possible. A positive test results in localized pain over the AC joint (Fig. 41.1) and is fairly specific for AC joint pathology.[4] In addition, direct manual pressure by the examiner on the superior surface of the AC joint should reproduce the patient's symptoms. A significant difference should be noted between the injured and noninjured sides.

The active compression test of O'Brien assists in excluding labral (SLAP [superior labral anterior posterior]) pathology as a possible pain generator (Fig. 41.2); the patient forward flexes the arm to 90 degrees with the elbow fully extended and adducted 15 degrees medial to the midline of the body with the thumb pointed downward. The examiner then applies a downward force to the arm while the patient resists. In the next position, the test is repeated with the arm in the same position, but the patient fully supinates with the palm facing the ceiling. If pain is produced in the first position and is reduced or eliminated in the second, a superior labral injury is favored over AC joint pathology.[4]

Studies (Labs, X-rays)

Laboratory studies are generally not helpful in the diagnosis of AC joint arthritis.

RADIOGRAPHIC EVALUATION

Although various imaging techniques have been utilized to study the AC joint, plain radiographs are still the most appropriate initial choice. Depending on the disease stage, AP radiographs may show degenerative

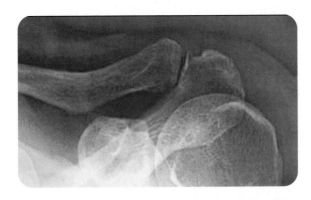

Figure 41.3 The Zanca view of the AC joint is obtained by angling the x-ray beam 10 to 15 degrees in the cephalic direction and decreasing the kilovoltage. This Zanca view better depicts the soft tissue and joint detail of the AC joint; however, the glenohumeral joint is no longer well visualized. (From Shaffer BS. Painful conditions of the acromioclavicular joint. *J Am Acad Orthop Surg* 1998;7:179.)

changes including subchondral cysts, sclerosis, osteophytes, and joint space narrowing. However, be careful to jump to this diagnosis based on radiographic findings alone, as many patients will have radiographic findings of AC arthritis without any objective physical exam findings to support the diagnosis. The Zanca view is particularly helpful in evaluating AC joint pathology[1] (Fig. 41.3).

If the differential diagnosis includes an os acromiale, an axial view of the shoulder should be completed. MRI, with its outstanding soft tissue resolution, can detect capsular hypertrophy, effusions, inferior osteophyte formation off of the distal clavicle, subchondral edema, and an os acromiale (Fig. 41.4). Although ultrasound is very sensitive for detecting the presence of joint inflammation, it is an operator-dependent diagnostic procedure that is rarely utilized in the evaluation of AC joint injuries or osteoarthritis. A bone scan should be considered in the patient with equivocal MRI findings and a confusing clinical picture[5] (Fig. 41.5).

OTHER DIAGNOSTIC MODALITIES

If after a thorough history and physical exam the AC joint is thought to be the cause of the patient's symptoms, an injection of a local anesthetic with steroids could prove both diagnostic and therapeutic. Although the AC joint is superficial, it can be very difficult to localize for injection, as there is significant variability in its orientation (Fig. 41.6). For these reasons, many clinicians prefer fluoroscopic guidance to improve accuracy (fluoroscopy, however, is not a practical option for most practitioners in the office). Within minutes of a successful injection, most patients with a

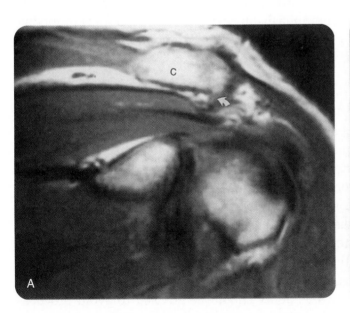
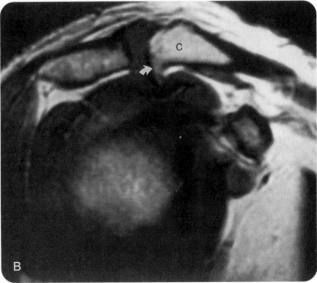

Figure 41.4 Oblique coronal **(A)** and oblique sagittal **(B)** images of the AC joint demonstrate a large spur (*white arrows*) on the undersurface of the distal clavicle. (C, clavicle.) (From Iannotti JP, Williams GR. *Disorders of the Shoulder: Diagnosis and Management.* Philadelphia: Lippincott Williams & Wilkins; 2006:915.)

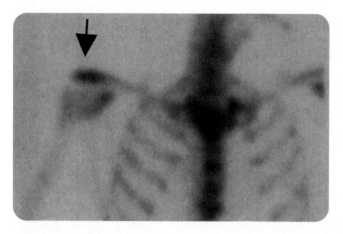

Figure 41.5 A bone scan usually demonstrates increased activity in the AC joint when a patient has symptomatic AC joint arthritis. (From Snyder S. *Shoulder Arthroscopy,* 2nd ed. Philadelphia: Lippincott William & Wilkins; 2002:209.)

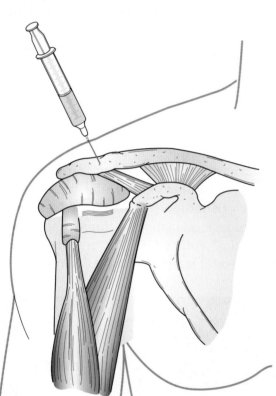

Figure 41.6 Direct injection into the AC joint through a superior approach. (From Shaffer BS. Painful conditions of the acromio-clavicular joint. *J Am Acad Orthop Surg* 1998;7:181.)

painful AC joint will experience a significant reduction in their pain. Continuation of symptoms after the injection suggests an additional diagnosis or an alternative diagnosis, the most common of which is rotator cuff impingement. In this situation, a second injection directed into the subacromial space may clarify the contribution of the rotator cuff to the patient's symptoms.[1]

Treatment

1. NSAIDs
2. Intra-articular injection of cortisone
3. Surgical excision of joint if pain persists

Unfortunately, treatment options for AC joint osteoarthritis are limited. Initial treatment is similar to that of osteoarthritis in other joints and include NSAIDs and an emphasis on activity modification. The patient should be reminded to avoid repetitive motions that exacerbate symptoms. Activity modification usually requires a change in the exercise routine for patients involved in a physical fitness program. Exercises to be avoided are push-ups, dips, flies, and bench presses. Physical therapy, unfortunately, has little to offer because therapeutic exercise and range of motion play only a minor role.[1] Appropriate treatment includes a stretching program designed to maintain active range of motion and strengthening in a painfree range of motion, with an emphasis on scapular stabilization. Pain modalities such as iontophoresis or phonophoresis may offer some benefit.

INTRA-ARTICULAR CORTICOSTEROIDS

If a diagnostic local anesthetic injection provides relief, the practitioner may want to consider therapeutic corticosteroid injections for the patient. Although there is no consensus regarding dosage, 10 to 20 mg of methylprednisolone may be injected by using the same techniques described previously. Current practice patterns limit intra-articular steroid injections to four per year,[2] and clinicians should be aware that the possible side effects of corticosteroid injections include skin blanching, localized fat atrophy, infection, and transient hyperglycemia in diabetics. Patients should be advised to avoid provocative activities for 2 to 3 days after the injection; pain relief can last up to several months.

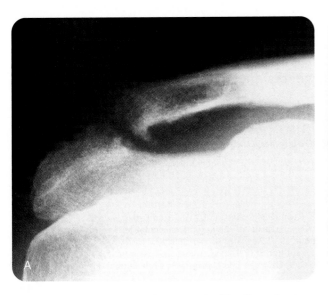
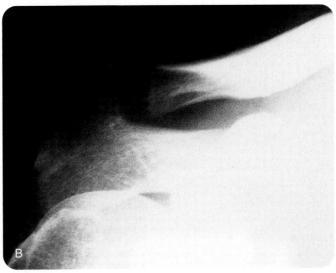

Figure 41.7 Preoperative **(A)** and postoperative **(B)** radiographs of a successful arthroscopic distal clavicle resection. (From Craig EV. *Master Techniques in Orthopaedic Surgery*, 2nd ed. Philadelphia: Lippincott Williams & Wilkins; 2003:32.)

SURGICAL INTERVENTION

If conservative measures fail to provide adequate pain relief and/or if the AC joint pathology is interfering with activities of daily living, surgical referral is recommended. As with any surgical referral, there is some debate regarding the duration of conservative treatment before surgical management. Multiple variables should be considered, including occupation, age, degree of activity restriction, shoulder dominance, and patient goals. Many authors feel that a minimum of 6 months of conservative treatment is warranted prior to entertaining surgery.[1] The decision to proceed with surgical intervention should be made by the patient and physician together after an appropriate attempt at conservative treatment has not produced an adequate alleviation of symptoms. Surgical options consist of open or arthroscopic distal clavicle resection (Fig. 41.7).

 Refer to Physical Therapy

WHEN TO REFER

- Patient not responding to conservative treatment after 3 to 6 months
- Glenohumeral instability
- Full-thickness rotator cuff tears
- Rheumatoid arthritis
- Symptomatic os acromiale
- Spinoglenoid notch cyst (Ganglion cyst of the shoulder)
- Recalcitrant adhesive capsulitis

Clinical Course

The clinical course of patients with AC joint arthritis is similar to other joints with osteoarthritis. The arthritis gradually becomes more severe, symptoms are usually intermittent, and it usually takes decades for them to become very severe. The symptoms will depend on activity. Surgical alternatives are satisfactory but should be reserved for patients failing conservative therapy for a prolonged period of time and have significant structural changes within the joint.

In conclusion, osteoarthritis of the AC joint is a commonly encountered yet often overlooked cause of shoulder pain. Although there are not an abundance of treatment options at this time, proper diagnosis and management may prevent further complications, including inappropriate management, worsening limitations in range of motion, and impaired function. Proper diagnosis may also limit costly diagnostic procedures and treatments when other diagnoses are being improperly considered.

> ### ICD9
> *716.91 Unspecified arthropathy involving shoulder region*

References

1. Shaffer BS. Painful conditions of the acromioclavicular joint. *J Am Acad Orthop Surg* 1998;7:176–188.
2. Buttaci CJ, Stitik TP, Yonclas PP, et al. Osteoarthritis of the acromioclavicular joint: a review of anatomy, biomechanics, diagnosis, and treatment. *Am J Phys Med Rehabil* 2004;83:791–797.
3. Arroyo JS, Flatow EL. Management of rotator cuff disease: intact and repairable cuff. In: Iannotti JP, Williams GR, eds. *Disorders of the Shoulder: Diagnosis and Management*. Philadelphia: Lippincott Williams & Wilkins; 1999:31–56.
4. Tokish JM. Clinical examination of the overhead athlete: the differential directed approach. In: Krishnan SG, Hawkins RJ, Warren RF, eds. *The Shoulder and the Overhead Athlete*. Philadelphia: Lippincott Williams & Wilkins; 2004:23–49.
5. Kneeland JB. Magnetic resonance imaging: general principles and techniques. In: Iannotti JP, Williams GR, eds. *Disorders of the Shoulder: Diagnosis and Management*. Philadelphia: Lippincott Williams & Wilkins: 1999:911–925.

42 Rotator Cuff Tear

Joseph A. Abboud

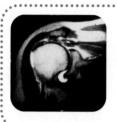

A 58-year-old man presents with shoulder pain, difficulty sleeping, and decreased strength and range of motion with attempted overhead activities.

CLINICAL POINTS

- The condition is much more frequently seen in older patients.

- Pain is the most common symptom.

- A complete tear may result in an inability to move the shoulder.

Clinical Presentation

Rotator cuff injuries are seen both in the young and old, but they are much more common in the older population. In younger patients, there usually is either a traumatic injury or the patient is demanding unusual use of the shoulder, as seen in professional baseball pitchers. As people age, the muscle and tendon tissue of the rotator cuff loses some elasticity, becomes more susceptible to injuries, and is often damaged while performing everyday activities. This is the reason that rotator cuff tears are more commonly seen in older patients.[1–5]

The most common symptom of a rotator cuff tear is pain. Often, the pain is felt over the outside of the shoulder and upper arm in the deltoid region. Patients will describe it as a generalized discomfort that is exacerbated with specific movements of the shoulder. Depending on the severity of the rotator cuff tear, there may also be a loss of motion. The patient also may complain of crepitus, catching, and stiffness.

If the injury is an incomplete tear, pain will likely be the most prominent symptom; decreased strength may be demonstrated but is usually not the patient's primary complaint. However, in a complete rotator cuff tear, the patient will likely be unable to move the shoulder through some normal motions. The diagnosis of a rotator cuff tear is best made by a physical examination where the specific muscles that form the rotator cuff can be isolated and tested.

PATIENT ASSESSMENT

1. Painful shoulder in older patients

2. May occur after trauma

3. Persistent weakness and inability to abduct or hold shoulder in abduction

4. MRI showing rotator cuff tear

Physical Findings

Approach the shoulder examination systematically in every patient with inspection, palpation, range of motion, strength testing, neurologic assessment, and performances of special shoulder tests. Also, include evaluation of the cervical spine and distal portions of the upper extremity. Inspect for scars, color, edema, deformities, muscle atrophy, and asymmetry. Palpate the bony and soft tissue structures, noting any areas of tenderness. Assess

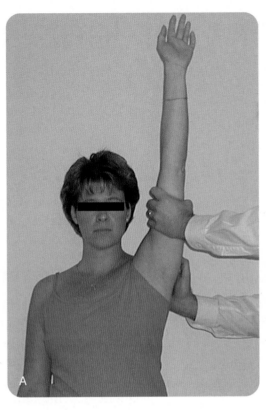
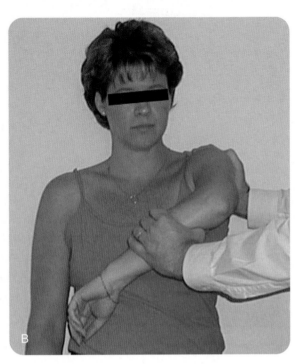

Figure 42.1 A: The Neer impingement sign is elicited by standing behind the patient and passively elevating the arm in the scapular plane while stabilizing the scapula. A positive test generally elicits pain in the 50- to 130-degree range of forward elevation. **B:** Hawkins sign—modification of the Neer sign. This test is performed by placing the arm in 90 degrees of forward flexion, with the elbow flexed 90 degrees. The examiner then passively internally rotates the arm maximally. A positive test is signified by production of pain.

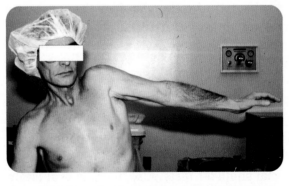

Figure 42.2 This patient is attempting to abduct his left arm. Notice how the shoulder is shrugged and the trunk is leaning to the right. This is a mechanism of compensation used by patients with rotator cuff tears to make up for a lack of rotator cuff strength with attempted abduction of the arm.

active and passive range of motion. Note any pain elicited and loss of motion.[1,2]

If a rotator cuff tear or subacromial impingement is suspected, then focus the examination and perform specific tests to reproduce the patient's symptoms. Patients with subacromial impingement have reproducible pain with the Neer and Hawkins tests (Fig. 42.1). Both of these tests bring the greater tuberosity, the biceps tendon, and the rotator cuff under the coracoacromial arch and reproduce painful symptoms.[2,6]

Patients with full-thickness tears of the rotator cuff may exhibit weakness during testing of the particular muscle involved, may have a difference between active and passive range of motion of the shoulder, and may have atrophy of the muscles involved if it is a chronic tear. During range-of-motion testing, patients will often initially shrug their affected shoulder when attempting to abduct their arms if a cuff tear is present, because they are using scapulothoracic motion to compensate for the inability of the cuff to abduct the arm[2] (Fig. 42.2).

Pain and weakness with the active compression test indicates weakness of the supraspinatus[2] (Fig. 42.3).

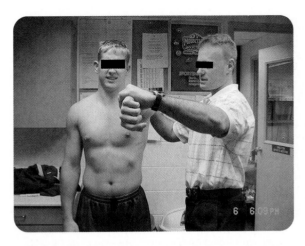

Figure 42.3 Active compression test (O'Brien test). This test is performed by having the patient place his or her arm forward, flexed to 90 degrees with 10 degrees of horizontal adduction and internal rotation (thumb down). A positive test is signified by pain on top of the shoulder when the arm is pushed in a downward direction, which is lessened when the test is repeated with the arm in external rotation (thumb up). Patients may also note weakness with this test as compared with that on the normal side. (From Tokish JM. Clinical examination of the overhead athlete: the differential directed approach. In: Krishnan SG, Hawkins RJ, Warren RF, eds. *The Shoulder and the Overhead Athlete*. Philadelphia: Lippincott Williams & Wilkins; 2004:33.)

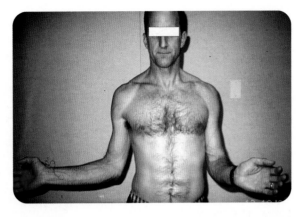

Figure 42.4 This patient demonstrates weakness with external rotation on his left side as compared with the right. Note that the patient is barely able to externally rotate past neutral on the left, while on the right he can actively externally rotate to approximately 45 degrees. This should lead the clinician to suspect a tear of the posterior rotator cuff.

Weakness or rupture of the external rotators of the shoulder should also be tested during the physical examination. Persons with large or massive cuff tears involving multiple tendons are often unable to actively externally rotate their arms[1–3,7] (Fig. 42.4).

Another way of testing the integrity of the external rotators is to place the arm at the side of the patient with the elbow bent to 90 degrees and the arm passively externally rotated; once the arm is released, it drifts back into internal rotation because of the unopposed action of the subscapularis (external rotation lag sign) (Fig. 42.5).

Similarly, the inability to actively externally rotate the abducted arm has been termed the *hornblower's sign* (Fig. 42.6).

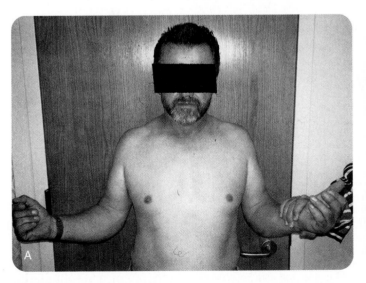

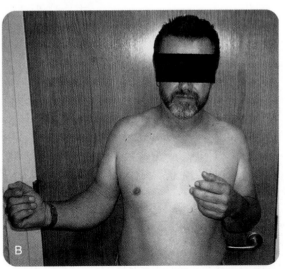

Figure 42.5 A: This patient, with a massive tear involving the posterior rotator cuff, can be passively externally rotated. **B:** When the arm is let go, it falls back into internal rotation, demonstrating severe weakness. (From Iannotti JP, Williams GR, eds. *Disorders of the Shoulder: Diagnosis and Management*. Philadelphia: Lippincott Williams & Wilkins; 2006:33.)

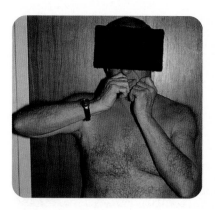

Figure 42.6 Hornblower's sign. In this patient, notice that the right arm must be elevated higher than the left to reach the mouth since active external rotation is impaired. (From Iannotti JP, Williams GR, eds. *Disorders of the Shoulder: Diagnosis and Management*. Philadelphia: Lippincott Williams & Wilkins; 2006:33.)

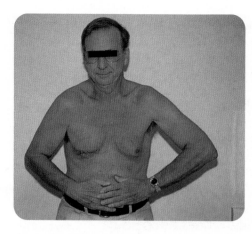

Figure 42.7 Positive abdominal compression test. The right elbow falls back when the patient tries to compress his abdomen. Notice that the left side is normal. (From Iannotti JP, Williams GR, eds. *Disorders of the Shoulder: Diagnosis and Management*. Philadelphia: Lippincott Williams & Wilkins; 2006:34.)

One test that is specifically used to identify weakness of the subscapularis tendon is the belly-press test, also called the *abdominal compression test* (Fig. 42.7). The test assesses the strength of internal rotation by having the patient place the hand of the affected side on the abdomen and then pressing the hand against the abdomen with the elbows in front of the torso. If the subscapularis is not intact, the patient cannot press against the abdomen and the elbow drops behind the torso.[2,8]

If there is a question as to the integrity of the rotator cuff with subacromial impingement, the author routinely injects the subacromial bursa with lidocaine, and after several minutes, the strength of the rotator cuff musculature is retested (Fig. 42.8). If the pain is no longer present but weakness persists, the diagnosis of compromised cuff integrity can be made with greater certainty.

Studies (Labs, X-rays)

Laboratory studies are generally not helpful in the diagnosis of rotator cuff tears unless there is concern about a septic shoulder.

RADIOGRAPHIC EVALUATION

Plain radiographs are used to determine the bony morphology of the acromion and to evaluate the position of the humeral head relative to the glenoid fossa and acromion. The author recommends three radiographic views of the involved shoulder in patients with suspected rotator cuff injury. The first is an AP view of the glenohumeral joint (Fig. 42.9). This view allows the clinician to examine the glenohumeral joint for

NOT TO BE MISSED

- Septic shoulder
- Brachial plexus injury
- Avascular necrosis of the humeral head
- Acromioclavicular separation
- Gout
- Calcific tendinitis
- Adhesive capsulitis
- Neurologic injuries (C5-C6) caused by repetitive trauma
- Spinoglenoid notch cyst (Ganglion cyst of the shoulder)

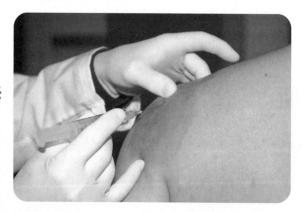

Figure 42.8 Subacromial injection. This injection is performed from the back by using the posterolateral border of the acromion as a landmark. The injection is placed into the subacromial space by advancing the needle directly under the acromion anteriorly and slightly medially. In exceptionally large individuals, the needle must be long enough to reach the anterior one third of the subacromial area because the pathology exists anteriorly. Alternatively, lateral and anterior injections techniques can be used in injecting the subacromial space. (From Tokish JM. Clinical examination of the overhead athlete: the differential directed approach. In: Krishnan SG, Hawkins RJ, Warren RF, eds. *The Shoulder and the Overhead Athlete*. Philadelphia: Lippincott Williams & Wilkins; 2004:39.)

- Referred pain of cardiac, pulmonary, or visceral origin
- Soft tissue or bone tumor
- Symptomatic os acromiale

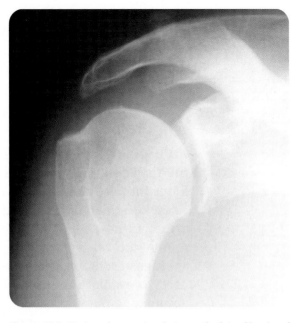

Figure 42.9 AP view shows osteophytes on the lateral border of the acromion. (From Tokish JM. Clinical examination of the overhead athlete: the differential directed approach. In: Krishnan SG, Hawkins RJ, Warren RF, eds. *The Shoulder and the Overhead Athlete*. Philadelphia: Lippincott Williams & Wilkins; 2004:149.)

evidence of degenerative disease. As well, the clinician can examine the acromioclavicular joint and assess the acromion for undersurface spur formation or degenerative changes.[1,2]

Normally, the space available for the cuff tendons between the humeral head and the acromion is estimated to be between 7 and 14 mm. With a space <7 mm, there is an increased likelihood of a large rotator cuff tear and a poorer prognosis (Fig. 42.10).

The second view is the axillary radiograph. Not only does this particular view allow verification that the shoulder is not dislocated, but it also is used to examine the glenoid and humerus. This view is also used to make the diagnosis of glenohumeral arthritis. In addition, an os acromiale is visible on this view (Fig. 42.11). An unstable os acromiale can hinge through the unfused segment and cause impingement symptoms.

The third view is a supraspinatus outlet view, which is used to assess the shape of the acromion, bony impingement that might be present, and

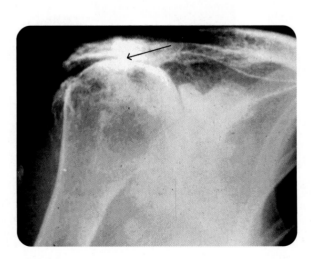

Figure 42.10 In this AP view, the space between the humeral head and the acromion is markedly diminished, suggesting a massive rotator cuff tear.

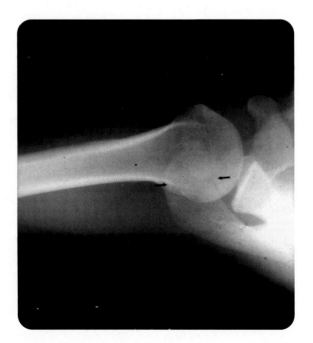

Figure 42.11 Axillary radiograph demonstrating an unfused acromial epiphysis (*arrows*).

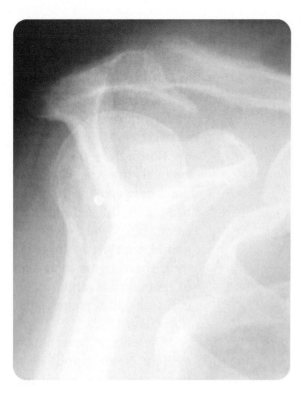

Figure 42.12 Supraspinatus outlet view shows the shape of the acromion. This patient has a type III acromion because of the osteophyte formation that impinges on the rotator cuff. (From Tokish JM. Clinical examination of the overhead athlete: the differential directed approach. In: Krishnan SG, Hawkins RJ, Warren RF, eds. *The Shoulder and the Overhead Athlete*. Philadelphia: Lippincott Williams & Wilkins; 2004:148.)

the space available for the rotator cuff (Fig. 42.12). Of the three acromial shapes visible on these radiographic views—flat (type I), curved (type II), or hooked (type III)—type III acromions have a greater association with abnormalities of the rotator cuff.[6]

TENDON IMAGING

Arthrograms are extremely accurate for the detection of full-thickness rotator cuff tears but are invasive procedures that do not give accurate information on tear size or the condition of the rotator cuff muscles. In addition, arthrograms do not reliably assess partial-thickness rotator cuff tears.[1]

High-resolution, real-time ultrasound has also been used to evaluate the integrity of the rotator cuff. The accuracy is operator dependent; therefore, ultrasound has not become a commonly employed method to assess the rotator cuff. However, it retains the advantages of being quick, inexpensive, safe, and tolerated by claustrophobics.[1]

MRI is the cuff-imaging study of choice in many centers (Fig. 42.13). The accuracy in detecting full-thickness cuff tears has been reported to be between 93% and 100%. Partial-thickness tears are less accurately detected and are more dependent on the technique used. The main advantage of MRI, however, is the wealth of information gained. The quality of the rotator cuff muscles, the size of the tear, involvement of the biceps tendon, and partial-thickness cuff tears can be clearly determined.[1]

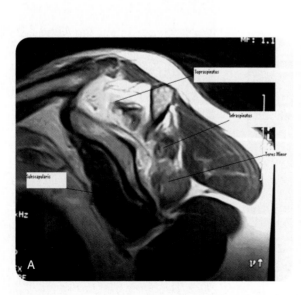

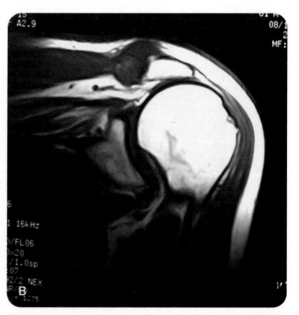

Figure 42.13 A: Sagittal T1 image of the shoulder medial to the glenoid showing the muscle bellies of the rotator cuff. Note the atrophy of the supraspinatus muscle belly. This is highly suggestive of a chronic rotator cuff tear. **B:** Coronal T1 image of the shoulder demonstrating a rotator cuff tear involving the supraspinatus tendon with retraction of the tendon to the glenoid margin.

Treatment

1. NSAIDs and analgesia
2. Physical therapy to strengthen rotator cuff muscles
3. Surgical repair for persistent pain and/or persistent weakness

A review of the literature suggests that nonoperative treatment of rotator cuff tears is successful in 33% to 92% of cases, with most studies reporting a satisfactory result in approximately 50% of patients.[1–5,7] The author's recommendation is nonoperative treatment for patients with rotator cuff disease who present with pain without dramatic or progressive weakness. Rotator cuff tears do not heal well with time. They tend to either enlarge or, at best, stabilize in size. The good news is that rotator cuff tears do not necessarily need to heal in order for the symptoms to resolve. Many people have rotator cuff tears but no symptoms of shoulder pain.[1]

Because many rotator cuff tears do not need surgery, the initial treatment is usually with conservative measures. While the size of the tear may not change with conservative treatment, the symptoms often diminish. In some cases, usually with a traumatic rotator cuff tear in a younger patient, early surgery should be recommended.

The first steps of rotator cuff treatment include the following:[1–5,7,9,10]

- *Physical therapy:* Physical therapy is the most important step in the treatment of a rotator cuff injury. Strengthening the rotator cuff muscles is important to maintain normal shoulder function. A few meetings with a physical therapist can help teach the patient exercises to help alleviate and prevent a recurrence of the shoulder pain.
- *NSAIDs:* Medications are most helpful at controlling the symptoms of a rotator cuff tear. Simple NSAIDs can be taken regularly for a short period and then can be used when symptoms of a rotator cuff tear flare up.
- *Cortisone injections:* Cortisone injections can be incredibly helpful at limiting the acute inflammatory process and allowing the patient to begin therapy. It is important to participate in the therapy and exercises even if the shoulder feels better after an injection. The therapy part of treatment will help to prevent a recurrence of symptoms.

These steps may help to relieve pain and strengthen the muscles around the joint.

However, conservative measures may not be effective in all patients. In general, a good effort at conservative therapy is first attempted, especially in older patients or in patients who have chronic injuries. In younger patients who have an acute, traumatic injury, surgery is sometimes considered early, as the likelihood that conservative treatment will help is low. Surgery is also considered in patients who have tried conservative treatment and still have difficulty with their shoulder.

There are several surgical procedures that are possible for rotator cuff treatment. The most common procedures include the following:

- *Open repair:* Prior to the use of the arthroscope, all rotator cuffs were repaired by looking directly at the torn tendon, through an incision

SECTION 8 Shoulder

about 6 to 10 cm in length. The advantage is that the rotator cuff tendons are easily seen by this method, but the incision is large, deltoid injury is possible, and the recovery can be more painful.

- *Mini-open repair:* The mini-open method of repairing a rotator cuff involves both the use of an arthroscope and a short incision to get access to a torn tendon. By using the arthroscope, the surgeon can also look into the shoulder joint to clean out any damaged tissue or bone spurs. The incision is about 3 to 4 cm, and the recovery is somewhat less involved than the open cuff repair.
- *Arthroscopic repair:* This is a more recent development in the treatment of rotator cuff tears. Arthroscopic repair has the advantage of less postoperative pain and muscle injury. However, this technique requires specialized surgical training and has been associated with somewhat higher rates of repair failure.

 Refer to Physical Therapy

Clinical Course

The clinical course of patients with rotator cuff tears is very variable and depends on such factors as the age of the patient, size of the lesion, duration of the tear, patient needs, patient expectations, and persistence of symptoms. The rotator cuff tear itself does not heal. Fortunately, most tears are small and are associated with minimal functional disability. Those that are associated with persistent symptoms may require surgical intervention.

If surgery is elected, the recovery time for rotator cuff surgery depends on several factors, including the surgical method used, the level of strength before the operation, and the severity of the rotator cuff tear. Some period of immobilization of the shoulder joint is needed to protect the newly placed sutures from being disrupted. Initially, the therapy is gentle so as not to affect the rotator cuff repair. After 4 to 6 weeks, more active lifting with the arm begins. Several months after the rotator cuff repair, physical therapy will become more intense in an effort to strengthen the rotator cuff muscles. Complete recovery usually requires at least 4 to 6 months.[1–3,5,7]

> *ICD9*
>
> *840.4 Rotator cuff (capsule) sprain*
> *726.10 Disorders of bursae and tendons in shoulder region, unspecified*
> *727.61 Complete rupture of rotator cuff*

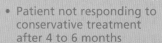 **WHEN TO REFER**

- Patient not responding to conservative treatment after 4 to 6 months
- If patient employment requires overhead use
- Glenohumeral instability (dislocation)
- Trauma-induced, full-thickness rotator cuff tear
- Any full-thickness rotator cuff tear in a patient <50 years of age
- Acute exacerbation of a chronic rotator cuff tear with sudden loss of forward elevation (pseudoparalysis of the arm)
- Recalcitrant adhesive capsulitis treated conservatively for at least 6 months

References

1. Arroyo JS, Flatow EL. Management of rotator cuff disease: intact and repairable cuff. In: Iannotti JP, Williams GR, eds. *Disorders of the Shoulder: Diagnosis and Management*. Philadelphia: Lippincott Williams & Wilkins; 1999.
2. Baker CL, Whaley AL, Baker M. Subacromial impingement and full thickness rotator cuff tears in overhead athletes. In: Krishnan SG, Hawkins RJ, Warren RF, eds. *The Shoulder and the Overhead Athlete*. Philadelphia: Lippincott Williams & Wilkins; 2004.

3. Iannotti JP. Full-thickness rotator cuff tears: factors affecting surgical outcome. *J Am Acad Orthop Surg* 1994;2:87–95.

4. Post M, Silver R, Singh M. Rotator cuff tear. Diagnosis and treatment. *Clin Orthop Relat Res* 1983;173: 78–91.

5. Williams GR Jr, Rockwood CA Jr, Bigliani LU, et al. Rotator cuff tears: why do we repair them? *J Bone Joint Surg Am* 2004;86:2764–2776.

6. Bigliani LU, Levine WN. Subacromial impingement syndrome. *J Bone Joint Surg Am* 1997;79:1854–1868.

7. Green A. Chronic massive rotator cuff tears: evaluation and management. *J Am Acad Orthop Surg* 2003; 11:321–331.

8. Lyons RP, Green A. Subscapularis tendon tears. *J Am Acad Orthop Surg* 2005;13:353–363.

9. McConville OR, Iannotti JP. Partial-thickness tears of the rotator cuff: evaluation and management. *J Am Acad Orthop Surg* 1999;7:32–43.

10. Tokish JM. Clinical examination of the overhead athlete: the differential directed approach. In: Krishnan SG, Hawkins RJ, Warren RF, eds. *The Shoulder and the Overhead Athlete*. Philadelphia: Lippincott Williams & Wilkins; 2004.

43 Shoulder Instability (Multidirectional and Unidirectional)

Fotios P. Tjoumakaris

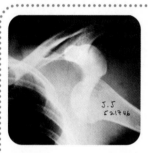

A 17-year-old high school football player presents with pain in the right shoulder and the history of a "pop" after trying to break up a play in the end zone. The patient required transfer to an emergency room for closed reduction of the shoulder. (Figure from Bucholz RW, Heckman JD. Rockwood and Green's Fractures in Adults, *5th ed. Philadelphia: Lippincott Williams & Wilkins; 2001.)*

Clinical Presentation

Instability of the glenohumeral joint is a common cause of disability and pain in the adolescent and young adult population. Patients can present to the clinician with a variety of symptoms, and in many instances, the description of instability can be quite vague. The main presenting symptoms are usually pain; varying degrees of instability or the sensation of joint subluxation; and occasionally, transient neurologic symptoms.[1] With unidirectional instability, the patient can typically localize the pain or instability to the position of shoulder abduction and external rotation and often can remember a specific event that may have brought on the symptoms. Unidirectional instability tends to afflict males more commonly than females and typically is the result of significant trauma to the shoulder. These patients may have had a dislocation in the past that required treatment in the form of an emergent closed reduction by medical personnel. With multidirectional instability, the classic presenting complaint is pain, and patients may experience symptoms during daily activities with seemingly insignificant provocation.[2] Patients with multidirectional instability of the shoulder are usually female and involved in athletic activities that repetitively cycle the glenohumeral joint (swimming, volleyball, etc.).

CLINICAL POINTS

- The condition is a common cause of disability and pain in adolescents and young adults.
- Unidirectional instability usually is more common in males.
- Multidirectional instability usually is more common in females.

Physical Findings

The physical examination of patients who are suspected of having instability can be deceiving. It is often advisable to begin the examination away from the shoulder to gauge the cooperation of the patient as well as to detect any concomitant pathology that may be contributing to or causing

SECTION 8 Shoulder

PATIENT ASSESSMENT

1. In males there may be a history of shoulder dislocation.

2. Females may experience a sense of pain and instability at extremes of motion and repetitive actions of the shoulder, like swimming.

3. Multidirectional instability is associated with general ligament laxity in females.

4. Recurrent dislocations may occur in males.

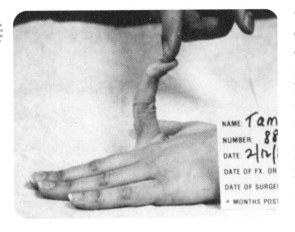

Figure 43.1 Example of metacarpophalangeal joint hyperextension in a patient with multidirectional instability. (From Bucholz RW, Heckman JD. *Rockwood and Green's Fractures in Adults*, 5th ed. Philadelphia: Lippincott Williams & Wilkins; 2001.)

the shoulder symptoms. The cervical spine should be examined first to rule out any abnormalities, such as radiculopathy or spondylosis that may be causing referred pain to the shoulder. A generalized assessment of the patient's ligamentous laxity can then be ascertained to determine if this may be a contributing factor to the instability. This is assessed by the presence of elbow hyperextension, metacarpophalangeal joint hyperextension, leg hyperextension or recurvatum, patella subluxation, and the ability of the abducted thumb to reach the forearm (thumb to forearm test) (Fig. 43.1). The presence of any or all of these tests may indicate an underlying connective tissue disorder such as Marfan or Ehlers-Danlos syndromes. This is vital information, as patients with these disorders are known to do poorly with surgical treatment.[3]

The patient should be inspected for muscle atrophy from both the front and back. In a relaxed patient, there may be an abnormal contour of the deltoid such as squaring, or the acromion may be prominent due to inferior subluxation of the involved shoulder[1] (Fig. 43.2). Muscle testing and a complete neurovascular examination of the upper extremity should be assessed and compared with the contralateral extremity. Nerve injuries (primarily those involving the axillary nerve) have been identified in 32% to 65% of patients with dislocations and are more common in older patients and those patients who sustain a concomitant fracture.[4] Range of motion of the shoulder is performed both actively and passively and compared with the contralateral extremity.[5] Strength deficits can be a result of pain during the examination or a sign that concomitant rotator cuff pathology exists. In patients over the age of 40, a traumatic dislocation may often be accompanied by acute rupture of the rotator cuff tendon; however, younger patients rarely have this concomitant injury, as capsular and labral pathology are more prevalent in this population. A range-of-motion deficit on examination may occasionally be due to the patient having been placed in a sling after a traumatic event. In the final portion of the examination, instability is assessed. The clinician should bear in mind that examination of the asymptomatic shoulder can serve as a control and may help to gain confidence from the patient prior to examination of the symptomatic extremity. In addition, it should be noted that laxity is

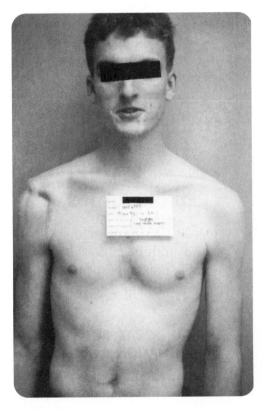

Figure 43.2 Abnormal contour of the deltoid with prominence of the acromion in a patient with multidirectional instability. (From Bucholz RW, Heckman JD. *Rockwood and Green's Fractures in Adults*, 5th ed. Philadelphia: Lippincott Williams & Wilkins; 2001.)

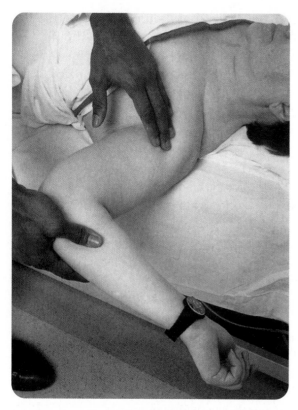

Figure 43.3 Apprehension test. The patient is supine, and the shoulder is in 90 degrees of abduction and external rotation. The arm is externally rotated until the patient experiences apprehension with either verbal cues, facial expression, or reflexive muscular contraction. (From Warren RF, Craig EV, Altchek DW. *The Unstable Shoulder*. Lippincott–Raven Publishers; 1999.)

not a synonym for instability; reproduction of symptoms during provocative maneuvers is key to confirming the diagnosis.

Inferior laxity is first assessed by applying traction with the arm at the side (sulcus test). A positive test is indicated by inferior translation of 1 to 2 cm with noticeable dimpling below the anterolateral acromion (sulcus sign). Anterior and posterior laxity is then assessed with the load and shift test in the supine position. In this test, the involved shoulder is placed slightly off of the examination table and held in slight abduction. The examiner grabs the proximal humerus and applies a gentle compressive force on the humeral head into the glenoid fossa while the free hand supports the elbow. The humeral head is then translated both anteriorly and posteriorly as far over the glenoid rim as possible. Medial translation of the head with this maneuver typically indicates that subluxation has occurred. The amount of subluxation is documented and compared with the uninvolved shoulder. Reproduction of the patient's symptoms with this maneuver is key to establishing a diagnosis of multidirectional instability.[6] Patients with unidirectional instability in the anterior plane will typically demonstrate anxiety as their shoulder is abducted and externally rotated while in the supine position (apprehension sign) (Fig. 43.3). This maneuver reproduces the sensation of an impending dislocation. Relief of apprehension with a posteriorly directed force on the humeral head in this same position is also a confirmatory test for anterior instability (relocation test) (Fig. 43.4).

Studies (Labs, X-rays)

Laboratory studies are generally not helpful in the diagnosis of shoulder instability.

RADIOGRAPHIC EVALUATION

Plain radiographs are the best initial diagnostic test to obtain when evaluating patients with instability. A standard shoulder series consisting of an AP, scapular

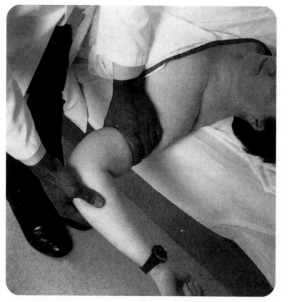

Figure 43.4 Relocation test. The arm is in the apprehension position and a posteriorly directed force is placed on the humeral head, relieving the symptoms of apprehension. (From Warren RF, Craig EV, Altchek DW. *The Unstable Shoulder*. Lippincott–Raven Publishers; 1999.)

NOT TO BE MISSED

- Associated neurovascular injury
- Associated rotator cuff tears
- Fracture of the proximal humerus or glenoid
- Chronic dislocation
- Cervical spine disorders
- Referred pain of cardiac, pulmonary, or visceral origin

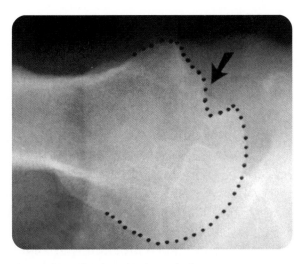

Figure 43.5 Axillary lateral radiograph after a traumatic posterior dislocation demonstrates an impression fracture of the anteromedial humeral head. (From Bucholz RW, Heckman JD. *Rockwood and Green's Fractures in Adults*, 5th ed. Philadelphia: Lippincott Williams & Wilkins; 2001.)

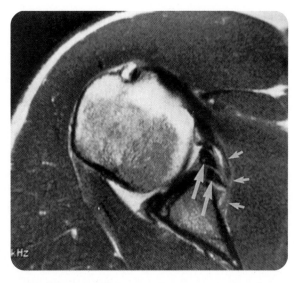

Figure 43.6 Axial MRI sequence through the anterior labrum demonstrates an anteroinferior labral tear in a 26-year-old man with an acute dislocation. (From Warren RF, Craig EV, Altchek DW. *The Unstable Shoulder*. Lippincott–Raven Publishers; 1999.)

Y, and axillary lateral view should be obtained. These images should first be checked for a concentric reduction of the humeral head into the glenoid fossa. The presence of any bony lesions and the contour of the humeral head should be documented (Fig. 43.5). An impression fracture of the posterolateral humeral head (Hill-Sachs lesion) is an indication of a prior anterior dislocation. Posterior or anterior glenoid bone loss may indicate posterior or anterior instability secondary to bone deficiency.

Oftentimes, plain radiographs will be normal. If this is the initial office visit for the patient, the clinician may choose to forego any additional testing. For patients who continue to experience symptoms despite initial treatment, an MR arthrogram of the shoulder may be obtained to further evaluate the integrity of the capsule, labrum, and articular structures (Fig. 43.6). Many centers use MRI as a preoperative test only, as the diagnosis is usually based on history and physical examination findings.[7] Ultrasound, although rarely utilized in diagnosis, can be used in the evaluation of the patient with suspected shoulder instability.

OTHER DIAGNOSTIC MODALITIES

Intra-articular injections of local anesthetic or corticosteroid are rarely, if ever, used within the setting of instability, as they have little utility in the diagnosis of this condition.

Treatment

1. Recurrent dislocations in males require surgical stabilization.
2. Multidirectional instability in females, related to ligament laxity, does well with muscle strengthening.
3. Age-related stiffening of the joints relieves symptoms.

SECTION 8 Shoulder

NONOPERATIVE

Treatment of shoulder instability is aimed at reducing the excessive translation of the humeral head with normal physiologic glenohumeral motion. In patients who have primarily multidirectional instability, physical therapy is the mainstay of treatment. Patients should be educated that the shoulder has become deconditioned and that a regular exercise program that strengthens the scapula stabilizers, rotator cuff muscles, and deltoid can help to regain neuromotor control. Phase I of the exercise program is aimed at restoring the strength of the deltoid and rotator cuff muscles. Once this is achieved, the patients are advanced to phase II with the addition of scapula stabilization exercises. Therapy should be carried out for a minimum of 6 months, after which the patient is given a maintenance program that should be continued indefinitely. Patients who present with significant discomfort and who have difficulty progressing during therapy can be given a short course of analgesic or NSAIDs. Approximately 90% of patients can expect a satisfactory result with therapy alone in the setting of multidirectional instability.[8] Patients who continue to experience symptoms despite compliance with a therapy program after 6 months may be candidates for surgical intervention. Patients should be counseled at the time of diagnosis that multidirectional instability will not typically persist into late adulthood, as the glenohumeral joint and surrounding capsular structures will stiffen with age.

In patients who present with primarily unidirectional instability, the treatment principles remain the same. Most patients in this setting have experienced a traumatic anterior dislocation (posterior dislocations are rare, occurring primarily in seizure and electrocution victims) and may require an initial period of sling immobilization to relieve symptoms. Sling immobilization, however, should be as brief as possible in order to regain full, active shoulder range of motion. Patients are started in a therapy program as soon as symptoms allow and continue this program until strength and range of motion are near symmetric to the uninvolved shoulder. Reports of success with therapy in this setting vary; however, most studies show that younger patients have a high likelihood of recurrence, which may be as high as 85%.[8] Older patients (>35–40 years) who sustain a dislocation are typically treated with conservative management alone, as recurrence in this patient population is less likely. Patients with anterior instability who continue to experience instability after a comprehensive rehabilitation program may be candidates for surgical intervention.

SURGICAL

If conservative measures fail to relieve the instability and the patient continues to have difficulty with activities of daily living, recreation, or occupational duties, surgical referral is recommended. When considering surgical intervention, multiple variables such as age, degree of activity restriction, hand dominance, patient expectations, and occupation all play a factor in predicting successful outcome. The decision to proceed with surgical intervention should be made by the patient and physician after all attempts at conservative management have not produced an adequate alleviation of symptoms. Surgical options consist of arthroscopic or open capsular shift (multidirectional instability) or anterior inferior glenohumeral ligament repair (Bankart repair for unidirectional anterior instability).

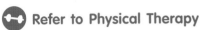 **Refer to Physical Therapy**

WHEN TO REFER

• Failure of conservative treatment after 6 months of rehabilitation
• Concomitant rotator cuff tears
• Associated fracture around the shoulder
• Suspected neurovascular injury
• Locked dislocation
• Frozen shoulder
• Ganglion cyst of the shoulder

Clinical Course

As note previously, the clinical symptoms of multidirectional instability resolve with age. The natural stiffening of the joints with age reduces the sense of instability. Therefore, unless significant disability persists after conscientious muscle-strengthening regimens, most patients can be treated conservatively, and their symptoms resolve with time.

Conclusion

Instability of the glenohumeral joint can present in a variety of ways, ranging from the sensation of pain with certain activities to the occurrence of a traumatic dislocation from a discrete event. Careful attention to the history and physical examination within these patients often leads to a successful diagnosis and treatment plan. The characteristics of patients with either multidirectional or unidirectional instability can be easily remembered with the help of the mnemonics *AMBRI* (Atraumatic Multidirectional Bilateral Rehabilitation Inferior shift) and *TUBS* (Traumatic Unidirectional Bankart Surgery).[9]

> *ICD9*
>
> *718.81 Other joint derangement, not elsewhere classified, involving shoulder region*

SECTION 8 Shoulder

References

1. Schenk TJ, Brems JJ. Multidirectional instability of the shoulder: pathophysiology, diagnosis, and management. *J Am Acad Orthop Surg* 1998;6:65–72.
2. Hawkins RJ, Abrams JS, Schutte J. Multidirectional instability of the shoulder: an approach to diagnosis. *Orthop Trans* 1987;11:246.
3. Jerosch J, Castro WHM. Shoulder instability in Ehlers-Danlos syndrome: an indication for surgical treatment? *Acta Orthop Belg* 1990;56:451–453.
4. Norris TR, Green R. Proximal humerus fractures and glenohumeral dislocations. In: Browner BD, Jupiter JB, Levine AM, et al., eds. *Skeletal Trauma.* Philadelphia: WB Saunders; 1998:1645.
5. Arroyo JS, Flatow EL. Management of rotator cuff disease: intact and repairable cuff. In: Iannotti JP, Williams GR, eds. *Disorders of the Shoulder: Diagnosis and Management.* Philadelphia: Lippincott Williams & Wilkins; 1999:31–56.
6. Hawkins RJ, Bokor DJ. Clinical evaluation of shoulder problems. In: Rockwood CA, Matson FA, eds. *The Shoulder.* Philadelphia: WB Saunders; 1990:149–177.
7. Steinbach LS. Magnetic resonance imaging of glenohumeral joint instability. *Semin Musculoskelet Radiol* 2005;9:44–55.
8. Burkhead WZ Jr, Rockwood CA Jr. Treatment of instability of the shoulder with an exercise program. *J Bone Joint Surg Am* 1992;74:890–896.
9. Thomas SC, Matsen FA III. An approach to the repair of glenohumeral ligament avulsion in the management of traumatic anterior glenohumeral instability. *J Bone Joint Surg Am* 1989;71:506–513.

CHAPTER 44 Glenohumeral Arthritis

Eric T. Ricchetti and Gautam P. Yagnik

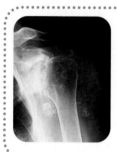

A 75-year-old retired male laborer presents with chronic right shoulder pain and stiffness.

Clinical Presentation

Glenohumeral arthritis occurs in up to 20% of adults and is much less common than arthritis of the knee or hip. The most common etiology of glenohumeral arthritis is osteoarthritis, but other diseases, such as rheumatoid or inflammatory arthritis, osteonecrosis, rotator cuff arthropathy, and posttraumatic or postsurgical arthritis, can also be a cause.[1–3] The different etiologies of glenohumeral arthritis may dictate potentially different treatment options.

Pain in the affected shoulder is the most common presenting complaint in patients with glenohumeral arthritis. Shoulder stiffness is also a frequent problem, and patients may note a sensation of crepitus with shoulder movement. Symptoms usually begin gradually and are chronic and progressive. Discomfort is typically worsened with activity, and patients may awaken at night from pain, particularly if they sleep on the affected shoulder.[1] Functional limitations may be evident, including an inability to perform overhead activities or reach behind the back or under the opposite axilla with the affected arm.[3]

In documenting the patient's history, it is important to characterize the onset and duration of symptoms as well as the degree of functional limitation and the patient's activity level.[4] All prior treatment modalities, including physical therapy regimens, use of NSAIDs, injections, and operative procedures on the shoulder should be documented. Additionally, obtaining the patient's overall medical history can provide information about disease severity or predisposing factors for glenohumeral arthritis, such as a history of steroid use in rheumatoid arthritis patients or radiation exposure in patients with osteonecrosis of the humeral head.[1,4]

Physical Findings

The physical examination should help in confirming or refuting the initial diagnosis that is made on the basis of the patient history. A careful

CLINICAL POINTS

- The condition occurs much less frequently than arthritis in the knee or hip.

- Pain is the most common presenting complaint.

- Onset is gradual and becomes chronic.

- History may provide important clues.

PATIENT ASSESSMENT

1. Older patients with long history of intermittent shoulder symptoms

2. Progressive pain and limitation in motion

3. X-rays show degenerative joint disease

examination of the cervical spine should first be performed to rule out any abnormalities, including radiculopathy and degenerative joint disease that may cause referred pain, stiffness, or weakness in the shoulder. The affected shoulder is then inspected for any prominence, atrophy, or asymmetry compared with the contralateral side as well as prior surgical scars. Mild shoulder atrophy may be present from disuse. Shoulder palpation is performed to define areas of tenderness. Although this is often nonspecific, posterior joint line tenderness is typical in osteoarthritis, while anterior and lateral tenderness is seen more frequently in inflammatory arthritis.[1] Muscle strength and range of motion are also assessed. Range of motion of the shoulder is performed actively and passively and compared with the asymptomatic side. Both active and passive motion are typically restricted in glenohumeral arthritis, usually in multiple planes. Decreased external rotation is commonly seen in osteoarthritis from chronic stiffness and anterior capsular contracture (Fig. 44.1).[4]

Specific patterns of restricted motion may also be related to prior trauma or surgery, such as a loss of external rotation in patients with previous surgical stabilization for anterior shoulder instability. Pain and crepitus in the glenohumeral joint may be elicited with active or passive motion.[3] Muscle-strength testing should assess the rotator cuff, deltoid, and other shoulder girdle muscles.[4]

Studies (Labs, X-rays)

Laboratory studies are generally not helpful in the diagnosis of glenohumeral arthritis unless septic shoulder is a concern.

RADIOGRAPHIC EVALUATION

Plain radiographs are the initial imaging study of choice. Radiographs should include a true AP view (Fig. 44.2) and an axillary lateral view (Fig. 44.3) to best see the classic features of arthritis.

Osteoarthritis will typically show joint space narrowing, osteophyte formation, sclerosis, and subchondral cysts, while rheumatoid arthritis will show joint space narrowing, osteopenia, bony erosions, subchondral cysts, and occasionally osteophyte formation.[2,3] Loose bodies may also be seen, typically in the axillary pouch. The axillary lateral view is particularly important in assessing the degree of joint space narrowing and the amount and location of glenoid erosion.[3]

Radiographs may also be helpful in identifying other shoulder abnormalities, such as osteoarthritis of the acromioclavicular joint, calcific tendinitis, and os acromiale.

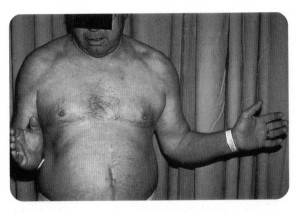

Figure 44.1 Decreased external rotation of the right shoulder from osteoarthritis of the glenohumeral joint. (From Iannotti JP, Williams GR. *Disorders of the Shoulder: Diagnosis and Management.* Philadelphia: Lippincott Williams & Wilkins; 1999:431.)

NOT TO BE MISSED

- Charcot or neuropathic arthropathy
- Septic shoulder
- Adhesive capsulitis
- Brachial plexus injury
- Peripheral nerve injury
- Radiculopathy
- Axillary-subclavian venous thrombosis
- Referred pain of cardiac, pulmonary, or visceral origin
- Soft tissue or bone tumor

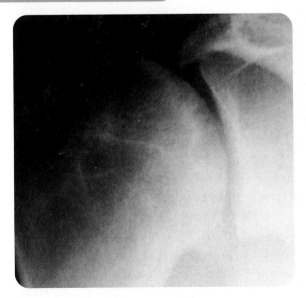

Figure 44.2 True AP view of the shoulder showing osteoarthritis. (From Iannotti JP, Williams GR. *Disorders of the Shoulder: Diagnosis and Management.* Philadelphia: Lippincott Williams & Wilkins; 1999:422.)

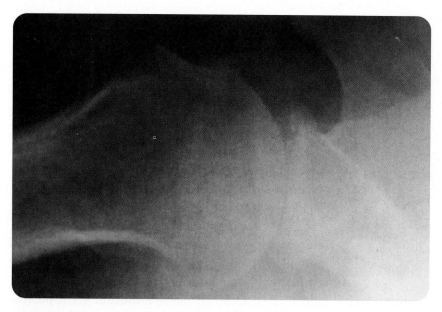

Figure 44.3 Axillary lateral view of the shoulder showing osteoarthritis. (From Iannotti JP, Williams GR. *Disorders of the Shoulder: Diagnosis and Management.* Philadelphia: Lippincott Williams & Wilkins; 1999:422.)

OTHER IMAGING MODALITIES

If the history, physical examination, and radiographs are consistent with glenohumeral arthritis, additional imaging studies are not needed. However, CT is useful in evaluating glenoid bone stock and wear when joint arthroplasty is being considered. Osteoarthritis, for example, typically leads to posterior glenoid erosion, while rheumatoid arthritis causes more central wear (Fig. 44.4).

MRI is useful in evaluating the status of the rotator cuff and other surrounding soft tissues.[1,3] Although rotator cuff tears are not commonly seen in osteoarthritis, they frequently occur in rheumatoid and inflammatory arthritis and are always present in rotator cuff arthropathy.[4]

Advanced imaging modalities may also be useful in ruling out other causes of a painful, stiff shoulder. MRI or bone scan may confirm a diagnosis of osteonecrosis of the humeral head by detecting more subtle changes not evident on plain radiographs, while electrodiagnostic studies and cervical spine radiographs or MRI may be needed if neuropathic arthritis is suspected.[3]

Treatment

1. Modified activity
2. Maintain range of motion
3. NSAIDs
4. Total shoulder replacement for advanced arthritis

The treatment of glenohumeral arthritis can vary depending on the specific etiology. However, initial management is typically nonoperative and includes modification of activity, the use of NSAIDs, the use of intra-articular corticosteroid injections, and physical therapy. At least 6 months of nonoperative treatment is recommended before surgical intervention is considered. Even in cases where surgery is inevitable, a period of nonoperative treatment can improve preoperative

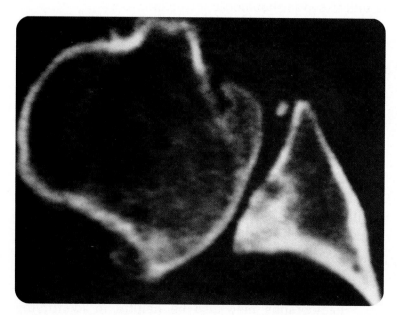

Figure 44.4 CT scan of glenohumeral osteoarthritis showing posterior glenoid erosion and joint space narrowing, humeral head osteophyte formation, and an anterior loose body. (From Iannotti JP, Williams GR. *Disorders of the Shoulder: Diagnosis and Management.* Philadelphia: Lippincott Williams & Wilkins; 1999:425.)

conditioning and shoulder function, which have been shown to correlate with better postoperative outcomes.[4–6]

The goals of nonoperative treatment are symptomatic relief and maintenance of function. Activity modification focuses on avoiding activities that place large loads on the glenohumeral joint. Intra-articular corticosteroid injections can provide short-term pain relief and are limited to four injections per year. Side effects include skin blanching, local fat atrophy, infection, and transient hyperglycemia in diabetics, and excessive injections can lead to further articular cartilage or rotator cuff degeneration.[4] Physical therapy is typically performed as a home program and is aimed at regaining motion and strength.[7] Exercises are first directed at regaining motion and flexibility by gentle, frequent stretching. As pain, inflammation, and/or stiffness resolve, more attention can be focused on strengthening the deltoid, rotator cuff, and other periscapular muscles. Aerobic activities that involve repetitive, nonimpact shoulder motion, such as swimming and walking, can also be encouraged to maintain flexibility.[4]

For patients failing nonoperative management, surgical options are considered. In young patients in the early stages of arthritis, arthroscopic shoulder debridement and capsular release may provide some short-term benefit in relieving pain and regaining motion. Arthroscopy is most useful in patients with mechanical symptoms from loose bodies or interposed soft tissue.[2,4,7] Arthroscopic or open synovectomy is a surgical option in patients with rheumatoid or inflammatory arthritis with severe synovitis but minimal articular degeneration.[4,7]

In the majority of patients with painful arthritis that is unresponsive to nonoperative treatment, however, definitive surgical intervention consists of shoulder replacement. While studies show both pain relief and improvement of function with shoulder arthroplasty, pain relief is more reliably achieved.[4,8] Therefore, pain, not function, should be the primary indication to operate. Shoulder replacement can be performed to replace both the humeral head and glenoid (total shoulder arthroplasty) or the humeral head alone (hemiarthroplasty), depending on the degree of glenoid degeneration, rotator cuff status, and age of the patient.[3] The humeral head replacement consists of a metal ball and stem prosthesis that is press fit or cemented into the humeral shaft, while the glenoid prosthesis, if used, is a polyethylene component cemented onto the remaining glenoid surface (Fig. 44.5).

Shoulder arthroplasty is contraindicated in patients with active infection, absent deltoid or rotator cuff function, Charcot or neuropathic arthropathy, and intractable shoulder instability.[2,8] Arthrodesis or surgical fusion of the glenohumeral joint may be an alternative option in some of these patients, such as those with arthritis accompanied by infection, those with significant loss of deltoid and/or rotator cuff function, and

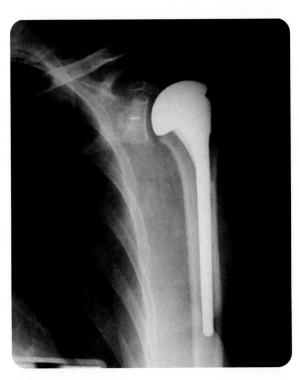

Figure 44.5 AP view of the shoulder showing a total shoulder replacement, consisting of the metal ball and stem prosthesis of the proximal humerus and a polyethylene glenoid component.

SECTION 8 Shoulder

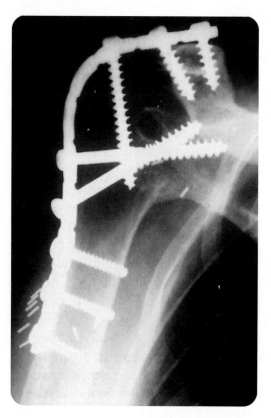

Figure 44.6 AP radiograph of the shoulder showing arthrodesis of the glenohumeral joint. (From Iannotti JP, Williams GR. *Disorders of the Shoulder: Diagnosis and Management*. Philadelphia: Lippincott Williams & Wilkins; 1999:510.)

those with failed prior surgery for arthritis or shoulder instability (Fig. 44.6).[3,7]

In rare cases of septic arthritis or failed prior shoulder arthroplasty, resection arthroplasty may be indicated.[4]

 Refer to Physical Therapy

Clinical Course

The clinical course of patients with glenohumeral arthritis is similar to other joints with osteoarthritis. The arthritis gradually becomes more severe, symptoms are usually intermittent, and it may take decades for symptoms to become significant. The symptoms will depend on activity. Surgical alternatives, such as total shoulder arthroplasty, are satisfactory but should be reserved for patients failing conservative therapy and with significant structural changes within the joint.

In summary, while glenohumeral arthritis is less common than arthritis of the joints of the lower extremity, it can be just as debilitating. Multiple etiologies exist, but initial management should consist of a minimum of 6 months of nonoperative treatment. For those patients who fail nonoperative management, shoulder replacement is typically indicated with the primary goal of relieving pain.

ICD9

716.91 Unspecified arthropathy involving shoulder region

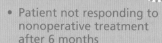

WHEN TO REFER

- Patient not responding to nonoperative treatment after 6 months
- Rheumatoid or inflammatory arthritis
- Osteonecrosis
- Rotator cuff arthropathy
- Posttraumatic or postsurgical arthritis (i.e., prior arthritis or instability surgery)
- Intractable shoulder instability
- Charcot or neuropathic arthropathy

References

1. Collins DN. Pathophysiology, classification, and pathoanatomy of glenohumeral arthritis and related disorders. In: Iannotti JP, Williams GR, eds. *Disorders of the Shoulder: Diagnosis and Management*. Philadelphia: Lippincott Williams & Wilkins; 1999:421–470.
2. Galatz LM. Shoulder reconstruction. In: Vaccaro AR, ed. *Orthopaedic Knowledge Update 8*. Rosemont, IL: American Academy of Orthopaedic Surgeons; 2005:295–306.
3. Shaffer B. The shoulder and the arm. In: Wiesel SW, Delahay JN, eds. *Principles of Orthopaedic Medicine and Surgery*. Philadelphia: WB Saunders; 2001:512–558.
4. Parsons IM 4th, Weldon EJ 3rd, Titelman RM, et al. Glenohumeral arthritis and its management. *Phys Med Rehabil Clin N Am* 2004;15(2):447–474.
5. Fehringer EV, Kopjar B, Boorman RS, et al. Characterizing the functional improvement after total shoulder arthroplasty for osteoarthritis. *J Bone Joint Surg Am* 2002;84(8):1349–1353.
6. Matsen FA 3rd, Antoniou J, Rozencwaig R, et al. Correlates with comfort and function after total shoulder arthroplasty for degenerative joint disease. *J Shoulder Elbow Surg* 2000;9(6):465–469.
7. Skedros JG, O'Rourke PJ, Zimmerman JM, et al. Alternatives to replacement arthroplasty for glenohumeral arthritis. In: Iannotti JP, Williams GR, eds. *Disorders of the Shoulder: Diagnosis and Management*. Philadelphia: Lippincott Williams & Wilkins; 1999:485–499.
8. Schenk T, Iannotti JP. Prosthetic arthroplasty for glenohumeral arthritis with an intact or repairable rotator cuff: indications, techniques, and results. In: Iannotti JP, Williams GR, eds. *Disorders of the Shoulder: Diagnosis and Management*. Philadelphia: Lippincott Williams & Wilkins; 1999:521–558.

45 Frozen Shoulder

Gautam P. Yagnik and Eric T. Ricchetti

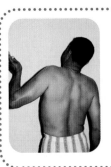

A 60-year-old diabetic man presents with a 3-week history of gradually worsening right shoulder pain and stiffness.

CLINICAL POINTS

- The characteristic feature is loss of both active and passive shoulder motion.

- Disease may be idiopathic or associated with medical conditions such as diabetes.

- Disease may last as long as 18 to 24 months.

- Patients are usually 40 years of age or older.

Clinical Presentation

Frozen shoulder, also known as *adhesive capsulitis* or *periarthritis of the shoulder*, is a common condition characterized by pain and loss of shoulder motion. Frozen shoulder is a syndrome or collection of symptoms with the hallmark feature being loss of both active *and* passive shoulder motion. The exact etiology remains unclear, and controversy exists about whether the underlying process is an inflammatory, fibrosing, or neurodystrophic condition. Regardless of the pathoanatomy, the final common pathway is a contracted joint capsule that restricts all planes of glenohumeral motion (Fig. 45.1).

The diagnosis of frozen shoulder is essentially one of exclusion and should not be made until other intrinsic causes of shoulder pain and stiffness have been ruled out. In most cases, the natural history of frozen shoulder is one of eventual resolution. In contrast, many intrinsic shoulder conditions that can also present with pain and stiffness, such as impingement syndrome, rotator cuff tears, and glenohumeral arthritis, may not improve without appropriate management.

Frozen shoulder is often classified into primary and secondary forms. Primary frozen shoulder is idiopathic, while secondary frozen shoulder is associated with other medical conditions. These conditions include cervical disc disease, central nervous system disorders, ischemic cardiac disease, pulmonary disease, diabetes mellitus, and thyroid dysfunction (Table 45.1). Diabetes mellitus has the highest association with frozen shoulder, and the incidence is two to four times higher in diabetic patients than in the normal population. Frozen shoulder occurs slightly more often in women than in men and is rare in patients under the age of 40.[1,2] Recurrence after resolution is rare.

Patients traditionally progress through three overlapping clinical phases over a period of 18 to 24 months. The initial or "inflammatory" phase (also known as the *freezing phase,* from a few weeks to 9 months)

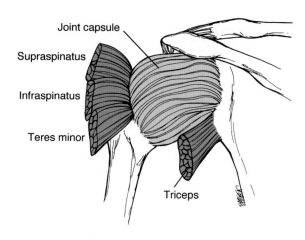

Figure 45.1 Normal shoulder joint capsule with rotator cuff muscles reflected. Regardless of the etiology, the common final pathway of frozen shoulder is a thickened, contracted joint capsule that restricts active and passive motion. (From Hendrickson T. *Massage for Orthopedic Conditions*. Philadelphia: Lippincott Williams & Wilkins; 2002.)

is characterized by the insidious onset of pain and stiffness around the shoulder. During the second or "adhesive" phase (also known as the *frozen phase*, from 4 to 12 months), the pain gradually subsides, but the stiffness persists. The final or "resolution" phase (also known as the *thawing phase*, from 5 to 24 months) is characterized by a spontaneous but gradual improvement in range of motion.

Because frozen shoulder represents a symptom complex rather than a specific diagnostic entity, a careful clinical history is crucial in making the diagnosis.[3] Patients typically present during the first clinical phase (inflammatory) and report the insidious onset of pain and shoulder stiffness. The pain can be of varying intensity, and rest and/or night pain are also commonly reported. Stiffness is reflected in the gradual loss of function. Patients report difficulty in performing overhead activities as well as activities behind their back. Since these symptoms closely resemble those found in rotator cuff pathology, it is important to combine this information with a good physical examination and imaging studies before a diagnosis of frozen shoulder is made.

Physical Findings

Since true frozen shoulder is primarily a clinical diagnosis, the physical examination is critical in ruling out other shoulder pathology and confirming the diagnosis of frozen shoulder. As with all suspected shoulder disorders, a careful examination of the cervical spine should be performed to rule out cervical pathology that may cause referred pain to the shoulder. On inspection, the patient's arm is often held in an adducted and internally rotated position. Mild disuse atrophy of the deltoid and supraspinatus may also be observed. Palpation of the shoulder often reveals diffuse nonspecific tenderness over the entire shoulder girdle.

PATIENT ASSESSMENT

1. Painful shoulder followed by loss of motion

2. Initially not responsive to conservative therapy

3. In time, pain resolves; stiffness resolves much later

4. May take 1 year to recover motion

Table 45.1 Medical Conditions Associated with Frozen Shoulder
• Diabetes mellitus
• Thyroid dysfunction
• ACTH deficiency
• Hypercholesterolemia
• Cardiac or pulmonary disease
• Parkinson disease
• Dupuytren disease
• Post cardiac or neurologic surgery

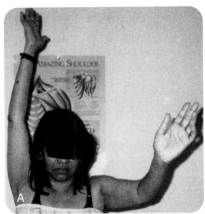
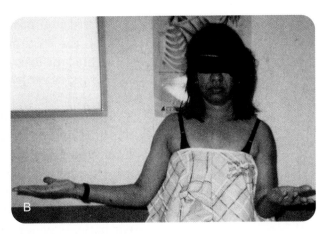
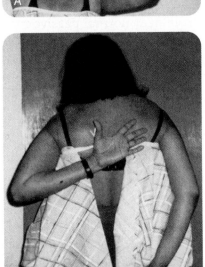

Figure 45.2 Globally restricted active and passive range of motion demonstrated by loss of forward elevation and external and internal rotation of the shoulder. (From Cuomo F. Diagnosis, classification and management of the stiff shoulder. In: Iannotti JP, Williams GR, eds. *Disorders of the Shoulder: Diagnosis and Management.* Philadelphia: Lippincott Williams & Wilkins; 1999:403.)

Assessing range of motion is the most important aspect of the physical examination. The key to diagnosis is documenting loss of *both* active and passive motion. While motion is lost in all planes of glenohumeral motion, near complete loss of external rotation is pathognomonic.[2] Examination and documentation of the range of motion in the unaffected shoulder is important for comparison purposes (Fig. 45.2).

Active range of motion is assessed with the patient standing and should be recorded in the following planes: forward flexion, abduction, internal and external rotation with the arm at the side, and with the arm abducted to 90 degrees. Patients with frozen shoulder will attempt to compensate for the loss of motion with increased scapulothoracic motion or excessive trunk lean. It is important for the examiner to be aware of and to control for these compensatory movements in order to avoid misdiagnosis.

In some situations, pain, rather than true soft tissue contracture, may limit active shoulder motion. The *impingement test*, which has been discussed in previous chapters, may be a useful adjunct in distinguishing impingement syndrome or rotator cuff pathology from frozen shoulder. For this test, 10 cc of 1% lidocaine is sterilely injected into the subacromial space, thereby eliminating pain and allowing for true assessment of

NOT TO BE MISSED

- Fracture
- Anterior and/or posterior dislocation
- Septic shoulder
- Brachial plexus injury
- Rotator cuff tears

active range of motion.[4] Increased motion following the injection can distinguish the motion loss due to pain from soft tissue contracture.[5]

Significant loss of passive shoulder motion further narrows the diagnosis. Passive range of motion should be assessed with the patient supine, which stabilizes the scapula and allows for a more accurate assessment of pure glenohumeral motion. Motion should be recorded in the following planes: forward flexion, abduction, internal and external rotation with the arm at the side, and with the arm abducted to 90 degrees. Limited passive range of motion distinguishes frozen shoulder from conditions like massive rotator cuff tears. Both frozen shoulder patients and massive rotator cuff tear patients demonstrate loss of active motion; however, massive cuff tear patients generally have near normal passive motion. Other conditions that may limit passive shoulder motion, such as glenohumeral arthritis, fractures, or dislocations, will be apparent on plain radiographs.

Studies (Labs, X-rays)

Laboratory studies are generally not helpful in the diagnosis of frozen shoulder unless there is a concern for septic shoulder.

RADIOGRAPHIC EVALUATION

Routine radiographs in patients with frozen shoulder are typically normal. The utility of plain films is to exclude other intrinsic causes of shoulder pain and stiffness, such as glenohumeral arthritis, calcific tendonitis, fractures, and/or dislocations. MRI may be useful in select cases if a rotator cuff tear is suspected.

Treatment

1. NSAIDs and analgesia as necessary
2. Range of motion activities to tolerance
3. Vigorous therapy after pain resolves
4. Rarely requires manipulation under anesthesia

Frozen shoulder can be effectively treated in the primary care setting. Patient education about the protracted natural history and eventual resolution can allay patient fears of permanent disability and encourage compliance with prescribed therapy. Although the natural history is one of resolution, patients should be cautioned that they might never regain full range of motion of the affected shoulder.

The goal of treatment is to relieve pain and to restore motion and function. Treatment should be tailored to the stage of the disease on presentation. Most patients present during the initial painful inflammatory phase. In these cases, treatment should be initially directed at pain relief. NSAIDs and acetaminophen or narcotics in severe cases are the primary means of analgesia. Intra-articular and subacromial corticosteroids may reduce synovitis and can be helpful in augmenting oral pain regimens.

Oral steroids have shown no long-term benefit and should not be used routinely.

Pain control is essential because it enables patients to more readily participate in an exercise program aimed at restoring motion.[3] Patients should be placed into a structured physical therapy program under the supervision of a knowledgeable physical therapist. The program should consist of active, assisted range-of-motion exercises as well as gentle, passive stretching exercises in all planes of motion.[3]

In patients who present during the adhesive phase, stiffness rather than pain is the primary problem. In these patients, a more aggressive therapy program aimed at restoring motion and function is generally better tolerated. Referral to an orthopaedic specialist is indicated in patients who fail to improve or in fact worsen despite 6 months of structured nonoperative therapy. In these refractory cases, patients may benefit from a manipulation under anesthesia or an open or arthroscopic capsular release.

 Refer to Patient Education

 Refer to Physical Therapy

WHEN TO REFER

- Fracture
- Anterior and/or posterior dislocation
- Septic shoulder
- Rotator cuff tears
- Patient not responding to conservative treatment after 6 months

Clinical Course

The clinical course of the patient with frozen shoulder is to gradually return to almost normal function. However, this is a difficult course, takes 6 to 12 months, and is associated with episodes of pain. After the initial symptoms begin to resolve, persistent effort must be directed to regaining motion.

In summary, regardless of the etiology of frozen shoulder, most patients will regain adequate motion and function when treated with a structured exercise program and appropriate analgesia. In patients who fail to improve after 6 months of organized therapy, referral to an orthopaedist for possible manipulation under anesthesia or capsular release is indicated.

> ### ICD9
> *726.0 Adhesive capsulitis of shoulder*

References

1. Chambler AF, Carr AJ. The role of surgery in frozen shoulder. *J Bone Joint Surg Br* 2003;85(6):789–795.
2. Dias R, Cutts S, Massoud S. Frozen shoulder. *BMJ* 2005;331(7530):1453–1456.
3. Cuomo F. Diagnosis, classification and management of the stiff shoulder. In: Iannotti JP, Williams GR, eds. *Disorders of the Shoulder: Diagnosis and Management*. Philadelphia: Lippincott Williams & Wilkins; 1999:397–417.
4. Arroyo JS FE, Ed. Management of rotator cuff disease: intact and repairable cuff. In: Iannotti JP, Williams GR, eds. *Disorders of the Shoulder: Diagnosis and Management*. Philadelphia: Lippincott Williams & Wilkins; 1999:31–56.
5. Warner JJ. Frozen shoulder: diagnosis and management. *J Am Acad Orthop Surg* 1997;5(3):130–140.

SECTION 8 Shoulder

Elbow

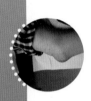
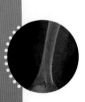

46 Lateral Epicondylitis

Matthew Garberina, Mitchell Fagelman, and Charles L. Getz

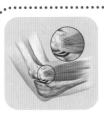

A 46-year-old male postal worker presents with right-sided lateral elbow pain. The patient is right-hand dominant and cannot recall a history of injury. His pain began about 3 months ago. He first noticed it while sorting mail at the office. The pain is worse at work and toward the end of the day. He is having more difficulty lifting catalogs and his bag. He takes some over-the-counter ibuprofen whenever he gets around to it. He is not particularly bothered with pain when he is not lifting objects. He reports no medical problems but acknowledges that he needs to lose weight and "get off of the couch."

CLINICAL POINTS

- Repetitive tasks involving the wrist frequently make pain worse.
- Pain may be related to activity (e.g., tennis) or occur at rest.
- Consideration of patient history allows identification of similar conditions.

Clinical Presentation

Runge first described lateral epicondylitis as "writer's cramp" in 1873 in the German literature. Over the years, the condition earned the moniker "tennis elbow," based on its observed prevalence in racquet sport participants. While up to 50% of all recreational tennis players will experience symptoms of lateral epicondylitis at some point, these individuals make up only 5% to 10% of the overall patient population with tennis elbow.

Patients with lateral epicondylitis often complain of diffuse lateral elbow pain of insidious onset. The patient may identify an injury or moment in time when the pain began. More commonly, there is no inciting event, and the pain has progressively worsened over time. The patient often describes worsening pain with repetitive tasks, especially those involving wrist extension and lifting. Radiating pain down the distal forearm often accompanies the proximal elbow pain. The degree of discomfort can range from the occasional activity-related dull ache to a constant, debilitating pain that is present even at rest. Occupations such as plumbing, meat cutting, and painting that involve repetitive motions are often seen in this patient population.

It is important for the physician to elicit any confounding aspects of the patient's history in order to identify conditions that may present similarly to lateral epicondylitis (Table 46.1). A history of neck pain or upper extremity numbness may indicate underlying cervical radiculopathy or posterior interosseous nerve compression. Complaints of persistent elbow stiffness are present in posttraumatic or primary elbow arthritis (although morning stiffness is a common complaint with tennis elbow). Histories of clicking, locking, or giving way are often components of chronic elbow instability. Finally, fracture about the elbow is possible with new-onset pain and recent injury.

Table 46.1 Differential Diagnosis of Lateral Epicondylitis

DIAGNOSIS	HISTORY	PHYSICAL EXAM	STUDIES
Cervical radiculopathy	Numbness and tingling in arm, hand, fingers	Positive Spurling Diminished reflexes Night pain	Cervical spine radiographs EMG MRI cervical spine
Radial head/ neck fracture	Trauma Fall on outstretched hand	Swelling Crepitus Block to motion	Elbow radiographs
Osteoarthritis	Remote trauma Prior surgery Systemic arthopathy	Deformity Stiffness	Elbow radiographs
Elbow instability	Prior dislocation Prior surgery Feeling of catching or giving way	Crepitus Apprehension with stress of the elbow	Elbow radiographs Elbow MRI
Nerve compression syndrome	Weakness Prior surgery without relief	Demonstrable weakness on exam of thumb, finger extensors	EMG

Nirschl[1] described specific risk factors for developing lateral epicondylitis. These include age >35 years, high-demand work or sport activities, and poor general fitness level. While tennis elbow patients can range in age from 12 to 80 years, the condition exists primarily in the fourth and fifth decades. About three fourths of patients experience pain in their dominant arm, and male–female ratios are about equal. Pain in tennis players is secondary to factors such as poor technique, improper racquet or grip size, extensive playing time, and use of a one-handed backhand stroke.[2]

The common extensor origin arises from the lateral epicondyle, and its muscles insert distally to extend the wrist and fingers. The muscles that make up this area include the extensor carpi radialis longus (ECRL), the extensor carpi radialis brevis (ECRB), the extensor digitorum communis (EDC), and the extensor carpi ulnaris (ECU). The primary tendon origin involved in lateral epicondylitis is the ECRB, with the EDC involved in approximately one third of patients.[1,2]

Physical Findings

The goal of the physical examination of a patient with suspected lateral epicondylitis is to identify the location of maximal tenderness through palpation and provocative tests. The main complaint of these patients is lateral elbow pain, which can be constant or activity related based on the disease severity. While the focus of the physical examination is the painful elbow, the physician must also evaluate the entire limb as well as the cervical spine. A Spurling test (axial compression applied to the extended neck

PATIENT ASSESSMENT

1. Gradual onset of pain over lateral epicondyle

2. Pain on extension of the wrist against resistance

3. Pain on simple tasks such as carrying a briefcase or playing tennis

4. Very persistent and resistant to therapy

deviated to the affected side) can elicit signs of C6-7 nerve root compression with radicular pain in that dermatome. Deep tendon reflexes are evaluated and compared with the opposite side. Strength testing of the entire limb is important to rule out both compressive neuropathy and possible rotator cuff pathology. Particular attention is paid to the presence of rotator cuff atrophy along the scapula. This can contribute to worsening lateral tendinosis and may require concomitant rehabilitation during treatment.

When specifically addressing the elbow, the examiner should evaluate range of motion, including rotation, and compare results with the opposite side. Palpate the posterolateral soft spot of the elbow to evaluate for a ballotable effusion. This finding, along with crepitus on range of motion, suggests possible osteochondral injury and should be correlated with a history of injury. When this portion of the examination is complete, the physician can focus on findings specific to lateral epicondylitis.

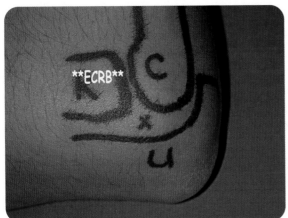

Figure 46.1 Point of maximal tenderness over origin of ECRB.

Tenderness to palpation is generally present over the origin of the conjoined tendon, specifically the ECRB. The point of maximal tenderness is usually 1 to 2 cm anterior and distal to the center of the lateral epicondyle (Fig. 46.1). The patient will likely have pain when the examiner resists active wrist or finger extension (Fig. 46.2). The sensory exam is predictably normal with lateral epicondylitis.[1,2]

Hand grip dynamometer testing will often show a decrease in grip strength compared with the opposite side. Two provocative tests specific for lateral epicondylitis include the chair-lift test and the handshake test. The chair-lift test is performed by having the patient attempt to lift a chair off of the ground with the shoulder adducted, elbow extended, and wrist pronated (Fig. 46.3). A positive test occurs when the patient develops pain distal to the lateral epicondyle. In severe cases, the patient often cannot lift the chair secondary to pain. In the handshake test, the examiner firmly grips the patient's hand and asks the patient to actively supinate the wrist

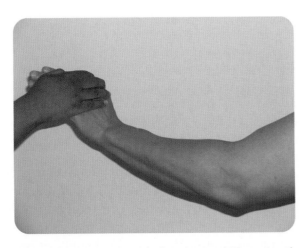

Figure 46.2 Provocative test for lateral epicondylitis—pain with resisted wrist extension.

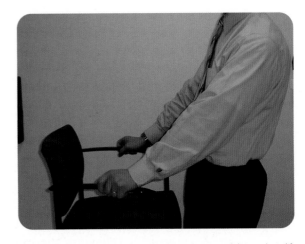

Figure 46.3 Provocative test for lateral epicondylitis—chair-lift test.

SECTION 9 Elbow

NOT TO BE MISSED

- Cervical radiculopathy
- Fracture
- Infection

against resistance. The test should first be performed with the elbow extended. Patients with lateral epicondylitis will have characteristic pain with this maneuver. The test should be repeated with the patient's elbow held in 90 degrees of flexion. The pain should be alleviated in this position. Equal pain intensity in both positions suggests severe lateral epicondylitis that has a less favorable prognosis with nonoperative treatment.[3]

Studies

No laboratory studies are necessary to confirm the diagnosis of lateral epicondylitis. Although up to 25% of patients with tennis elbow will have lateral calcification seen on x-ray, there is some controversy as to whether initial radiographic evaluation is indicated. Lateral calcific changes offer no prognostic guidance, and the changes often reverse with treatment. For the sake of a thorough workup, some authors recommend AP, lateral, and axial radiographs to rule out fracture, loose bodies, or arthropathy. However, lateral epicondylitis is a clinical diagnosis and should be made on the basis of a proper history and physical examination.

MRI studies can identify diseased tissue adjacent to the lateral epicondyle. High T2 signal intensity in the tendinous origin of the ECRB has correlated well with active granulation tissue found at surgery.[4] One proposed advantage of MRI is the identification of a granulation focus deep to the ECRB that can be surgically removed without standard detachment of the common extensor origin. Further investigation is required to determine the timing and defined role of MRI in the treatment algorithm for lateral epicondylitis.

EMG may be indicated in patients with suspected nerve compression syndromes, especially those involving the posterior interosseous nerve. This study is helpful in patients with continued pain despite surgical treatment.

In summary, if the patient history and physical examination exclude prior trauma, surgery, systemic arthropathy (e.g., rheumatoid arthritis), clinical stiffness, instability, or crepitus, the physician can likely refrain from initial radiographs on patients with clear-cut lateral epicondylitis.

Treatment

1. NSAIDs
2. Occasional injection of cortisone
3. Consider surgical release of tendon if refractory to therapy after 6 to 10 months

The initial goals of treatment in patients with lateral epicondylitis are control of pain and inflammation. While an actual inflammatory component has not been established, local tissues can experience secondary myositis or tendinitis. Primary use of ice, relative rest, and NSAIDs can alleviate the initial symptoms and facilitate early rehabilitation. No study has shown definitive pain relief or tendon repair with the use of NSAIDs, but they work well anecdotally in patients who can tolerate them. The observed benefit may be secondary to a decrease in regional inflammation as well as their analgesic effects. The physician may prescribe NSAIDs over the initial 2-week treatment period, longer if necessary, with the goal of increasing the patient's therapeutic potential.[2]

Activity modification is an important component of acute treatment of tennis elbow. It is not advisable to completely immobilize the patient's elbow or wrist, but adjustments in activities of daily living contribute to pain relief. Patients should limit participation in racquet sports, and laborers should decrease performance of repetitive tasks, heavy lifting, and use of vibratory equipment. This may require communication with the patient's employer. The use of a counterforce brace, applied to the forearm just distal to the common extensor origin, can dissipate forces across the elbow and transfer them to areas other then diseased tissue.

Once the patient experiences pain relief, physical therapy becomes the most important component to tendon healing. Therapy initially involves active and passive range-of-motion exercises, aimed at restoring a full, painless motion arc. Early motion enhances tendon healing and tensile strength by facilitating collagen alignment and organization.[2] On achieving full motion, the patient is progressed to resistance-based exercises, the mainstay of physiotherapy for lateral epicondylitis.

The first resistive isometric tasks involve concentric exercises at low resistance. Over time, the resistance and repetitions are increased. The therapist simultaneously builds the patient's opposing muscle groups, such as the wrist flexors, to balance the force couples across the elbow. In advanced stages of therapy, low-velocity eccentric exercises are felt to further facilitate final tendon healing.[2] On a case-specific basis, occupational therapy consultation may be helpful in teaching the patient job-specific exercises to reduce forces on the common extensor origin. Also, tennis players are slowly brought back to sport, initially performing simulated strokes with proper technique, then advancing to low-intensity ball striking before attempting full play. There is a small amount of data supporting the use of adjunctive treatments, such as acupuncture, ultrasound, or extracorporeal shock wave therapy.

Although the use of corticosteroid injections is common, some authors question their usefulness.[2] This is secondary to a lack of localized inflammatory response as well as a suspicion that intratendinous injection furthers tendon degeneration. There is evidence of acute-pain relief with corticosteroid injection, but there is a high recurrence rate of pain.[2,5] Some authors suggest a prognostic benefit, noting that patients who require multiple injections are more likely to fail nonoperative treatment. A commonsense approach is to consider corticosteroid injection a helpful adjunct in initial pain control but not a sole means of treatment. In patients with pain levels that preclude adequate initial treatment, a corticosteroid injection is helpful in facilitating early physiotherapy.[2]

The choice and dose of corticosteroid is often arbitrary and not scientifically established. After sterilizing the area, a mixture of 1 cc of 2% lidocaine and 1 cc of traimcinolone (Kenalog) (40 mg/1 cc) can be injected deep to the ECRB, anterior and distal to the lateral epicondyle. This often

SECTION 9 Elbow

WHEN TO REFER

- After the patient has failed a well-structured conservative treatment regimen over a period of 3 to 6 months

correlates with the point of maximal tenderness. Superficial injection can result in skin depigmentation and subdermal atrophy. Intratendinous injection could accelerate tendinosis. A short, 25-gauge needle with a small (3 cc) syringe allows the physician to inject the medication with minimal force applied to the plunger. As the length of the needle and capacity of the syringe increase, more force is necessary to administer the medication.

Surgical treatment is considered after the patient has failed a well-structured nonoperative regimen that includes appropriate physiotherapy and activity modification. Some suggest up to a year of conservative treatment, while others feel that 3 to 6 months is adequate to determine which patients will respond nonoperatively.[1,2] It is estimated that approximately 5% of community patients with lateral epicondylitis will require operative intervention.[1,2] A reasonable algorithm for the primary care physician is to start the patient on an initial regimen of relative rest, ice, NSAIDs, activity modification, and progressive therapy. Re-evaluation of the patient should occur in 6 weeks. If necessary, a corticosteroid injection can be administered to help advance therapy. Another re-evaluation occurs at the 3- to 6-month period. If the patient is regressing or has plateaued at an unacceptable level, referral to an orthopaedic surgeon is reasonable.

 Refer to Patient Education

 Refer to Physical Therapy

Clinical Course

Historically, lateral epicondylitis is expected to resolve with proper treatment in 90% to 95% of cases. Most relapses are felt to be secondary to inadequate rehabilitation or insufficient activity modification. There is reason to believe that this estimate of recovery may be overly optimistic. Coonrad and Hooper[6] followed 1,000 patients with tennis elbow and received follow-up on 339. They were able to avoid surgery in 278 patients (83%).[6] More recent studies suggest that prognosis is more closely correlated with manual labor and degree of pain on presentation than the treatment regimen initiated. Furthermore, patients may have prolonged symptoms to some degree up to 40% of the time.

Initial pain level and job requirements offer the physician a window into the difficulty in fully restoring function in patients with tennis elbow. Based on the disease process and multiple clinical studies, physiotherapy appears to be the mainstay of treatment. Adjunctive use of bracing and NSAIDs, along with judicious use of corticosteroid injections, allows the physician to fully treat or properly refer patients with lateral epicondylitis.

ICD9
726.32 Lateral epicondylitis

References

1. Nirschl RP. Elbow tendinosis/tennis elbow. *Clin Sports Med* 1992;11:851–870.
2. Kraushaar BS, Nirschl RP. Current concepts review: tendinosis of the elbow/tennis elbow. *J Bone Joint Surg Am* 1999;81:259–278.
3. Paoloni JA, Appleyard RC, Murrell GA. The Orthopaedic Research Institute–Tennis Elbow Testing System: a modified chair pick-up test–interrater and intrarater reliability testing and validity for monitoring lateral epicondylosis. *J Shoulder Elbow Surg* 2004;13:72–77.
4. Potter HG, Hannafin JA, Morwessel RM, et al. Lateral epicondylitis: correlation of MR imaging, surgical and histopathologic findings. *Radiology* 1995;196:43–46.
5. Smidt N, van der Windt DA, Assendelft WJ, et al. Corticosteroid injections, physiotherapy, or a wait-and-see policy for lateral epicondylitis: a randomised controlled trial. *Lancet* 2002;359:657–662.
6. Coonrad RW, Hooper R. Tennis elbow: its course, natural history, conservative and surgical management. *J Bone Joint Surg Am* 1973;55:1177–1182.

SECTION 9 Elbow

Matthew Garberina, Mitchell Fagelman, and Charles L. Getz

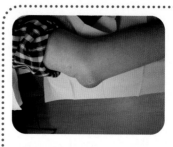

A 46-year-old male carpet layer presents with a 2-week history of left posterior elbow swelling. He has minimal pain and full range of motion. He thought it would just "go away." When the swelling persisted, his wife insisted that he see a doctor about his "infected elbow." He reports no fever, chills, or history of trauma to the elbow.

CLINICAL POINTS

- Pain and discomfort vary.
- The majority of cases are aseptic.
- Patients are likely to be in their fourth to sixth decades of life.
- Patients may have jobs that involve repetitive elbow motion.

Clinical Presentation

A bursa is a synovial cavity, and its function is to reduce friction between adjacent tissues. Diarthrodial joint cavities develop during the first trimester and cavitate over time with joint motion. Conversely, superficial bursae involute after birth and reform over bony prominences when the overlying skin is subject to friction and pressure.[1] The lining of bursae is similar to the synovial lining of a joint cavity. This capsule is surrounded by loose areolar tissue and small vascular structures. Normally, the cavity contains no appreciable fluid, and the space is acellular.[1,2] Bursitis is a condition characterized by accumulation of fluid and cells within the bursal cavity.

The olecranon bursa is the only bursa about the elbow. It lies subcutaneously over the olecranon process.[3] Patients with olecranon bursitis present with swelling and pain over the posterior elbow. It rarely occurs bilaterally. It is a common condition, accounting for approximately 3 out of every 1,000 outpatient visits.[2] Often, the symptoms began days to weeks prior to the patient seeking medical attention. Olecranon bursitis is generally categorized as either septic or aseptic, based on the results of aspirate culture. Aseptic cases are more common (70% of cases)[3] and are further divided into three groups: idiopathic, traumatic, and crystal induced.

The patient with olecranon bursitis may report a direct blow to the area or a history of repetitive trauma, such as constant leaning on the elbow. These insults, either acute or multiple, result in synovial damage with increased vascular permeability. This leads to intrabursal hemorrhage and fluid transudation.[2] Certain populations are at risk for olecranon bursitis. It is most common in the fourth to sixth decades of life. It is often seen in individuals whose occupations require repetitive elbow motion, such as mining, gardening, and mechanical work.[4] Also, a history of systemic disease, such as chronic renal failure or rheumatoid arthritis, predicts a more chronic clinical course.

Patients with aseptic olecranon bursitis present with varying degrees of pain. While bursal pressures are highest in full flexion and lowest in full extension, increased pressures alone may not explain pain associated with this condition. More likely, the discomfort is secondary to the stretching of receptors at the attachment of the bursa to the underlying bony and tendinous structures. Extreme levels of pain, along with a history of fever and chills, should alert the physician to the possibility of septic bursitis. The physician should also seek a history of abrasion or penetrating trauma to the posterior elbow that may predispose to septic bursitis.

Physical Findings

Patients with olecranon bursitis will have physical findings of localized bursal swelling and fluctuance over the dorsal aspect of the elbow (Fig. 47.1). The amount of fluid present varies from a few to 40 mL. Patients will usually have a painless range of motion, though they may have some pain at full flexion. Significant stiffness or deformity suggests an underlying destructive or degenerative process, such as rheumatoid or osteoarthritis.[5] Also, patients with rheumatoid arthritis or gout may have a concomitant "sympathetic effusion" with diffuse synovitis of the elbow joint.[6]

In aseptic olecranon bursitis, the bursal sac may or may not have tenderness with palpation. There is often mild peribursal edema and warmth. Occasionally, there is mild cellulitis. Patients with aseptic bursitis will generally not have systemic complaints such as fever or chills. In contrast, patients with septic olecranon bursitis always have a tender bursal sac. The peribursal edema, warmth, and cellulitis are more pronounced. Systemic symptoms are present more commonly with an infected bursa. It is estimated that about half of these patients will have a visible abrasion or laceration adjacent to the inflamed area.[4]

Aspiration of the bursal sac is indicated in patients with olecranon bursitis on initial presentation. This is necessary to definitively rule out septic or crystal-induced bursitis, as physical findings between septic and aseptic bursitis are often similar. Fluid aspirate also guides clinical treatment as well as improves the appearance of the elbow.

Studies

Routine elbow radiographs are unnecessary when there is no history of significant trauma and no stiffness on joint examination.[3] MRI does not definitively differentiate between septic and aseptic bursitis and therefore is also not indicated in the workup of this condition. The most important test is the analysis of the bursal fluid.[2,3,4,6]

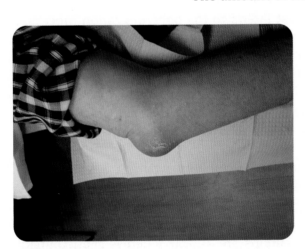

Figure 47.1 Clinical picture of olecranon bursitis—erythema, swelling, and fluctuance over the posterior aspect of the olecranon.

SECTION 9 Elbow

Table 47.1 Characteristics of Bursal Fluid in Patients with Septic and Aseptic Olecranon Bursitis

CHARACTERISTIC	ASEPTIC BURSITIS	SEPTIC BURSITIS
Fluid appearance	Straw colored or serosanguinous	Varies; straw colored, serosanguinous, or purulent
WBC per μL	<1,500	1,500 to 200,000
Predominant cell type	Mononuclear cells	Polymorphonuclear cells
Ratio of bursal fluid to serum glucose	>50%	<50%
Gram stain	Negative	Positive in 70%
Culture results	Negative	Positive

From Johnson G. A follow-up of one hundred cases of fractures of the head of the radius with a review of the literature. *Ulster Med J* 1962;31:51.

After sterilizing the area just lateral to the bony olecranon process, a 22-gauge needle attached to a 10 mL syringe is introduced into the bursal sac.[7] A lateral rather than a direct posterior approach is felt to lessen the chance of leaving a conduit for subsequent bursal infection, as persistent pressure on the elbow may introduce microorganisms through the dorsal wound.[6,8] Fluid is aspirated and visually analyzed. Frank pus clearly indicates septic bursitis. More commonly, the fluid is straw-colored, pink, or serosanguineous.[2–4]

The bursal aspirate is sent to the laboratory, where it is analyzed for cell count and manual differential, Gram stain, culture and sensitivities, glucose level, and presence of crystals. In contrast to pyarthrosis, septic bursitis is considered when WBC counts >1,500 are found in the bursal fluid. Average cell counts in aseptic bursitis are <1,000, whereas septic bursitis has cell counts in the range of 1,500 to 200,000. The predominant cell type in aseptic bursitis is mononuclear cells (T cells in particular),[2] whereas polymorphonuclear cells predominate in septic bursitis. Glucose levels are generally <50% of serum levels in septic bursitis and >50% (average 80%) in aseptic bursitis. Gram stain is negative in aseptic cases but is only positive in 70% of cases of septic bursitis.[2,3,6] Therefore, a negative Gram stain does not eliminate a diagnosis of septic bursitis, and clinical findings consistent with infection warrant antibiotic treatment until culture results are finalized. Positive cultures reveal *Staphylococcus aureus* and *S. epidermis* in 90% of cases. The analysis of bursal fluid is summarized in Table 47.1.

Treatment

1. Aspiration and injection with cortisone if fluid is clear
2. Repeat aspiration and injection of cortisone

Aseptic bursitis is treated with initial aspiration, followed by application of a compressive dressing. Once septic bursitis is ruled out with negative culture results, recurrence of bursal fluid can be treated with repeat aspiration followed by injection of 20 mg of methylprednisolone acetate. The benefits of steroid injection were demonstrated in a prospective, randomized study.[7] Intrabursal methylprednisolone was found to be more effective than NSAIDs or placebo. Patients treated with steroids had a rapid and sustained decrease in bursal swelling. The postinjection problems of subsequent septic bursitis and skin atrophy were not observed, although these complications were reported in a retrospective study.[8] These improved results may be secondary to use of a lateral injection point followed by covering the site with a sterile dressing.

Evidence of an inflamed, painful bursa, with or without a positive Gram stain, requires empiric antibiotic treatment. Use of a penicillinase-resistant penicillin (dicloxacillin 500 mg four times a day/ciprofloxacin 750 mg twice a day in patients with penicillin allergy) is used for 2 weeks, with follow-up exams to evaluate efficacy of treatment. Repeat bursal aspiration is performed as needed. Supportive treatment with warm soaks and compressive wraps is helpful. A history of prior septic bursitis, unusual organisms on culture, or presence of gouty tophi or rheumatoid nodules portend to a more protracted clinical course. The presence of unrelenting peribursal edema or cellulitis, high fever, or other signs of systemic toxicity requires more aggressive treatment, with hospital admission and use of intravenous antibiotics.[9] Nafcillin or cefazolin are adequate, with penicillin-allergic patients receiving vancomycin. Identification of crystals on fluid analysis prompts treatment with NSAIDs or Colchicine.

Recalcitrant olecranon bursitis can be treated with either open or endoscopic bursal excision.[9] Surgical results are less impressive in patients with rheumatoid arthritis. The benefits of endoscopic bursal resection are decreased infection and quicker recovery time.[9] However, conservative treatment is the mainstay for both septic and aseptic olecranon bursitis.

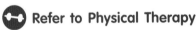 **Refer to Physical Therapy**

Clinical Course

Most cases of septic and aseptic olecranon bursitis that are treated properly resolve without complication. Patients can expect improvement over a period of 1 to 3 weeks. In septic bursitis, bacteremia is rare.[3] Cases that are resistant to treatment require more aggressive treatment: intravenous antibiotics or corticosteroid injections in septic and aseptic bursitis, respectively. The patient is advised to avoid trauma to the area and repetitive tasks involving elbow motion. If the patient's occupation requires pressure on the olecranon bursa, protective pads are helpful. Patients should be followed and reassured over the course of their treatment. Surgical consultation is rarely necessary.

WHEN TO REFER

- After the patient has failed treatment consisting of NSAIDs, aspiration, and/or oral antibiotic treatment

ICD9

726.33 Olecranon bursitis

References

1. Canoso JJ, Yood RA. Reaction of superficial bursae in response to specific disease stimuli. *Arthritis Rheum* 1979;22(12):1361–1364.
2. Smith DL, Bakke AC, Campbell SM, et al. Immunocytologic characteristics of mononuclear cell populations found in nonseptic olecranon bursitis. *J Rheumatol* 1994;21(2):209–214.
3. McAfee JH, Smith DL. Olecranon and prepatellar bursitis: diagnosis and treatment. *West J Med* 1988;149(5):607–610.
4. Canoso JJ. Idiopathic or traumatic olecranon bursitis: clinical features and bursal fluid analysis. *Arthritis Rheum* 1977;20(6):1213–1216.
5. Nirschl RP. Elbow tendinosis/tennis elbow. *Clin Sports Med* 1992;11:851–870.
6. Ho G, Tice AD. Comparison of nonseptic and septic bursitis: further observations on the treatment of septic bursitis. *Arch Intern Med* 1979;139:1269–1273.
7. Smith DL, McAfee JH, Lucas LM, et al. Treatment of nonseptic olecranon bursitis: a controlled, blinded, prospective trial. *Arch Intern Med* 1989;149:2527–2530.
8. Weinstein PS, Canoso JJ, Wohlgethan JR. Long-term follow-up of corticosteroid injection for traumatic olecranon bursitis. *Ann Rheum Dis* 1984;43:44–46.
9. Ogilvie-Harris DJ, Gilbart M. Endoscopic bursal resection, the olecranon bursa and prepatellar bursa. *Arthroscopy* 2000;16(3):249–253.

48 Radial Head and Neck Fractures

Matthew Garberina, Mitchell Fagelman, and Charles L. Getz

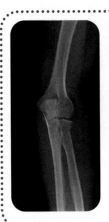

A 55-year-old right-hand–dominant man presents 24 hours after a fall onto an outstretched hand. He complains of elbow pain that began immediately after the fall. He was seen in the emergency department the previous day, where elbow radiographs were taken. The study was reported as negative. The patient was placed into a sling and instructed to follow-up with his primary medical doctor.

CLINICAL POINTS

- The majority of patients are between 30 and 40 years of age.
- The condition is more commonly seen in women.
- Impact that causes elbow fracture transmits forces from the wrist through the forearm.
- Symptoms include elbow pain and inability to use the arm.

Clinical Presentation

Fractures are a frequent source of elbow pain. Radial head and neck fractures are common after a fall onto an outstretched hand and account for one third of elbow fractures. Of these, approximately 20% involve the radial neck, usually in children.[1] Most fractures occur in patients between 30 and 40 years of age and are more commonly seen in women (2:1).[1,2]

Following a radial head or neck fracture, a patient will complain of elbow pain and an inability to use the arm. Although neurovascular injury is rare, patients may also complain of numbness or tingling in the arm or hand. Depending on the mechanism of the injury, some patients may complain of wrist discomfort in addition to elbow pain. Focusing on the entire upper extremity injury is important. However, the astute clinician will also evaluate for cervical or other extremity injury as well.

The forces across the elbow that cause fractures and/or dislocation are transmitted through the forearm from the wrist on impact. An axially loaded, pronated forearm transmits the greatest amount of force to the radial head. Osseous congruence and intact ligaments provide the necessary stability to resist elbow dislocation. Forces applied to the elbow are termed *varus* if they apply compression medially and tension laterally. A *valgus* force, by contrast, has tensile forces medially and compressive forces laterally.[3–5] The bony congruence of the elbow resists the compressive forces, while the ligaments counter joint gapping caused by tensile forces. The capitellum is the portion of the distal humerus that articulates laterally with the radial head to resist lateral compression of a valgus load (Figs. 48.1, 48.2). The radial head is considered the most important secondary restraint to valgus stress across the elbow.[6] The anterior band of the medial collateral ligament is the primary constraint.

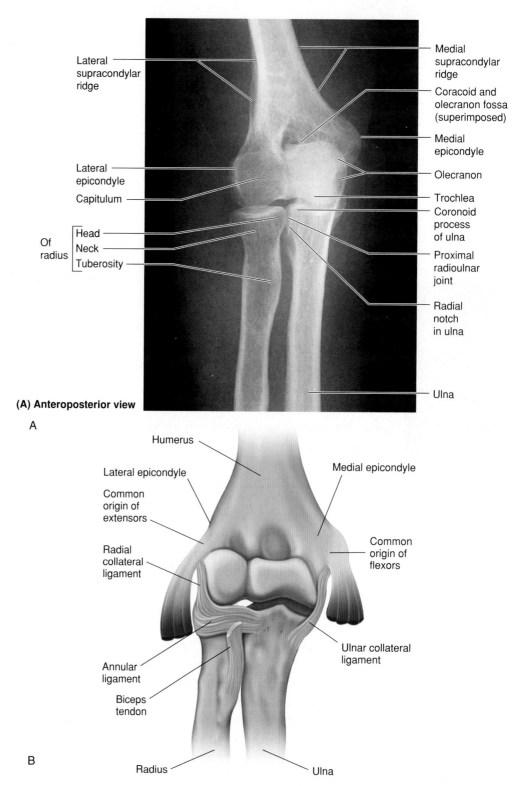

(A) Anteroposterior view

A

B

Figure 48.1 A: AP x-ray—elbow anatomy. (From Moore KL. *Clinically Oriented Anatomy*, 4th ed. Philadelphia: Lippincott Williams & Wilkins; 1999.) **B:** AP view—soft tissue structures around the elbow. (From Premkumar K. *The Massage Connection*. Philadelphia: Lippincott Williams & Wilkins; 2003.)

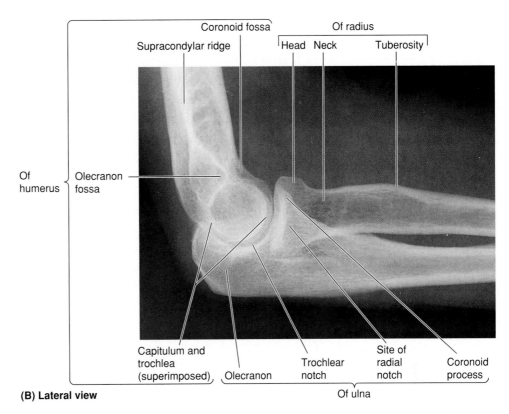

Figure 48.2 Lateral x-ray—elbow anatomy. (From Moore KL. *Clinically Oriented Anatomy*, 4th ed. Philadelphia: Lippincott Williams & Wilkins; 1999.)

SECTION 9 Elbow

A fall onto an outstretched arm typically places a valgus load across the elbow. The force also tends to drive the forearm posterior to the upper arm. Depending on the force applied and position of the arm at impact, a variety of injuries may occur (Table 48.1). Radial head and neck fractures tend to occur with greater degrees of elbow flexion at impact. In contrast, falls with a direct blow to the elbow are more frequently associated with fractures of the olecranon and distal humerus.

Physical Findings

Examination of the injured elbow is systematic and comprehensive. The injured arm is typically held close to the body with the elbow flexed to about 45 degrees. The arm is held in this partially flexed position to maximize joint

PATIENT ASSESSMENT

1. Fall onto outstretched arm
2. Pain on lateral aspect of elbow associated with swelling
3. X-rays show radial neck fracture
4. Nondisplaced fractures can be overlooked on plain films

Table 48.1 **Common Injuries to the Elbow after a Fall**		
FRACTURE	**SOFT TISSUE**	**OTHER**
Distal humerus	Medial collateral ligament	Elbow dislocation
Medial/Lateral epicondyle	Lateral collateral ligament	—
Olecranon process	Flexor/Extensor muscles	—
Coronoid process	—	—
Radial head/Neck	—	—

volume and reduce the joint pressure and pain created by the fracture hemarthrosis. Inspection of the skin is performed first, with particular attention paid to bruising and lacerations. Fractures associated with a break in the skin (open fractures) require immediate surgical consultation. Bruising can be located over a bony or ligamentous injury. The final major component of the initial inspection is to observe the amount of swelling. The presence of significant swelling is more indicative of a serious injury and usually is seen with more severe fractures or ligamentous injuries.

A thorough neurovascular exam distal to the elbow is critical for evaluating these injuries. This is accomplished by palpating both the radial and ulna arteries at the wrist and performing a capillary refill test of the hand. Distal motor and sensory functions of the median, radial, and ulnar nerves are determined. Although neurovascular injuries are uncommon in isolated radial head or neck fractures, significant fracture displacement associated with higher-energy injuries may cause more neurovascular injuries.[7]

Palpation of bony landmarks should begin in areas that seem to be the least affected. This approach adds to patient comfort, allows relaxation for a more reliable exam, and prevents missing less obvious injuries. The elbow is subcutaneous, and therefore the medial and lateral epicondyles, olecranon, capitellum, and radial head can all be easily palpated. Gentle pronation and supination of the forearm makes locating the radial–capitellar joint easier. The entire elbow is often swollen, painful, and somewhat uncomfortable to palpation. However, the location of a fracture will be markedly painful when touched. When a radial head fracture is present, palpation laterally at the radial head will be the most painful part of the elbow exam. Any other areas that are extremely painful may correspond to a ligament injury or fracture.

If the patient's pain level allows, the elbow is then gently ranged in flexion/extension and pronation/supination. The range of motion that is comfortable for the patient is noted but may be severely limited by a painful elbow hemarthrosis. Aspiration of the elbow joint followed by an injection of 5 cc of lidocaine can improve the patient's pain and give a more reliable exam. However, aspiration is challenging in inexperienced hands and should be referred to an orthopaedist. Although the exam may be difficult, it is also important to document whether or not a mechanical block to pronation and supination is present. Finally, careful examination of the wrist must be done following a fall onto an outstretched hand. Tenderness to palpation could signify wrist injury and should warrant wrist radiographs.

Studies

A complaint of elbow pain after a fall requires evaluation with plain radiographs. Lateral, AP, and oblique x-rays of the elbow will show most fractures (Fig. 48.3). Fractures of the radial neck can result in an incongruent radial head–capitellum articulation. In normal elbows, the radial head and capitellum should be aligned on every view.

Occasionally, nondisplaced radial head or neck fractures can be missed on plain films. If radiographs are negative and there is pain to palpation over the lateral aspect of the elbow, other studies may be ordered. CT is

NOT TO BE MISSED

- Elbow dislocation
- Elbow infection
- Vascular injury
- Ipsilateral wrist injury

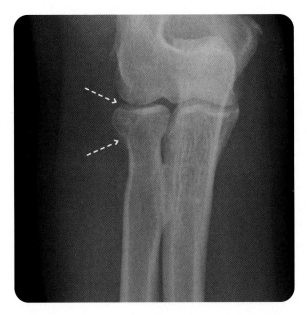

Figure 48.3 AP x-ray revealing nondisplaced radial head fracture.

a very good study to show bony abnormalities and is generally well tolerated by patients. In addition to evaluating the radial head and neck, the remainder of the bony anatomy of the elbow is well visualized. MRI is another excellent study that can show occult fractures as well as ligamentous injuries of the elbow. MRI is the authors' preferred study to evaluate for occult fractures because of the added information obtained about the soft tissue structures of the elbow.

Treatment

1. Aspiration of hemarthrosis
2. Brief immobilization
3. Gentle activities for first 6 weeks
4. Displaced fractures require surgical interventions

Treatment of radial head and neck fractures depends on the nature and severity of the injury. Nondisplaced radial head and neck fractures can often benefit from aspiration of the hemarthrosis and injection of 5 cc of lidocaine into the elbow. After a brief period of immobilization (1–2 days), the elbow can be used for nonweight-bearing activities of daily living. Therapy consisting of active-assisted range-of-motion and edema control are started within a week of injury. At 6 weeks following injury, patients can use the arm for light lifting (<5 pounds) and continue with therapy if any stiffness is noted. Activity restrictions are discontinued at 3 months postinjury. During the first 6 weeks after an injury, the patient is seen for follow-up every 2 weeks. At 6 weeks, the patient can be seen on a monthly basis.

When nondisplaced radial head or neck injuries are combined with medial bruising or medial tenderness, a medial collateral ligament injury is assumed. To support the injured structures on both the medial and lateral sides, a hinged elbow brace is worn in the first 6 weeks for activities of daily living and during therapy.

Displaced or fragmented radial head and neck fractures are candidates for surgery. The decision to perform fracture repair or radial head replacement will depend on the size and displacement of the fragment. Furthermore, a fracture associated with a concurrent elbow dislocation may be an indication for surgery. In each of these cases, referral to an orthopaedist is warranted.

Clinical Course

The outcome following radial head and neck fractures depends on the severity of the fracture and injury to other elbow structures. Most pain from nondisplaced fractures of the radial head that are treated nonoperatively will be completely resolved by 4 to 6 months. However, many

SECTION 9 Elbow

patients continue with some low level of discomfort in the elbow for many years and may have mild loss of elbow extension.

Radial neck fractures are somewhat more difficult to predict. Patients with nondisplaced fractures are started on early range-of-motion exercises to prevent elbow stiffness. However, this will likely cause motion at the fracture site and the potential for fracture displacement. Therefore, radial neck fractures require closer radiographic monitoring for displacement and development of a nonunion. Radiographs are performed every 2 weeks following the initial injury for the first month and then monthly until the fracture has united. Activity is restricted to no lifting, pushing, or pulling with the injured arm until fracture healing has occurred.

Although radial head and neck fractures may not appear to be severe injuries, especially when nondisplaced, these are not benign injuries in adults.[7] Even with nondisplaced fractures, a loss of terminal extension will occur in up to 13% of patients. Radial neck nonunion is a frequent occurrence but often does not produce any symptoms.

More severe radial head and neck fractures (displaced/comminuted fractures) are associated with other complications, including elbow instability, heterotopic ossification, loss of strength, elbow arthritis, and neurologic injury. Therefore, patients with these injuries should seek immediate orthopaedic care.

 Refer to Physical Therapy

> ### *ICD9*
>
> *813.05 Fracture of head of radius, closed*
> *813.06 Fracture of neck of radius, closed*
> *813.15 Fracture of head of radius, open*
> *813.16 Fracture of neck of radius, open*

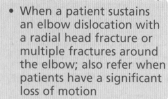

WHEN TO REFER

- When a patient sustains an elbow dislocation with a radial head fracture or multiple fractures around the elbow; also refer when patients have a significant loss of motion

References

1. Castberg T, Thing E. Treatment of fractures of the upper end of the radius. *Acta Chir Scand* 1953;105:62–69.
2. Johnson G. A follow-up of one hundred cases of fractures of the head of the radius with a review of the literature. *Ulster Med J* 1962;31:51.
3. Hotchkiss RN, Weiland A. Valgus stability of the elbow. *J Orthop Res* 1987;5:372–377.
4. Morrey BF, An K. Articular and ligamentous contributions to the stability of the elbow joint. *J Sports Med* 1983;11:315–319.
5. Pribyl CR, Kester MA, Cook SD, et al. The effect of the radial head and prosthetic radial head replacement on resisting valgus stress at the elbow. *Orthopedics* 1986;9:723–726.
6. Morrey BF, Tanaka S, An K. Valgus stability of the elbow. A definition of primary and secondary constraints. *Clin Ortho Relat Res* 1991;265:187–195.
7. Morrey BF. Radial head fracture. In: Morrey BF, ed. *The Elbow and Its Disorders*. Philadelphia: WB Saunders; 2000:341–364.

Wrist

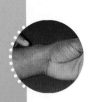

49 Carpal Tunnel Syndrome

David Bozentka

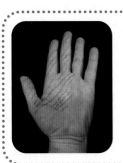

A 50-year-old woman presents with activity-related hand numbness of the thumb, index, long, and ring fingers.

CLINICAL POINTS

- Presenting symptoms include numbness and tingling of the hand.
- Pathology involves compression of the median nerve at the wrist.
- Etiology may be anatomic, physiologic, and/or positional.

Clinical Presentation

Carpal tunnel syndrome is the most common peripheral compression neuropathy. The symptoms are related to compression of the median nerve at the wrist. Patients will present with complaints of numbness and tingling of the hand. The median nerve sensory distribution includes the thumb, index, long, and radial half of the ring finger. To differentiate from other compression neuropathies, it is helpful to have the patient determine whether the numbness occurs in this distribution. Patients with carpal tunnel syndrome will often note diffuse hand numbness. In the mild to moderate stages of the syndrome, the patient will note that the paresthesias are intermittent. As the neuropathy progresses to the more severe stages, the numbness will become more constant.

Nocturnal symptoms are common. Patients will often complain of awaking and having to shake their hand in an attempt to relieve their symptoms, termed the *shake sign*. Pain often occurs about the volar aspect of the wrist and can radiate proximally. Occasionally, the symptoms radiate to the shoulder and rarely to the neck region due to carpal tunnel syndrome. The symptoms are aggravated by activities such as talking on the telephone, reading a book, or driving. Patients will complain of dropping objects, often noting that they need to carefully watch as they grasp small objects to ensure adequate grip.

The carpal canal is made up of carpal bones, which form a "C"-shaped ring dorsally and the transverse carpal ligament that lies volarly. The transverse carpal ligament runs across the canal, attaching to the scaphoid and trapezium radially and pisiform and hook of the hamate ulnarly. The thenar and hypothenar musculature arise from the transverse carpal ligament and insert on the thumb and small finger, respectively. The median nerve and nine flexor tendons run within the canal (Fig. 49.1). In general, compression of the median nerve at the wrist occurs, related to the canal being too small or the contents being too large for the tunnel.

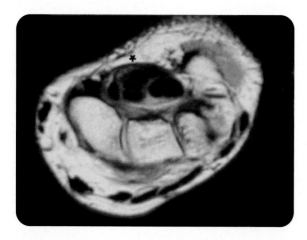

Figure 49.1 MRI wrist T1-weighted image axial cut at the level of the carpal canal. The transverse carpal ligament is located just below the *asterisk*.

There are multiple etiologic factors that may lead to the development of carpal tunnel syndrome. These factors are classified as anatomic, physiologic, and positional.[1] Anatomic factors include anomalous muscles in the canal, distal radius fractures, or a hematoma following an injury in an anticoagulated patient. Physiologic factors are further divided into metabolic, inflammatory, and fluid changes. The metabolic factors leading to the neuropathy may include diabetes mellitus, alcoholic neuropathy, and hypothyroidism. The inflammatory causes include factors such as rheumatoid arthritis, gout, or infection. The fluid changes that are associated with hemodialysis, and pregnancy may also be related. Certain positional changes of the wrist can lead to compression of the median nerve. By holding the wrist in flexion or extension, the size of the carpal canal decreases, thus placing the nerve at risk for a compression neuropathy. These etiologic factors should be entertained prior to concluding that the neuropathy is idiopathic.

The differential diagnosis for patients with carpal tunnel syndrome includes sensory motor polyneuropathy, such as in diabetes. Proximal sites of nerve compression can also lead to similar symptoms. A patient with a C6 or C7 radiculopathy will often have numbness in the median nerve distribution. Pronator syndrome, related to median nerve compression in the proximal forearm, will also manifest with similar symptoms and should be ruled out.

Physical Findings

On physical examination, it is important to assess the entire upper extremity including the cervical spine to rule out other potential etiologic factors. An evaluation for carpal tunnel syndrome should include certain provocative maneuvers as well as a thorough motor and sensory evaluation.

Common provocative maneuvers to confirm the diagnosis of a median nerve compression at the wrist include the Phalen maneuver, Tinel sign, and carpal canal compression test.[2,3] These tests are considered positive if the symptoms develop in the median nerve distribution. The Phalen maneuver is performed by placing the patient's wrist in full flexion for 1 minute (Fig. 49.2). The reverse Phalen maneuver involves placing the

PATIENT ASSESSMENT

1. Pain or dysesthesias in thumb, index, and long fingers
2. Difficulty grasping small objects
3. Worse at night
4. Examination shows diminished sensation in the median nerve distribution
5. Examination shows muscle atrophy
6. Occasional history of trauma

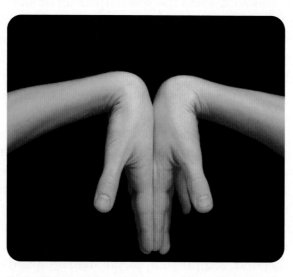

Figure 49.2 The Phalen maneuver is performed by having the patient flex the wrists for 1 minute.

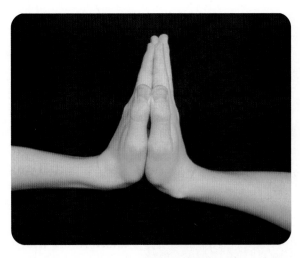

Figure 49.3 The reverse Phalen maneuver is performed by having the patient extend the wrist for 1 minute.

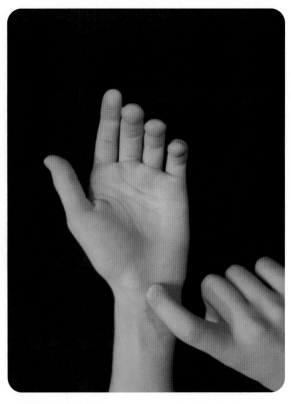

Figure 49.4 The Tinel sign for carpal tunnel syndrome is performed by percussing over the median nerve at the wrist.

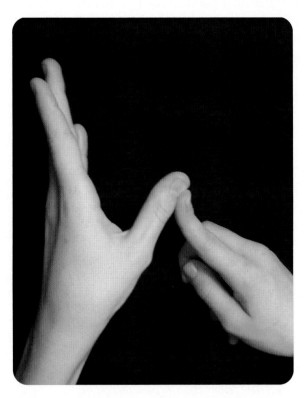

Figure 49.5 The strength of the abductor pollicis brevis muscle is tested by having the patient actively palmarly abduct the thumb against resistance.

patient's wrists in extension (Fig. 49.3). The time at which symptoms develop and the anatomic distribution of the paresthesias during the maneuvers are documented. The Tinel sign is performed by percussing over the median nerve at the wrist (Fig. 49.4). The median nerve lies centrally in the volar wrist deep to the palmaris longus tendon. The examiner's index finger or a reflex hammer is used to tap over this area. The carpal canal compression test is considered the most sensitive and specific provocative maneuver for carpal tunnel syndrome. The maneuver is performed by compressing the median nerve at the wrist and documenting the time and location in which symptoms develop.

On observing the patient's hand, it is important to assess for thenar atrophy. Atrophy occurs in patients with a severe neuropathy and is best assessed with the hands held adjacent to each other and the palms perpendicular to the floor. The strength of the abductor pollicis brevis is also tested by having the patient palmarly abduct the thumb against resistance (Fig. 49.5). The strength is compared with that of the contralateral side and is graded by using the standard manual muscle test grading of zero to five.

The sensory component of the median nerve can be evaluated by using several methods. The distribution of abnormal light touch should be documented. In addition, two-point discrimination is an objective test that can be readily performed in the office. The tips of a

NOT TO BE MISSED

- Cervical radiculopathy
- Pronator syndrome
- Diabetic polyneuropathy
- Acute carpal tunnel syndrome

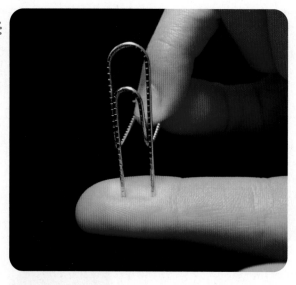

Figure 49.6 Two-point discrimination can be readily evaluated in the office by using a paper clip. Normal two-point discrimination is between 5 and 7 mm.

paper clip can be bent to various widths for the evaluation (Fig. 49.6). Normally, a patient can discriminate the two tips of the paper clip when they are placed between 5 and 7 mm apart.

A patient with a very severe carpal tunnel syndrome will have altered sweat patterns. The palmar skin in the median nerve distribution will tend to be very dry, and a pen or pencil will slide smoothly over the abnormally dry skin. Typically, a pen or pencil slid across the normal glabrous skin will not move smoothly but will skip across the skin due to the normal sweat patterns.

Studies

The possible etiologic factors for carpal tunnel syndrome are considered at the time of the examination. If clinically indicated, laboratory studies are considered to rule out these medical conditions. For example, a fasting blood glucose and thyroid function tests may be helpful in ruling out a neuropathy related to diabetes and thyroid disorder. X-rays typically do not change the treatment decisions in patients with carpal tunnel syndrome. Therefore, x-rays are not routinely obtained unless a patient has a history of trauma or arthritic symptoms in addition to the neuropathic symptoms.

An EMG-NCV is helpful in confirming the diagnosis and in determining the severity of carpal tunnel syndrome. The study is performed following a course of nonoperative treatment in those patients considered to have a mild to moderate neuropathy. The electrodiagnostic studies are performed at the time of the initial evaluation in those patients suspected of having a severe carpal tunnel syndrome.

Treatment

1. NSAIDs
2. Splints worn at night
3. Occasional intracarpal tunnel injection of cortisone
4. Surgical release for persistent, progressive symptoms or neurologic deficits

Patients who develop carpal tunnel syndrome related to specific medical conditions should maximize the medical management of these conditions.

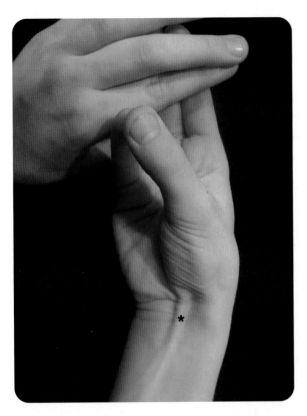

Figure 49.7 The palmaris longus tendon, denoted by the *asterisk*, is identified by having the patient oppose the thumb to the small finger while flexing the wrist against resistance.

Treatment for patients in the mild to moderate category of severity includes use of a volar wrist splint. The splint is worn at night and occasionally throughout the day during activities that aggravate the symptoms. Wrist-immobilizing devices should hold the wrist in neutral or a more functional position of slight extension. There are a wide variety of splints available. Most patients are treated with an over-the-counter prefabricated splint. For comfort of fitting, it may be beneficial to have an occupational therapist fabricate a custom-molded, forearm-based orthoplast splint.

The patient's activities are modified so that aggravating factors are limited. Frequent breaks should be taken while performing repetitive activities. The assistance of an occupational therapist may be beneficial to review stretching exercises, offer ergonometric tips, and perform a workplace evaluation. A strengthening program is contraindicated for patients with carpal tunnel syndrome, as this may aggravate the process. NSAIDs are often prescribed on a short-term basis for symptomatic relief.

Injections are not routinely performed, because they typically only provide temporary relief of symptoms. Approximately 25% of patients will have long-term relief of their symptoms following an injection.[4] The injection is performed with a combination of 1 mL methylprednisolone acetate (Depo-Medrol) (40 mg/mL) and 1 mL lidocaine (Xylocaine) without epinephrine. A 25-gauge needle 1 ½ inch in length is used. The needle is placed within the ulnar bursa and not the median nerve. The location of the injection is ulnar to the palmaris tendon to protect the median nerve and radial to the flexor carpi ulnaris tendon to prevent injury to the ulnar neurovascular bundle. The palmaris longus tendon is located centrally about the volar wrist and is identified by having the patient oppose the thumb and small finger while flexing the wrist. The palmaris longus tendon will become prominent with this maneuver (Fig. 49.7). The needle enters the skin at a 45-degree angle at the distal wrist crease proximal to the border of the glabrous skin of the palm (Fig. 49.8). To confirm placement in the ulnar bursa, the digits are mildly passively flexed and extended with the needle in place. The needle will move with the flexor tendons proximally and distally if placement is correct. The patient is asked to notify the physician of any dysesthesias during the injection to prevent injection into the nerve. If dysesthesias are noted, the needle is repositioned prior to injecting. The risks of the injection are reviewed with each patient. Patients with diabetes may notice a blood sugar elevation and should monitor their blood sugar regularly following the injection. Patients

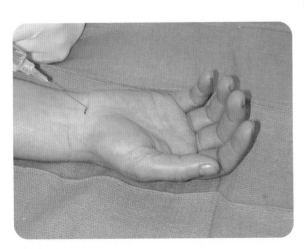

Figure 49.8 A carpal canal injection is performed by placing the needle ulnar to the palmaris longus tendon at the volar wrist crease.

must also be aware of a possible flare reaction. A small percentage of patients will notice increased pain, swelling, and mild redness for several days following an injection, which is treated with ice, immobilization, and analgesics.

Surgical treatment is considered for patients who have persistent or progressive symptoms despite a course of nonoperative treatment. The length of time that nonoperative treatment is continued is variable but in general is maximized after approximately 3 months. Surgical treatment is recommended initially for patients with a severe neuropathy, who will have abnormal two-point discrimination >7 mm and weakness of abductor pollicis brevis strength and will be documented by EMG-NCV. Nonoperative treatment is not successful once the disease has reached the severe stages, and surgical release is performed to limit progressive nerve injury. In addition, surgical treatment is performed urgently for patients with an acute progressive carpal tunnel syndrome that often occurs following trauma.

In conclusion, carpal tunnel syndrome is the most common peripheral compression neuropathy. There are multiple etiologic factors that need to be considered. Nonoperative treatment is often successful, with surgical treatment recommended for patients who have persistent and progressive symptoms.

 Refer to Patient Education

 Refer to Physical Therapy

Clinical Course

In most patients, the majority of symptoms from carpal tunnel syndrome resolve in 3 to 6 months. However, some patients will have persistent pain or progressive neurologic deficits with diminished sensation or muscle weakness. These patients will require a surgical release.

> *ICD9*
>
> *354.0 Carpal tunnel syndrome*

WHEN TO REFER

- Surgical treatment is considered for patients with a severe neuropathy or for those who have had persistent symptoms despite nonoperative management.

References

1. Szabo RM, Steinberg DR. Nerve compression syndromes at the wrist. *J Am Acad Orthop Surg* 1994; 2:115–123.
2. Braun RM, Davidson K, Doehr S. Provocative testing in the diagnosis of dynamic carpal tunnel syndrome. *J Hand Surg Am* 1989;14:195–197.
3. Koris M, Gelberman RH, Duncan K, et al. Carpal tunnel syndrome: evaluation of a quantitative provocational diagnostic test. *Clin Orthop* 1990;251:157–161.
4. Gelberman RH, Aronson D, Weisman MH. Carpal-tunnel syndrome: results of a prospective trial of steroid injection and splinting. *J Bone Joint Surg Am* 1980;62:1181–1184.

50 De Quervain Tendinitis

David Bozentka

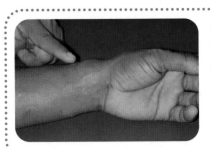

A 30-year-old woman developed radial-sided wrist pain and swelling 6 months following the delivery of her first child.

CLINICAL POINTS

- Wrist pain is a common complaint.
- The onset of symptoms may be sudden or gradual.
- Women are more likely to be affected than men.
- Chronic overuse of the wrist may lead to the condition.

Clinical Presentation

Tendinitis involving the first extensor compartment is named after Fritz de Quervain, who reported five cases in 1895.[1] Patients with this tenosynovitis describe pain and swelling about the radial aspect of the wrist that is aggravated by use of the wrist and thumb. The symptoms may develop suddenly or are gradual in onset. The pain often radiates proximally and distally along the forearm and thumb. It is aggravated by lifting, grasping, and pinch activities while relieved with rest. Some patients note paresthesias along the dorsal aspect of the thumb and index finger due to the proximity of the dorsal radial sensory nerve branches. Occasionally, patients will describe triggering, snapping, or catching that occurs with motion of the thumb.[2]

The dorsal wrist is separated into six fibro-osseous compartments, and de Quervain tenosynovitis develops within the first extensor compartment. Since this is a confined space, the process is considered an entrapment tendinitis, also termed *stenosing tenosynovitis*. The first compartment can be found by locating the volar tendons that make up the snuffbox (Fig. 50.1). Two tendons traverse within the first dorsal compartment, which is located in the region of the radial styloid. The extensor pollicis brevis is the more dorsal of the two tendons and inserts on the base of the thumb proximal phalanx. The abductor pollicis brevis tendon lies more volar, often has two or more slips, and inserts on the base of the thumb metacarpal (Fig. 50.2). There is often a septum between the two tendons, which may lead to limited improvement following an injection and persistent pain following surgical treatment if not identified.

De Quervain tenosynovitis occurs in women more commonly than in men, most often occurs in middle age, and develops due to various factors. Most often, patients give a history of chronic overuse of the wrist. The activities include use of the thumb and specifically radial and ulnar deviation of the wrist. The symptoms can develop during pregnancy and

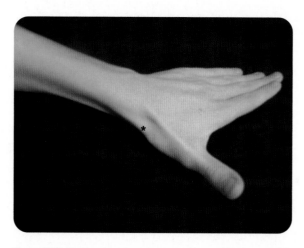

Figure 50.1 The first dorsal compartment, denoted by the *asterisk*, can be found by locating the volar tendons of the wrist snuffbox.

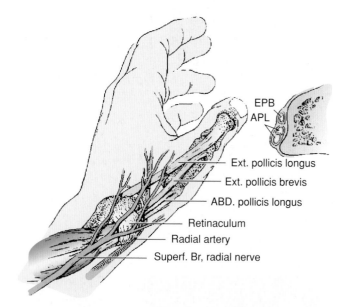

EPB
APL
Ext. pollicis longus
Ext. pollicis brevis
ABD. pollicis longus
Retinaculum
Radial artery
Superf. Br, radial nerve

Figure 50.2 The diagram demonstrates the extensor tendons of the first dorsal compartment. EPB, exterior pollicis brevis, APL, abductor pollicis longus. (From Froimson AI. Tenosynovitis and tennis elbow. In: Green DP, ed. *Operative Hand Surgery*, 2nd ed. New York: Churchill Livingstone; 1988:2118.)

commonly in new mothers due to infant care. Hormonal factors and awkward hand positioning with infant lifting may be related. Patients often note a traumatic event. Direct trauma to the tendon sheath may predate the symptoms, or a wrist fracture may lead to increased stresses across the tendons. The disease occurs more commonly in patients with diabetes mellitus. An inflammatory arthritis such as rheumatoid arthritis may also be related to the development of the process.

Physical Findings

PATIENT ASSESSMENT

1. Pain at the base of the thumb
2. Aggravated with lifting, grasping, or pinching
3. Tenderness along tendons at base of thumb
4. Painful thickening over tendons at base of thumb
5. Painful Finkelstein test (thumb in fist)

On physical examination, swelling is localized to the radial aspect of the wrist. On palpation, patients will have tenderness localized along the tendons of the first dorsal compartment. The tendon sheath will appear thickened and prominence will be noted, which can feel as hard as bone. Occasionally, a small ganglion cyst can be palpated about the extensor retinaculum associated with the tenosynovitis. Wrist range of motion becomes limited as the tenosynovitis progresses in severity. The limitation in motion will occur with flexion, extension, and most significantly ulnar deviation. There are several provocative maneuvers that can be performed in confirming the diagnosis of de Quervain tenosynovitis. These maneuvers are considered positive if they reproduce pain in the region of the first dorsal compartment. The Finkelstein maneuver is performed by having the patient make a fist around the thumb, and the wrist is ulnar deviated (Fig. 50.3). Another maneuver, termed the *hitchhiker sign*, involves having the patient actively radially abduct the thumb against resistance (Fig. 50.4). Brunelli described a similar maneuver that is performed by having the patient actively radially abduct the thumb with the wrist in radial

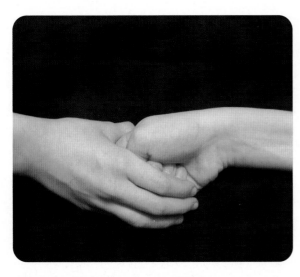

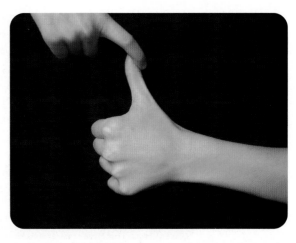

Figure 50.4 The hitchhiker sign is performed by having the patient actively radially abduct the thumb against resistance.

Figure 50.3 The Finkelstein maneuver is performed by having the patient make a fist around the thumb and ulnarly deviating the wrist.

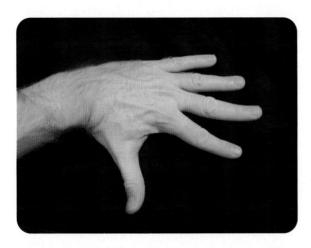

Figure 50.5 The Brunelli test is performed by having the patient actively radially abduct the thumb with the wrist in radial deviation.

deviation[1] (Fig. 50.5). To specifically evaluate for triggering, the patient performs a maneuver with resisted palmar abduction of the thumb followed by adduction and flexion.

The exam should also include maneuvers to differentiate other common causes of radial-sided wrist pain. Patients with thumb carpometacarpal (CMC) arthritis will have localized tenderness more distally at the CMC joint. A thumb CMC grind will reproduce the patient's pain with thumb CMC arthritis. This maneuver involves grasping and rotating the thumb metacarpal while placing an axial load. Crepitation and pain in the CMC joint will occur. Intersection syndrome, a tenosynovitis of the second extensor compartment, leads to pain just proximal to the area of involvement in de Quervain tenosynovitis. Intersection syndrome occurs in the region 4 cm proximal to the radial carpal joint. In this region, the first extensor compartment muscles cross superficial to the extensor carpi radialis brevis and longus tendons of the second extensor compartment. On examination, crepitation will be noted in this region while performing the Finkelstein maneuver. Patients with radial carpal arthritis will have limited wrist range of motion and tenderness at the radial carpal joint rather than the first dorsal extensor compartment.

Studies

The diagnosis of de Quervain tenosynovitis is made after a through history and physical examination. Occasionally, an MRI will be obtained if the diagnosis is in question (Fig. 50.6). On MRI, edema around the tendons of the first dorsal compartment will be noted on the T2-weighted images.

NOT TO BE MISSED

- Thumb CMC arthritis
- Intersection syndrome
- Flexor carpi radialis tendinitis
- Scaphoid fracture
- Radial carpal arthritis

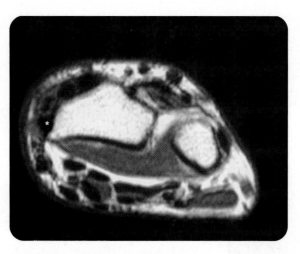

Figure 50.6 MRI T1-weighted axial view of the wrist, with the *asterisk* denoting the first dorsal compartment.

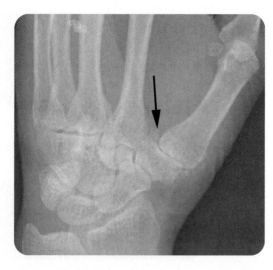

Figure 50.7 The wrist x-ray shows evidence of thumb CMC degenerative joint disease (*arrow*).

These changes are best visualized on the axial views. X-rays are not necessary to determine the diagnosis, although they may show calcific deposits within the region. X-rays are more helpful in ruling out other etiologic factors for radial-sided wrist pain. Arthritic changes about the thumb CMC joint (Fig. 50.7), radial carpal joint, and scaphoid–trapezium–trapezoid region are evaluated on the films. If diabetes or rheumatoid arthritis is suspected, the appropriate laboratory tests are ordered.

Treatment

1. Corticosteroid injection into first dorsal compartment over tendons
2. Splint
3. Surgical release if refractory to conservative care

After the diagnosis of de Quervain tenosynovitis has been made, patients are treated with a variety of nonoperative modalities. The causative activity is modified. Avoidance of repetitive activities and frequent breaks are recommended. A thumb spica wrist splint is used to rest the thumb and wrist. The splint may be prefabricated or custom-molded from orthoplast. The thumb interphalangeal joint does not necessarily need to be immobilized, as the extensor pollicis longus tendon that inserts on the distal phalanx is not affected (Fig. 50.8). The splint is worn on a consistent basis for several weeks until the acute symptoms have improved. The splint is then worn during activities that may aggravate the process. A short course of NSAIDs is helpful in controlling the symptoms. A corticosteroid injection of the first dorsal compartment is performed for patients with persistent symptoms. In a prospective study, Weiss and colleagues[3] have shown better results

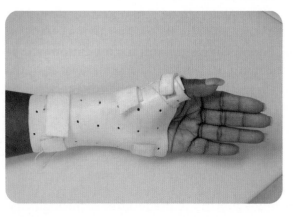

Figure 50.8 A short-arm thumb spica splint can be fabricated for patients with de Quervain tenosynovitis. The thumb interphalangeal joint does not need to be immobilized, as the tendons involved in the tendinitis do not insert onto the distal phalanx.

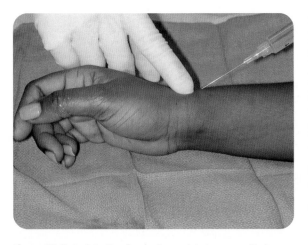

Figure 50.9 An injection for de Quervain's tenosynovitis is performed by palpating the tendons while placing the needle from proximal to distal into the first dorsal compartment.

following a corticosteroid injection than splint immobilization. A long-acting corticosteroid is injected directly into the sheath while palpating the first dorsal compartment (Fig. 50.9). Following the injection, swelling related to the injected fluid is often seen along the distal aspect of the compartment as a sausage shape. Patients should be aware of the risk of altered pigmentation and skin atrophy following an injection in this area. A consultation with a physical or occupational therapist is considered for hydrocortisone iontophoresis, stretching, and review of ergonometric tips.

 Refer to Patient Education

 Refer to Physical Therapy

Clinical Course

The nonoperative treatment of de Quervain tenosynovitis has been reported to be successful in 51% to 90% of patients.[3,4,5] Patients with persistent symptoms despite a course of nonoperative treatment are candidates for surgical treatment. Nonoperative treatment is not as successful when triggering of the first dorsal compartment occurs; therefore, surgical management is considered earlier in this setting than when other etiologic factors are involved. Surgical treatment involves release of the first dorsal compartment retinaculum under local anesthesia.

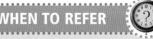

WHEN TO REFER

- Persistent pain despite nonoperative modalities, including the use of a thumb spica splint, NSAIDs, and a corticosteroid injection

ICD9

727.04 Radial styloid tenosynovitis

References

1. Ahuja NK, Chung CK. Fritz de Quervain, MD (1868–1940): stenosing tenosynovitis at the radial styloid process. *J Hand Surg Am* 2004;29:1164–1170.
2. Albertson GM, High WA, Shin AY, et al. Extensor triggering in de Quervain stenosing tenosynovitis. *J Hand Surg Am* 1999;24:1311–1314.
3. Weiss A-PC, Akelman E, Tabatabai M. Treatment of de Quervain disease. *J Hand Surg Am* 1994;19:595–598.
4. Harvey FJ, Harvey PM, Horsley MW. De Quervain's disease: surgical or nonsurgical treatment. *J Hand Surg Am* 1990;15:83–87.
5. Witt J, Pess G, Gelberman RH. Treatment of de Quervain tenosynovitis: a prospective study of the results of injection of steroids and immobilization in a splint. *J Bone Joint Surg Am* 1991;73:219–222.

SECTION 10 Wrist

51 Ganglion Cyst

David Bozentka

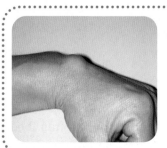

A 20-year-old woman has developed a prominence about the dorsal radial aspect of the wrist. It is not painful and does not limit activities.

CLINICAL POINTS

- The majority of soft tissue masses of the hand and wrist appear to be ganglion cysts.

- Cysts may develop at joints, tendons, or nerves.

- Cysts contain thick, gelatinous material.

- Women are three times more likely to be affected than men.

Clinical Presentation

Ganglion cyst is the most common soft tissue mass of the hand and wrist. Of all soft tissue masses of the hand and wrist, between 50% and 70% are diagnosed as ganglions cysts. The cysts most commonly occur in the second to fourth decades of life. Women are three times more likely than men to develop a ganglion cyst. Most ganglion wrist cysts are asymptomatic and are often present for months to years prior to evaluation. Approximately 10% of patients will give a history of preceding trauma.[1,2] Patients with a cyst may have discomfort that is often described as an ache. Small cysts of the dorsal wrist in the region of the scapholunate ligament tend to be more painful than large cysts. It has been proposed that pain associated with these dorsal wrist cysts is related to impingement of the terminal branch of the posterior interosseous nerve branch, which innervates the dorsal wrist capsule. Therefore, these patients may note pain particularly when the wrist is held in full extension. Volar wrist ganglion cysts occasionally arise from the carpal canal and can lead to compression of the median nerve (Fig. 51.1). In this setting, symptoms of carpal tunnel syndrome may develop, with numbness occurring in the median nerve distribution. Similarly, cysts arising from the volar ulnar carpus may lead to compression of the ulnar nerve at the Guyon canal. These patients may present initially with symptoms of clumsiness and difficulty with fine manipulation due to ulnarly innervated intrinsic muscle weakness. The motor symptoms develop prior to the sensory symptoms because the motor fibers of the nerve are dorsal and the sensory fibers are more volar in the cross-sectional makeup of the ulnar nerve in this region.

Ganglion cysts can arise from a variety of locations, including joints, tendons, and nerves. Wrist joint cysts arise most commonly dorsally from the region of the scapholunate ligament (Fig. 51.2). These dorsal cysts account for approximately 60% to 70% of all ganglion cysts of the hand

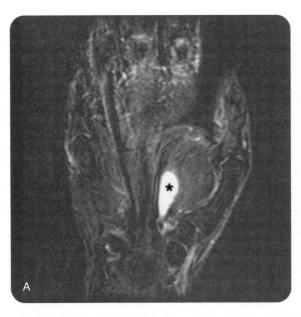
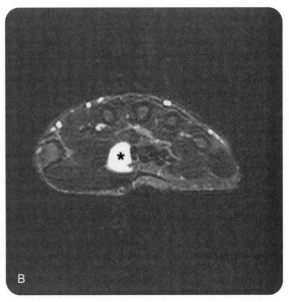

Figure 51.1 MRI wrist T2-weighted images coronal **(A)** and axial **(B)** views demonstrating a ganglion cyst (*asterisk*) arising from the carpal canal, which led to compression of the median nerve.

and wrist. Approximately 20% of wrist cysts arise from the volar aspect of the wrist.[1] These volar cysts most often arise from the radiocarpal joint or scaphotrapezial joints. Volar radial cysts typically lie just radial to the flexor carpi radialis tendon and are often adherent to the radial artery (Fig. 51.3). Ganglion cysts may also arise from the ulnar aspect of the wrist, including the ulnar carpus and distal radial ulnar joint.

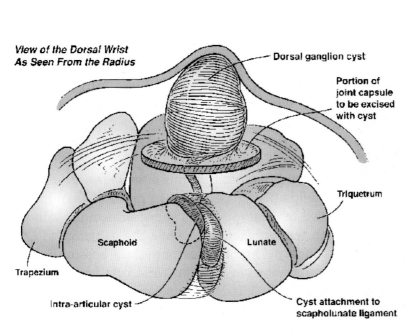

Figure 51.2 Diagrammatic representation of a dorsal wrist ganglion cyst arising from the dorsal scapholunate interval. (From Minotti P, Taras J. Ganglion cysts of the wrist. *J Am Soc Surg Hand* 2002;20(2):104.)

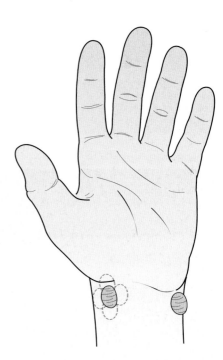

Figure 51.3 Diagrammatic representation of common locations for volar wrist to arise, including the volar radial and ulnar wrist. (Minotti P, Taras J. Ganglion cysts of the wrist. *J Am Soc Surg Hand* 2002;20(2):105.)

The histologic features of a ganglion cyst from the dorsal wrist, volar wrist, dorsal distal interphalangeal joint, and tendon sheath are similar. The outer layer of a ganglion cyst is composed of randomly oriented collagen fibers with a few fibroblasts and mesenchymal cells. There is no synovial tissue within the cyst and no epithelial lining. The thick, gelatinous material contains glucosamine, hyaluronic acid, albumin, and globulin. Injection studies have shown that fluid communicates from the wrist into the cyst but not from the cyst back into the wrist.

There are multiple theories regarding the pathogenesis of ganglion cysts. A herniation of synovial tissue through the wrist capsule has been proposed, although the lack of synovial tissue within the cyst is not consistent. It has been proposed that the leakage of synovial fluid from a rent in the joint capsule may cause an irritation of the surrounding tissue. The local tissue reacts by forming a pseudocapsule. The ganglion fluid develops related to the irritation of the synovial fluid and this tissue. An alternative theory considers mucinous degeneration as the main factor. The breakdown products of collagen collect in pools, leading to the formation of the cyst. Microtrauma involving repetitive stretching of the capsular tissues may also lead to the formation of hyaluronic acid by the mesenchymal cells and fibroblasts.[1,3]

Physical Findings

Ganglion cysts are well-circumscribed, compressible subcutaneous structures. They are firm, rubbery, and often lobulated structures that transilluminate. Small dorsal wrist ganglion cysts may not be palpable unless the wrist is fully flexed. Cysts are typically nontender structures that are not adherent to the skin. Ganglions are slightly moveable but have a pedicle or stalk, which leads to adherence of the cyst to the joint capsule. Occult dorsal wrist ganglion cysts are not palpable, but tenderness is elicited while palpating the dorsal scapholunate interval, which lies just distal to the Lister tubercle of the radius.[4] Pain may be reproduced with the wrist placed in maximal extension. In evaluating a volar radial wrist cyst, it is important to perform an Allen test to determine patency of the radial artery.

The differential diagnosis includes an active tenosynovitis (Figs. 51.4, 51.5). On physical examination, an active tenosynovitis will move proximally and distally with tendon excursion while the ganglion will remain stationary. Carpometacarpal (CMC) bossing, which lies more distal than a dorsal wrist cyst from the scapholunate interval, is often misdiagnosed as a ganglion cyst (Fig. 51.6). The prominence in CMC bossing is due to the bone at the base of the index and long finger metacarpals, and in 50% of patients, a small ganglion may arise from the CMC joint.

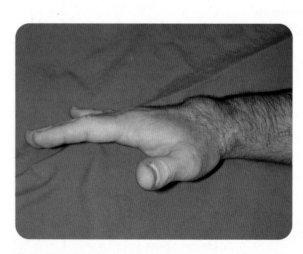

Figure 51.4 Photograph of a patient with extensor tenosynovitis about the dorsal wrist. The prominence becomes more evident with extension of the fingers.

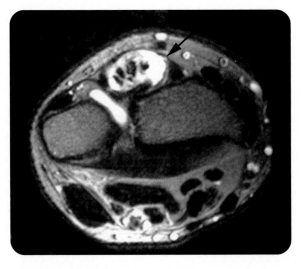

Figure 51.5 MRI T2-weighted axial image of the wrist with edema surrounding the fourth extensor compartment consistent with an active extensor tenosynovitis.

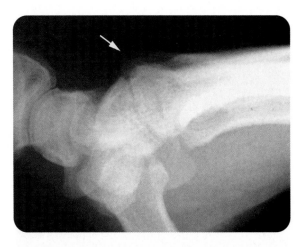

Figure 51.6 A lateral wrist x-ray, with an *arrow* localizing the CMC boss, often misdiagnosed as a ganglion cyst.

SECTION 10 Wrist

Studies

The diagnosis of a ganglion cyst is typically made following a thorough history and physical examination. An aspiration can confirm the diagnosis if gelatinous material consistent with a cyst is obtained. Laboratory studies are not required in the assessment of ganglion cysts. X-rays are unremarkable. MRI is the study of choice to verify the diagnosis. A ganglion cyst will demonstrate high signal intensity on the T2-weighted images. MRI is very helpful in the evaluation of the patient with dorsal radial wrist pain related to a small, nonpalpable ganglion cyst. Ultrasound has been used in the diagnosis of ganglion cysts but is operator dependent. Although less expensive than MRI, ultrasound provides less information in ruling out alternative etiologic factors.

Treatment

1. Some spontaneously resolve
2. Aspiration and injection with cortisone
3. Recurrences can be removed surgically

Asymptomatic ganglion cysts are observed. Studies have shown up to 50% spontaneous resolution of ganglion cysts, with a higher rate in children. Other options include closed compression, aspiration, or surgical excision. Aspiration can be both diagnostic and therapeutic in nature. The gelatinous material aspirated from the cyst will confirm the diagnosis, and 80% of patients will have at least temporary relief of their symptoms. Unfortunately, recurrence is common, and the cyst will recur in >50% of cases following aspiration.[1] A large-bore 18-gauge needle is used to drain the thick, gelatinous fluid, and a corticosteroid can be injected. Dorsal cysts may be aspirated with no significant risk of neurovascular injury. Volar

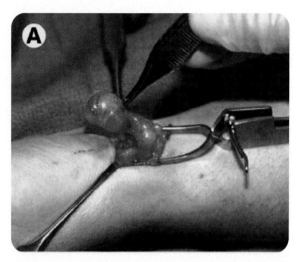

Figure 51.7 Intraoperative photo of a cyst being removed from the dorsal wrist. (Minotti P, Taras J. Ganglion cysts of the wrist. *J Am Soc Surg Hand* 2002;20(2):105.)

radial carpal cysts lie adjacent to the radial artery and its venae comitantes. Aspiration of volar radial carpal cysts risks injury to the vascular structures.

SURGICAL INTERVENTION

Surgical treatment is considered for patients who have a symptomatic cyst despite nonoperative treatment modalities. Cosmesis is often a consideration when the cysts become quite large. The surgical options include an open excision in which the cyst and stalk are removed with a cuff of adjacent capsule (Fig. 51.7). Alternatively, arthroscopic treatment can be performed for certain cysts.

 Refer to Physical Therapy

Clinical Course

A ganglion cyst is the most common soft tissue mass of the wrist and hand. The cysts are usually asymptomatic, and some resolve spontaneously, but occasionally, a cyst will lead to a nerve compression syndrome. Typically, treatment is observation, and if symptomatic, aspiration or excision is considered.

ICD9

727.41 Ganglion of joint
727.42 Ganglion of tendon sheath
727.43 Ganglion, unspecified
727.49 Other ganglion and cyst of synovium, tendon, and bursa

WHEN TO REFER

- Symptomatic cyst despite nonoperative treatment
- Associated nerve palsy

References

1. Minotti P, Taras JS: Ganglion cysts of the wrist. *JASSH* 2002;2:102–107.
2. Nelson CL, Sawmiller S, Phalen G: Ganglions of the wrist and hand. *JBJS* 1972;54:1459–1464.
3. Thornburg LE: Ganglions of the hand and wrist. *J Am Acad Ortho Surg* 1999;7:231–238.
4. Steinberg BD, Kleinman WB. Occult scapholunate ganglion: a cause of dorsoradial wrist pain. *J Hand Surg Am* 1999;24:225–231.

Hand

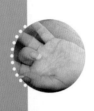

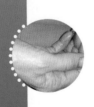
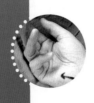

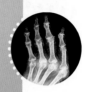
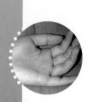

52 Trigger Finger

Jonas L. Matzon and David R. Steinberg

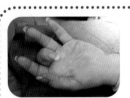

A 52-year-old woman with a past medical history of diabetes mellitus presents with pain in her palm and occasional locking of her long finger.

CLINICAL POINTS

- The inability to smoothly extend or flex the finger is common.

- Pathology is at the metacarpal joint.

- Condition is most common in people >40 years of age.

PATIENT ASSESSMENT

1. Triggering of finger on flexion and extension

2. Tender nodule

3. Common in women and associated with repetitive motion

4. On examination, can feel tender nodule trigger on flexion and extension of the finger

Clinical Presentation

Trigger finger, or stenosing flexor tenosynovitis, is a very common problem seen by primary care physicians, orthopaedic surgeons, and hand surgeons. Patients typically present with a tender nodule located on the palm at the metacarpal head and the inability to smoothly extend or flex the digit. Their complaints are sometimes vague, consisting of aching in the palm and morning stiffness of one or more digits. As the flexor tenosynovitis becomes more severe, patients have increased pain at the nodule and increased triggering that occurs during flexion or prevents them from fully extending the finger. Although the pathology is at the metacarpal joint, patients frequently perceive the triggering as occurring at the proximal interphalangeal (PIP) joint. Early in the disease process, symptoms may improve as the day progresses, but this improvement stops when the tenosynovitis becomes more severe and locking occurs.

Stenosing flexor tenosynovitis results from localized tenosynovitis of the superficial and deep flexor tendons adjacent to the A1 pulley at the metacarpal head. This inflammation causes hypertrophy of the A1 pulley, which leads to discrepancy between the tendon and the tendon sheath. The two types are nodular, with thickening of the tendon on the distal edge of the A1 pulley, and diffuse, with thickening of the entire flexor tenosynovium (more commonly seen in rheumatoid arthritis). It can affect any digit but most commonly affects the ring finger, thumb, and long finger.[1] It is more common in women than men by an approximate 4:1 ratio and occurs most often in people >40 years old. It is associated with medical conditions such as diabetes mellitus, hypothyroidism, gout, renal disease, and rheumatoid arthritis. Patients who develop trigger digits are more likely to be affected by carpal tunnel syndrome and de Quervain stenosing tenosynovitis.

Physical Findings

The diagnosis of trigger finger is usually suspected from the clinical presentation and can be easily confirmed on the physical examination.

SECTION 11 Hand

273

NOT TO BE MISSED

- Impingement of the collateral ligaments on a prominent metacarpal head condyle (locked metacarpophalangeal [MCP] joint)
- Dupuytren disease
- Infection
- Dislocation

Patients usually have a lump or nodule at the A1 pulley that moves with the flexor tendon and that can be readily palpated. In patients with more severe tenosynovitis, the examiner can feel the digit "trigger" as it is flexed and extended. Some patients will present with the digit locked in flexion and may require manipulation to restore full extension.

Based on the physical exam, trigger fingers can be classified based on severity. Grade 0 is mild crepitus in a nontriggering finger, grade 1 is uneven movement of the digit, grade 2 is clicking without locking, grade 3 is locking of the digit that is either actively or passively correctable, and grade 4 is a locked digit.[2]

Studies

Laboratory and radiographic studies are generally not helpful in the diagnosis of trigger finger. They should be obtained when there is a history of trauma (acute or remote) or for trigger thumbs, in which there is a higher association with degenerative changes.[3]

Treatment

1. Corticosteroid injection into tendon sheath (very successful)
2. Surgical release of tendon pulley for failures of injection

Treatment of trigger finger is based on the severity of the disease and the time of presentation in relation to symptom onset. If symptoms are mild and infrequent, observation and avoidance of inciting activities may be sufficient. However, most patients who present with a chief complaint of triggering require some treatment.

In the early stages of tenosynovitis, treatment should consist of NSAIDs and massage. Paraffin or other heat treatments can be effective when multiple fingers are involved. Some physicians advocate the use of custom finger splints, which hold the metacarpalphalangeal joint in 10 to 15 degrees of flexion while allowing the proximal and distal interphalangeal joints to move freely (Fig. 52.1). The splint should be worn continuously for an average of 3 to 6 weeks, and therefore this form of therapy is highly dependent on patient compliance.[4] Corticosteroid injections are the next form of nonoperative treatment. They have a success rate of approximately 50% to 90%, but there is a high rate of recurrence.[5] Water-soluble steroids such as betamethasone sodium phosphate and acetate suspension are preferred because they do not precipitate, leaving a residue. Although protocols vary, a 25- to 27-gauge needle is used to inject 0.5 to 1.0 mL of corticosteroid and 0.5 to 1.0 mL of 1% lidocaine (Xylocaine) into the tendon sheath. The injection can be performed from either a lateral or palmar approach, with care being taken to avoid the neurovascular bundle)

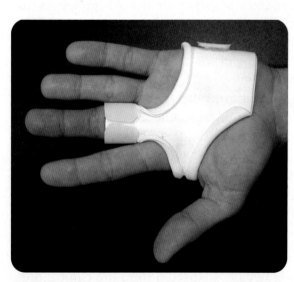

Figure 52.1 Custom-molded, hand-based trigger finger splint immobilizing the MCP joint.

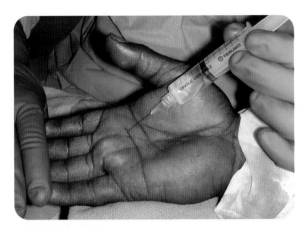

Figure 52.2 Standard technique for injection of a flexor tendon sheath.

(Fig. 52.2). Refer to Chapter 72 for more information. Complications such as depigmentation, fat necrosis, flare reaction, and hyperglycemia should be discussed with patient. Injections are less likely to be successful in patients with triggering for >6 months, diffuse tenosynovitis, and diabetes mellitus. Usually, lack of improvement after two or three injections constitutes failure of nonoperative management.

While stenosing tenosynovitis is relatively responsive to nonoperative treatment, a fixed digit or failure of corticosteroid injections is an indication that surgery is necessary. Operative treatment of nodular tenosynovitis involves either open or percutaneous release of the A1 pulley (Fig. 52.3). Both procedures are generally safe and effective. The main risk is neurovascular injury to the digital nerves or vessels, but this complication occurs infrequently. While percutaneous release avoids a scar and can be done in the office setting, it has a higher rate of incomplete pulley release and nerve injury, particularly in the thumb and index and small fingers. Diffuse flexor tenosynovitis requires an extensive tenosynovectomy with preservation of all pulleys (including A1).

 Refer to Patient Education

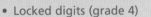
WHEN TO REFER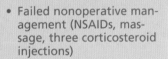

- Locked digits (grade 4)
- Failed nonoperative management (NSAIDs, massage, three corticosteroid injections)

Clinical Course

Most patients with trigger fingers can be treated conservatively, with avoidance of irritation and corticosteroid injection. If three injections fail

SECTION 11 Hand

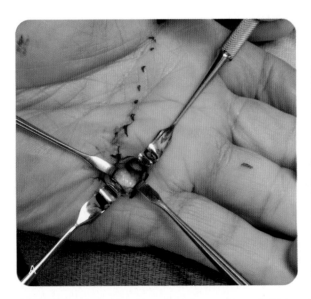
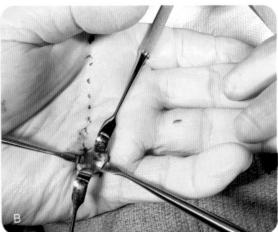

Figure 52.3 Intraoperative open trigger finger release. **A:** Thickened sheath overlying the flexor tendon. **B:** Tendon can be seen easily after incision through the A1 pulley.

and symptoms persist more than 3 to 6 months, then surgical release is very successful.

> *ICD9*
>
> *727.03 Trigger finger (acquired)*

References

1. Freiberg A, Mullholland RS, Levine R. Nonoperative treatment of trigger fingers and thumbs. *J Hand Surg Am* 1989;14:553–558.
2. Patel MR, Moradia VA. Percutaneous release of trigger digit with and without cortisone injection. *J Hand Surg Am* 1997;22:150–155.
3. Katzman BM, Bozentka DJ, Steinberg DR, et al. The utility of obtaining radiographs in patients with trigger finger. *Amer J Orthop* 1999;28(12):703–705.
4. Ryzewicz M, Wolf JM. Trigger digits: principles, management, and complications. *J Hand Surg Am* 2006;31:135–146.
5. Patel MR, Bassini L. Trigger fingers and thumb: when to splint, inject, or operate. *J Hand Surg Am* 1992;17:110–113.

CHAPTER 53 Ganglia of the Hand

Jonas L. Matzon and David R. Steinberg

A 58-year-old woman presents with an unsightly finger mass.

CLINICAL POINTS

- Masses of the finger are common.
- Patients typically are young adults.
- Ganglia contain thick, mucinous fluid.

PATIENT ASSESSMENT

1. Tender masses in flexor sheath in palm at the level of the PIP joint or distal joint.
2. First recognized with grasping objects or making tight fists
3. Rarely painful

Clinical Presentation

While ganglia of the wrist are more common, ganglion cysts of the hand may also be encountered by the primary care physician. Patients typically present with a finger mass that fluctuates in size and may be painful (depending on its location). Hand ganglia typically manifest in one of three forms: flexor sheath cyst, proximal interphalangeal (PIP) mass, or mucous cyst.

The flexor sheath ganglion (volar retinacular or "seed" ganglion) usually arises between the A1 and A2 pulleys of the flexor tendon sheath chief. Most patients are young adults who complain of pain when grasping objects or making a tight fist. Ganglia of the PIP joint usually affect middle-aged adults and may arise either from the extensor mechanism or directly from the PIP joint capsule. Patients may recall blunt trauma to the dorsal joint that initiated the process. They may be bothered by the appearance of the mass or complain of a tight joint when attempting to make a fist. Mucous cysts often present in older adults and commonly are associated with osteoarthritis of the distal interphalangeal (DIP) joint. These are rarely painful. Patients are often concerned with cosmesis or with drainage when these occasionally rupture spontaneously.

Ganglia consist of thick, mucinous fluid comprised of glucosamine, hyaluronic acid, albumin, and globulin that is surrounded by an acellular fibrous wall. However, the pathogenesis of ganglia is controversial. Some physicians believe that ganglions result from herniation of the synovial lining and collection of joint fluid. Others speculate that ganglia arise from synovial fluid leakage and subsequent irritation of the surrounding soft tissue and formation of a capsule. A few authors believe that ganglia may originate from mucoid degeneration of connective tissue and subsequent cyst formation.[1]

Physical Findings

The clinical presentation of ganglia is classic, and diagnosis can usually be made on the basis of history and physical examination. The hand should

NOT TO BE MISSED

- Infection
- Osteoarthritis
- Tenosynovitis
- Giant cell tumor
- Lipoma
- Soft tissue sarcoma

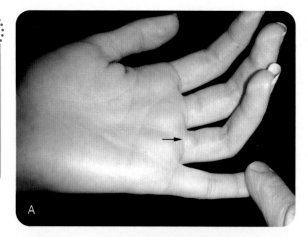

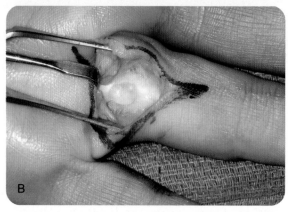

Figure 53.1 A: Flexor sheath ganglion at the base of the ring finger. **B:** Intraoperative appearance of the flexor sheath ganglion, in this case arising from the less common location of the distal aspect of the A2 pulley.

be inspected and palpated in standard fashion. A flexor sheath ganglion usually presents as a small, firm, mobile volar mass at the level of the proximal digital flexion crease (Fig. 53.1). These are occasionally seen in conjunction with a trigger digit. A good neurovascular examination of the finger must be performed to ensure that the mass is not causing any digital nerve compression. The PIP ganglion arises over the dorsolateral aspect of the joint and is relatively fixed in position (Fig. 53.2A). The mucous cyst presents as an immobile dorsal mass anywhere between the DIP joint and eponychial fold (cuticle). The skin over the cyst may be attenuated. Ridges or pitting of the nail may occur secondary to pressure on the germinal matrix (Fig. 53.3). The mucous cyst should be evaluated for warmth and erythema to rule out infection if there is any history of drainage.

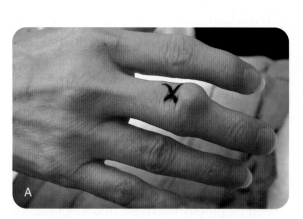

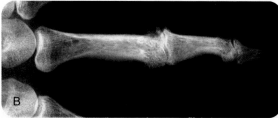

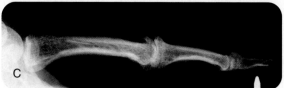

Figure 53.2 A: Clinical appearance of the PIP joint ganglion of the long finger. **B:** PA radiograph of associated PIP arthritis. **C:** Lateral radiograph of associated PIP arthritis.

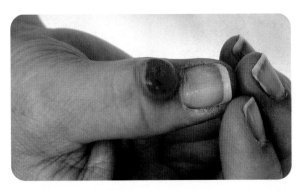

Figure 53.3 Large mucous cyst of the thumb, with attenuated skin and early nail changes.

Studies

Laboratory tests are generally not helpful in the diagnosis of ganglion cyst. However, if there is any suspicion of associated infection (e.g., draining mucous cyst), it is reasonable to check a CBC, CRP, and ESR.

Although a ganglion cyst is usually a clinical diagnosis, imaging is useful when the diagnosis is not obvious. Radiographs of the hand will document any significant arthritis (Fig. 53.2B,C). Ultrasonography and MRI, while occasionally helpful in the diagnosis of wrist ganglia, are rarely indicated for ganglion cysts of the digits.

Treatment

1. Aspiration and corticosteroid injections
2. Excision if they recur

Treatment of ganglions is dependent on the patient's age, symptoms, and wishes. Most ganglions can be treated successfully by nonoperative measures, with spontaneous resolution occurring up to 50% of the time. The key when using this treatment option is reassuring the patient regarding the benign nature of the mass. This is the treatment of choice in children, who have an even higher rate of spontaneous resolution.[2]

While conservative management is a viable option, it is a difficult one for patients to accept if they are symptomatic. In this case, there are several considerations. Closed rupture, at one time a common form of treatment, can still be performed today with firm massage. It is not commonly advocated because recurrence rate is extremely high; it should not be performed on a mucous cyst with attenuated skin due to risk of skin slough. Intermittent splinting of the DIP joint may decrease arthritic pain (Chapter 73). The next consideration is needle aspiration, which serves two functions. First, it allows withdrawal of diagnostic fluid that can be sent to pathology for definitive diagnosis. Second, it may give the patient some pain relief. However, it is associated with long-term recurrence rates of approximately 50%. It should be performed cautiously (if at all) and under sterile conditions for mucous cysts; the paucity of soft tissues in this area increases the risk of developing septic arthritis of the DIP joint.[3]

For patients with persistent pain and symptoms, the treatment of choice is open surgical excision. It is important to excise the cyst, its stalk, and a sleeve of normal capsule, because this decreases recurrence rates to approximately 5%.[4] Débridement of associated osteophytes of the PIP or DIP joints also minimizes risk of recurrence. Postoperatively, the patients are briefly splinted. Overall, the procedure is well tolerated, with the major complication being recurrence.

WHEN TO REFER

- Persistent pain or symptoms
- Mucous cyst associated with painful joint or impending skin breakdown
- Desire to have ganglion excised
- Unsure of benign nature of mass

Clinical Course

If asymptomatic, ganglia cysts in the hand can be treated conservatively. They may persist for long periods of time and spontaneously resolve. However, many do cause symptoms, and then they can be aspirated and injected or excised. Recurrences can occur.

ICD9

727.42 Ganglion of tendon sheath

References

1. Thornburg L. Ganglions of the hand and wrist. *J Am Acad Orthop Surg* 1999;7:231–238.
2. Donthineni-Rao R. Tumors. In: Beredjiklian PK, Bozentka DJ, eds. *Review of Hand Surgery*. Philadelphia: Elsevier; 2004:189–205.
3. Steinberg DR. Management of the arthritic hand. In: Chapman MW, ed. *Chapman's Orthopaedic Surgery*, 3rd ed. Philadelphia: Lippincott Williams & Wilkins; 2001:1943–1956.
4. Nelson CL, Sawmiller S, Phalen GS. Ganglions of the wrist and hand. *J Bone Joint Surg Am* 1979;54:1459.

CHAPTER 54 Heberden Nodes

Jonas L. Matzon and David R. Steinberg

 A 63-year-old male laborer presents with chronic pain in the distal aspect of his index finger.

CLINICAL POINTS

- Patients complain of deep, achy pain that is aggravated by activity.
- Decreased range of motion may eventually result.
- Enlargement of the distal interphalangeal (DIP) joint is characteristic.

PATIENT ASSESSMENT

1. Related to osteoarthritis of the DIP joints of the fingers
2. Common in women
3. Nodules on the sides of the joints
4. Tender at first but painless later
5. Associated with enlargement of the DIP joints
6. Associated with limitation in motion of the DIP joints
7. X-ray changes of degenerative joint disease

Clinical Presentation

Osteoarthritis is an idiopathic, degenerative condition that frequently occurs in the hand. Most commonly involved, in descending order, are the DIP joint, the carpometacarpal (CMC) joint of the thumb (Chapter 55), the proximal interphalangeal (PIP) joint, and the metacarpophalangeal (MCP) joint. Patients usually present complaining of joint pain and joint deformity or enlargement. Pain is usually described as deep and achy and is worse with activity. Over time, as the joints enlarge, patients often describe decreased range of motion, crepitation, and morning stiffness. This diffuse enlargement of the DIP joint, due to osteophytes, synovitis, and capsular thickening, is referred to as a *Heberden node*. The Bouchard node describes the analogous condition of the PIP joint. Some patients may also notice a slowly enlarging, discrete subcutaneous mass over the distal DIP joint, which is firm and minimally mobile. This is usually consistent with a mucous cyst (Chapter 53).

Physical Findings

The clinical presentation of hand arthritis is relatively straightforward. A careful and complete examination of the hand should be performed. First, the hand should be inspected for deformity, with special attention being paid to the PIP and DIP joints and the nails. Usually, marked enlargement of the joints is present. Passive and active range of motion of all joints of the hand should be assessed. During this testing, any pain and/or crepitation should be noted. Oftentimes, range of motion is markedly decreased and accompanied by some mild pain and crepitation. However, pain with micromotion in any joint and associated signs of infection such as purulent drainage, erythema, and warmth is extremely concerning for septic arthritis. Next, the joints should be palpated for tenderness. Finally, all of the joints should be assessed for range of motion and varus/valgus instability to rule out associated collateral ligament attenuation. If concern exists regarding a systemic inflammatory condition, other joints

SECTION 11 Hand

281

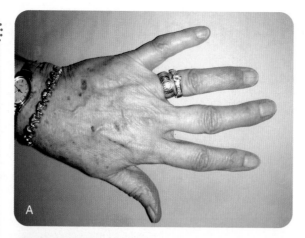

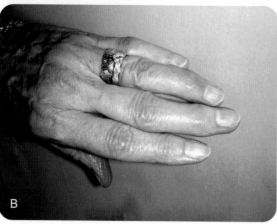

Figure 54.1 A: Clinical appearance of erosive osteoarthritis, with significant involvement of the long and small finger PIP joints and multiple DIP joints **(B)**.

should also be assessed. A more aggressive form of degenerative arthritis is erosive osteoarthritis, which can affect both PIP and DIP joints (Fig. 54.1 and 54.4). It can be differentiated from inflammatory arthritis by lack of systemic symptoms as well as absence of MCP joint involvement.[1]

Studies

Along with clinical history, radiographs are the most important tool for diagnosing arthritis of the hand. X-rays should at minimum include PA, lateral, and oblique views of the hand. If the patient is only complaining of pain in one digit, then the radiographs can be centered on the area of interest and only involve a PA and lateral view of the specific finger (Fig. 54.2). When viewing the x-rays, the four radiographic signs of osteoarthritis are joint space narrowing, osteophyte formation, sclerosis, and subchondral cysts (Fig. 54.3). More severe joint destruction is seen in cases of erosive osteoarthritis (Fig. 54.4). All radiographic findings must be correlated with clinical history and examination before determining a diagnosis.

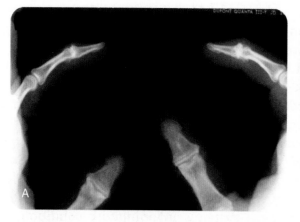

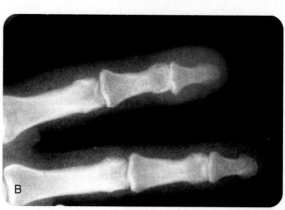

Figure 54.2 A: Lateral and **(B)** PA radiographs of a presenting patient with isolated Heberden nodes.

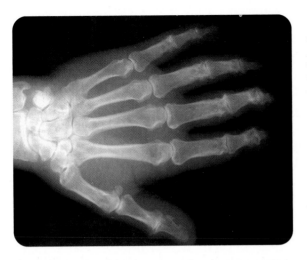

Figure 54.3 More advanced radiographic changes in multiple DIP joints with standard osteoarthritis.

Laboratory values are important in ruling out other diagnoses. If multiple joints are involved or patients present with inflammatory conditions of other organ systems (i.e., rashes, conjunctivitis, urethritis), rheumatologic labs including RF, ANA titer, anti-dsDNA titer, and HLA-B27 antigen should be ordered. Rheumatology consultation should be considered if any of these laboratory values are positive. If infection is a concern, CBC, ESR, and CRP should be checked.

Treatment

1. Modify activities
2. Occasional NSAIDs
3. Rarely, fusion of the DIP joint

Osteoarthritis of the hand is a common problem in the general population, and treatment is adapted to each patient based on the severity of the problem. Management usually begins with activity modification and NSAIDs, which often decrease pain to a tolerable level. Occasionally, this can be supplemented with a corticosteroid injection, but injections should be limited to three in one location (Chapter 72). A hand therapist can fashion orthoplast splints, apply paraffin and other modalities, and provide adaptive aids to assist with activities of daily living.

SECTION 11 Hand

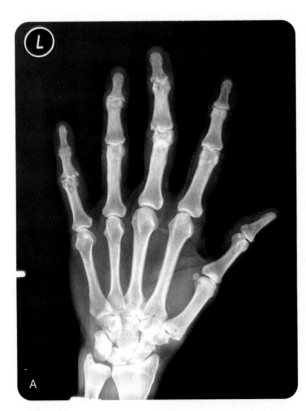

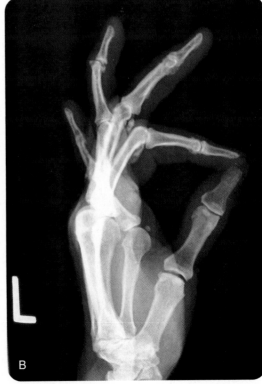

Figure 54.4 A: PA and lateral **(B)** radiographs of the patient from Figure 54.1 with erosive osteoarthritis.

WHEN TO REFER

- Failure of conservative management[4]
- Septic arthritis[4]
- Unstable interphalangeal joints interfering with hand function[4]
- Mucous cyst associated with painful joint or impending skin breakdown[4]

Failure to control pain and disability with these conservative options mandates consideration of surgical options. At the DIP joint, mucous cysts can be aspirated or surgically excised with débridement of phalangeal osteophytes. Otherwise, definitive treatment of osteoarthritis at the DIP joint is arthrodesis (fusion) in 0 to 15 degrees of flexion. At the PIP joint, mucous cysts are less common but are treated in the same fashion. However, definitive treatment of osteoarthritis at the PIP joint includes not only arthrodesis in 30 to 45 degrees of flexion but also arthroplasty.[2] Which digits are best served by fusion and which by arthroplasty remains a point of controversy.[2-6]

Clinical Course

The nodes reflect the degree of arthritis in the hand. As with all osteoarthritis, it progresses slowly and is only symptomatic with activity. In the hand, the nodes are cosmetically unpleasing and probably cause more concern than the symptoms. Most patients eventually accept the appearance and learn to manage the functional disability of the arthritis.

ICD9

715.04 Osteoarthrosis, generalized, involving hand

References

1. Marmor L, Peter JB. Osteoarthritis of the hand. *Clin Orthop* 1969;64:164.
2. Linscheid RL. Implant arthroplasty of the hand: retrospective and prospective considerations. *J Hand Surg Am* 2000;25:796–816.
3. Naidu S, Temple JD. Arthritis. In: Beredjiklian PK, Bozentka DJ, eds. *Review of Hand*. Philadelphia: Elsevier; 2004:171–187.
4. Steinberg DR. Management of the arthritic hand. In: Chapman MW ed. *Chapman's Orthopaedic Surgery*, 3rd ed. Philadelphia: Lippincott Williams & Wilkins; 2001:1943–1956.
5. Steinberg DR. Osteoarthritis of the hand. In: Fitzgerald RH, Kaufer H, Malkani AL, eds. *Orthopaedics*. St. Louis: Mosby; 2002:1830–1836.
6. Wright PE. Arthritic hand. In: Canale ST, ed. *Campbell's Operative Orthopaedics*, Vol. 4. Philadelphia: Elsevier; 2003:3689–3737.

CHAPTER 55

Osteoarthritis at the Base of the Thumb (Carpometacarpal Joint)

Jonas L. Matzon and David R. Steinberg

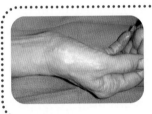

A 55-year-old right-hand–dominant female laborer presents with chronic pain at the base of her thumb that worsens with pinch.

CLINICAL POINTS

- Onset is usually insidious.
- The condition may not have a traumatic stimulus.
- More severe disease makes activities of daily living increasingly difficult.

PATIENT ASSESSMENT

1. Most common site for symptomatic arthritis in the body, occurring at the base of the thumb
2. More common in women
3. Increased incidence with age
4. Made worse with activities that utilize the thumb
5. Pain at the base of the thumb
6. Swelling and tenderness at the base of the thumb
7. X-rays show degenerative joint disease

Clinical Presentation

Osteoarthritis of the base of the thumb is the most common arthritis in the hand that requires surgical management. Approximately 25% of women and 10% of men will ultimately develop radiographic evidence of osteoarthritis of the thumb carpometacarpal (CMC) joint. The reason for this high incidence is the unusual anatomy of the joint, which has a saddle joint architecture with little intrinsic osseous stability. This allows the thumb to move in three planes of motion (flexion–extension, abduction–adduction, and opposition) but also subjects it to high forces. Other risk factors associated with thumb CMC osteoarthritis are age, female gender, obesity, mechanical stress, hypermobility, and traumatic injuries.[1]

Most patients present with radial-sided hand or thumb pain that started insidiously without trauma and has been ongoing for at least a few months. The pain is exacerbated by daily activities that utilize the thumb, such as writing and turning door knobs and is improved with rest and pain medications. As the disease progresses, it becomes more and more difficult to perform tasks of daily living.

Physical Findings

The diagnosis of CMC arthritis can usually be made by correlating the history, physical examination, and radiographs. On physical exam, inspection may reveal a prominence at the dorsoradial base of the thumb metacarpal. Palpation of this prominence will usually produce tenderness. Depending on the severity of the disease, pain may be produced by palpating the scaphotrapezial joint as well. Range of motion should be performed in all planes and compared with the contralateral side. It may be decreased secondary to pain or increased early in the disease secondary

NOT TO BE MISSED

- De Quervain tenosynovitis
- Metacarpophalangeal (MCP), intercarpal, or radiocarpal arthritis
- Compression of radial sensory nerve (Wartenberg syndrome)
- Trigger thumb

to soft tissue insufficiency. Provocative maneuvers include the CMC grind test, which involves axial thumb loading with metacarpal rotation to produce pain and trapeziometacarpal joint distraction, which stretches an inflamed capsule to reproduce symptoms. The Finkelstein maneuver (forced ulnar deviation of the wrist with flexed thumb), which is considered pathognomonic for de Quervain tenosynovitis, may also be positive in this condition.

Studies

Laboratory studies are generally not helpful in the diagnosis of CMC arthritis. Radiographic studies are necessary to evaluate the stage of disease. Three views of the base of the thumb are the minimum x-rays that are required. More advanced views include a basal joint stress view, which is a PA 30-degree oblique view centered on both thumbs and taken with the patient pressing the opposing thumb tips together. These x-rays can be used to stage the disease.[2] In stage I, there is no joint destruction, but joint space widening secondary to synovitis may occur (Fig. 55.1). Stage II involves mild joint space narrowing with osteophytes >2 mm (Fig. 55.2). Stage III involves significant trapeziometacarpal joint space narrowing and osteophytes >2 mm (Fig. 55.3). Stage IV involves pantrapezial arthritis (trapeziometacarpal and scaphotrapezial joint involvement) (Fig. 55.4). It is important to correlate x-ray findings to patient symptoms because

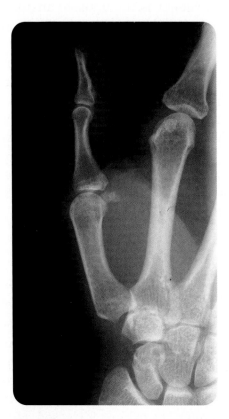

Figure 55.1 Stage I thumb CMC osteoarthritis, manifested by slight joint space widening.

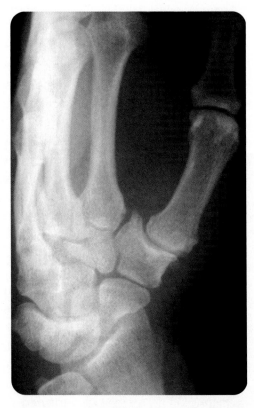

Figure 55.2 Stage II thumb CMC osteoarthritis, with small peripheral osteophytes and mild lateral subluxation of the joint.

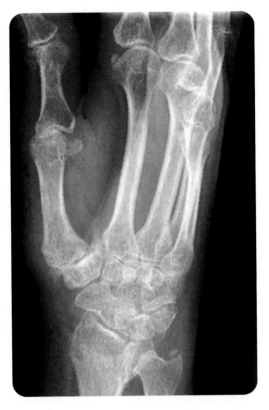

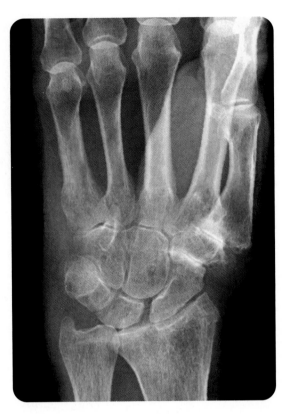

Figure 55.3 Stage III thumb CMC osteoarthritis, with significant loss of joint space and larger osteophytes.

Figure 55.4 Stage IV thumb CMC osteoarthritis, with severe involvement of both the CMC and scaphotrapezial joints.

SECTION 11 Hand

treatment decisions are based predominantly on symptoms. More advanced imaging such as CT, MRI, or ultrasound is not helpful.

Treatment

1. NSAIDs
2. Intra-articular cortisone injections
3. Splinting in thumb spica
4. Late stages require surgical management for relief of pain

Treatment of CMC arthritis starts with conservative management regardless of the stage of disease. The patient is advised to modify activities that exacerbate the pain, which may involve alternating hand use and also switching to bigger grips for pens, golf clubs, and such. The patient is also started on a short 3-week course of NSAIDs. Furthermore, the patient is given a thumb spica splint to wear at all times for approximately 3 weeks and then part-time for another 3 weeks. Finally, the physician may consider corticosteroid injection into the CMC joint (Chapter 72). The combined treatment of splinting for 3 weeks and a single corticosteroid injection has shown reliable long-term relief in thumbs with Eaton stage I disease.[3]

If nonoperative management fails and the patient continues to have persistent pain and disability, operative treatment is indicated regardless of the stage of disease. However, the stage of disease influences which

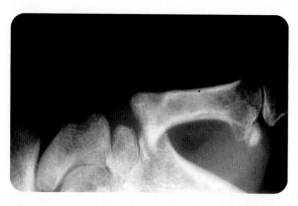

Figure 55.5 Postoperative radiograph of trapezial resection/ligament reconstruction (LRTI). Base of the metacarpal was also resected. Reconstructed joint space has been maintained.

procedure is performed. The surgical options include open versus arthroscopic CMC synovectomy and debridement, metacarpal osteotomy, ligament reconstruction, trapeziectomy with or without tendon interposition, trapeziectomy with ligament reconstruction and tendon interposition (LRTI), trapeziometacarpal arthrodesis, and prosthetic arthroplasty[2,4,5] (Fig. 55.5). Overall, surgical management results in decreased pain and increased grip and pinch strength. The major risks are injury to the superficial radial nerve and the radial artery. The surgeon must also address any compensatory hyperextension deformity of the MCP joint.

Clinical Course

The clinical course of patients with CMC joint arthritis is similar to other joints with osteoarthritis. The arthritis gradually becomes more severe, symptoms are usually intermittent, and it usually takes decades for them to become very severe. The symptoms will depend on activity. Surgical alternatives are satisfactory but should be reserved for patients failing conservative therapy for a prolonged period of time and having significant structural changes within the joint.

ICD9

715.14 Osteoarthrosis, localized, primary, involving hand
715.24 Osteoarthrosis, localized, secondary, involving hand
715.34 Osteoarthrosis, localized, not specified whether primary or secondary, involving hand

WHEN TO REFER

- Failure of nonoperative treatment
- Symptomatic stage III or IV disease
- Severe compensatory MCP joint hyperextension deformity

References

1. Haara MM, Heliovaara M, Kroger H, et al. Osteoarthritis in the carpometacarpal joint of the thumb: prevalence and associations with disability and mortality. *J Bone Joint Surg Am* 2004;86:1452–1457.
2. Eaton RG, Glickel SZ. Trapeziometacarpal osteoarthritis: staging as a rationale for treatment. *Hand Clin* 1987;3:455–471.
3. Day CS, Gelberman RH, Patel AA, et al. Basal joint osteoarthritis of the thumb: a prospective trial of steroid injection and splinting. *J Hand Surg Am* 2004;29:247–251.
4. Barron OA, Glickel SZ, Eaton RG. Basal joint arthritis of the thumb. *J Am Acad Orthop Surg* 2000;8:314–323.
5. Naidu S, Temple JD. Arthritis. In: Beredjiklian PK, Bozentka DJ, eds. *Review of Hand Surgery*. Philadelphia: Elsevier; 2004:171–187.

56 Dupuytren Contracture

Stephan G. Pill and David R. Steinberg

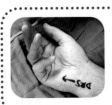

A 60-year-old diabetic male presents with gradual onset of stiffness and inability to straighten his left small and ring fingers.

Clinical Presentation

Dupuytren contracture is a relatively common disorder of the hand that is characterized by progressive fibrosis and contracture of the palmar fascia. It most commonly affects middle-aged men of northern European descent and has been associated with tobacco use and alcohol intake,[1] diabetes mellitus, epilepsy, and, possibly, HIV infection. Although most cases are sporadic, an autosomal dominant form with variable penetrance exists. Patients with inherited forms are typically younger and may also present with plantar fibromatosis (Leder-hosen disease) and penile fibrosis (Peyronie disease).

Initially, there is painless thickening of the palmar fascia that may go unnoticed. These nodules may cause transient pain that is usually self-limited. They coalesce into thick, longitudinal cords, causing a progressive loss of full extension and joint stiffness. The scarring process results in the formation of thick cords in the pretendinous bands of the palmar fascia that extend into the digits, skin dimpling, and flexion contracture at the metacarpophalangeal (MCP) and proximal interphalangeal (PIP) joints (Fig. 56.1). The ulnar side of both hands is involved in most patients, with the ring and small fingers usually affected earliest. Web space contractures can also occur, predominantly the thumb–index web space (Fig. 56.2). Patients usually complain of finger stiffness of the involved fingers. They may have difficulty reaching their hand into a pants pocket or grabbing large objects.

Physical Findings

Dupuytren contracture is a clinical diagnosis based on the history of painless stiffness of the fingers and physical examination. An early sign is skin dimpling over the flexor tendon just proximal to the flexor crease of the finger. Passive extension of the affected fingers will exaggerate the dimple as the tendon courses over the head of the metacarpal. The nodules are visible or palpable, overlying the flexor tendons, and there may be

CLINICAL POINTS

- Complaints of stiffness of involved fingers is common.
- The ulnar side of both hands is usually affected.
- Disease may be acquired or inherited.

PATIENT ASSESSMENT

1. Progressive fibrosis and contracture in the palmar fascia
2. Middle-aged man
3. Usually, painless thickening of the palmar fascia
4. Progressive loss of extension

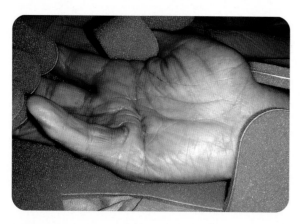

Figure 56.1 Dupuytren cord, causing dimpling of palmar skin and 30-degree MCP flexion contracture.

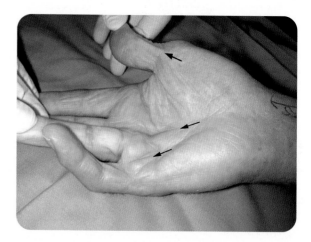

Figure 56.2 Multiple cords (*arrows*) involving the thumb, MCP contracture of the ring finger, and PIP contracture of the small finger.

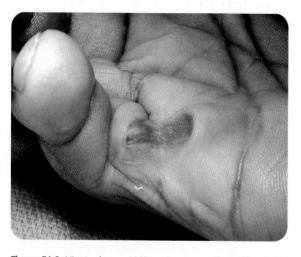

Figure 56.3 Ninety-degree MCP contracture, with significant skin involvement that will require dermatofasciectomy.

thickening of the palm. The range of motion of the MCP and PIP joints is reduced, and a flexion contracture may be present. Bilateral involvement is present in about 50% of cases. More advanced cases may involve significant portions of skin (Fig. 56.3).

Differential Diagnosis

Flexor tenosynovitis
Diabetic cheiroarthropathy
Camptodactyly
Traumatic scars
Ulnar neuropathy/Claw deformity
Volkmann ischemic contracture
Intrinsic joint disease

NOT TO BE MISSED

- Kanavel signs of suppurative flexor tenosynovitis:

  1. Tenderness along the flexor tendon sheath

  2. Pain with passive extension

  3. Flexed finger

  4. Fusiform swelling of the finger

- Complex regional pain syndrome (previously known as *reflex sympathetic dystrophy*)

- Palmar fascial fibrosis: all fingers equally affected, frequently associated with a malignant neoplasm

Studies

Laboratory tests and diagnostic imaging are not necessary, as the diagnosis of Dupuytren contracture can be made by taking a careful history and physical examination. Radiographs may be helpful in long-standing contractures to ensure that the joints remain in good condition.

Treatment

1. Early painless nodules require no treatment.
2. With >30 degrees of PIP contracture, consider excision of the palmar fascia.

Initial management is focused on preventing progression of the disease. For mild disease, daily passive hyperextension stretches can be prescribed along with avoiding tight-grasping activities. For patients with persistent painful nodules and local tenderness, intralesional injection with triamcinolone acetonide, cortisone, or lidocaine hydrochloride may reduce symptoms. Injections are particularly effective in patients with recent onset of the disease, as long-standing scar tissue does not respond as well to injection. Small, painless nodules and MCP joint contractures of <30 degrees can generally be observed.

A multitude of nonsurgical therapies have been tried (and discarded) with marginal success rates for treating the flexion contractures. These include injections of corticosteroid and hyaluronic acid, prophylactic external beam radiation therapy, continuous slow skeletal traction, and ultrasound therapy. Enzymatic fasciotomy with clostridial collagenase injections has shown encouraging results, particularly in dealing with MCP joint flexion contracture.[2] Clinical trials are currently being performed.

Surgery is an option for patients who have considerable functional impairment, MCP joint contractures >30 degrees, or any PIP contracture. A variety of surgical options are available.[3] A partial or complete palmar fasciectomy is the procedure of choice. More than 80% of patients can expect a full recovery, although recurrence rate is about 10% per year.[4] Skin flaps must be handled with care to promote wound healing and decrease scar formation. Release of MCP joint contractures often yields satisfactory results with excellent restoration of motion. However, patients with PIP joint involvement and those with recurrent disease tend to have less successful surgical outcomes. Although these patients initially do well after surgery, the recurrence rate is high, particularly among younger patients. The need for amputation is rare, and it is reserved for severe, long-standing contractures of the small finger. In the medically compromised patient, limited open fasciotomy or percutaneous release under local anesthesia have met with some success. Dermatofasciectomy may be used for patients with diffuse disease or skin involvement[5] (Fig. 56.3). The wounds are then covered with full-thickness skin grafts or are allowed to heal by secondary intention. Complications of these surgeries include hematoma formation, neurovascular injury, scar contracture, stiffness, and complex regional pain syndrome.

Clinical Course

Dupuytren contracture runs a variable course. Some patients maintain a high level of function for many years. In others, fibrous bands radiate distally and cause severe contraction and dysfunction (Fig. 56.4). In general,

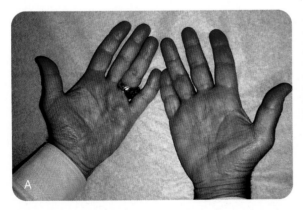
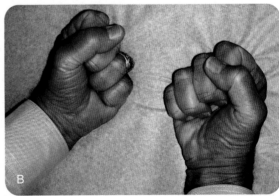

Figure 56.4 Postoperative result after release of bilateral small and ring finger contractures: digital extension **(A)** and flexion **(B)**.

SECTION 11 Hand

WHEN TO REFER

- MCP joint contractures >30 degrees
- Progressive PIP contracture
- Impending skin breakdown/ Infection
- Significant functional impairments resulting from the deformity or persistent discomfort with conservative therapy

patients with inherited forms tend to have more severe disease, higher recurrence, and poor outcomes. Recurrence of flexion contractures can be minimized if the postoperative protocol includes nighttime use of a forearm-based extension splint (out to the fingertips) for 3 months after surgery.

ICD9

728.6 Contracture of palmar fascia

References

1. Godtfredsen N, Lucht H, Prescott E, et al. A prospective study linked both alcohol and tobacco to Dupuytren's disease. *J Clin Epidem* 2004;57(8):858–863.
2. Badalamente MA, Hurst LC, Hentz VR. Collagen as a clinical target: nonoperative treatment of Dupuytren's disease. *J Hand Surg Am* 2002;27:788–798.
3. Skoff HD. The surgical treatment of Dupuytren's contracture: a synthesis of techniques. *Plast Reconstruct Surg* 2004;113(2):540–544.
4. McGrouther DA. Dupuytren's contracture. In: Green DP, Hotchkiss RN, Pedersen WC, et al., eds. *Green's Operative Hand Surgery*, 5th ed. Philadelphia: Elsevier Churchill Livingstone; 2005:159–185.
5. Armstrong JR, Hurren JS, Logan AM. Dermofasciectomy in the management of Dupuytren's disease. *J Bone Joint Surg Br* 2000;82(1):90–94.

(57) Finger Dislocation

Stephan G. Pill and David R. Steinberg

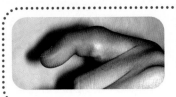

A 17-year-old male presents with severe pain and finger deformity after "jamming" his small finger while playing basketball.

CLINICAL POINTS

- The proximal interphalangeal joint (PIP) of the finger is the most commonly dislocated joint in the body.

- The Patient is reluctant to move the finger.

- Dislocations can occur in any direction.

PATIENT ASSESSMENT

1. Occurs after moderate trauma

2. Generally, hyperextension injury

3. X-rays to rule out fracture

Clinical Presentation

Dislocations of the finger are relatively common and occur when the bones of the finger are displaced from their normal position. The PIP joint of the finger is the most commonly dislocated joint in the body.[1] Improper treatment can cause long-term morbidity, and the severity is often underestimated at the time of injury. The patient most commonly presents with a history of trauma leading to finger deformity and reluctance to move the finger. The most common mechanism of injury is hyperextension, resulting in a dorsal dislocation and injury to the volar plate and the collateral ligaments.[2] However, dislocations can occur in any direction, and determining the exact mechanism of injury helps to identify other structures that may be injured. The exact location of tenderness can be helpful in localizing the injured structures. Perhaps more common is the "jammed finger," in which a lesser degree of force may result in only a sprain of the ligaments and joint capsule and/or a tendon avulsion.

Physical Findings

Patients present with deformity and swelling of the involved finger. The finger is usually deformed in either hyperextension or dorsal translation of the middle phalanx, as seen in a dorsal PIP dislocation (Introductory figure, Fig. 57.1). These are usually associated with damage to the volar plate. The location of tenderness depends on the direction of dislocation. In a dorsal dislocation, the volar plate is usually tender, and full active range of motion (ROM) is typically lacking. A volar PIP dislocation is usually associated with rupture of the central slip (extensor tendon attachment to the base of the middle phalanx) (Fig. 57.2). A careful examination is important to rule out extensor or flexor tendon avulsion injuries. Instability to varus and valgus stressing may be present and is more reliably demonstrated after digital block anesthesia. A careful evaluation for angulation is important to rule out damage to one or both of the collateral

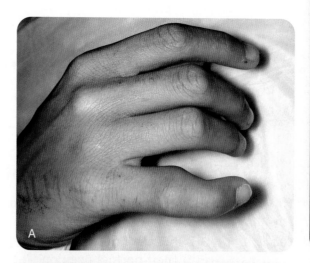

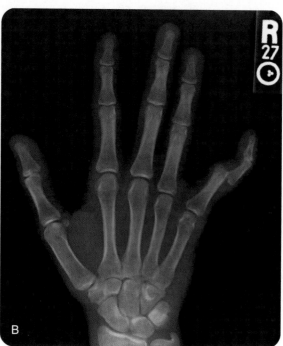

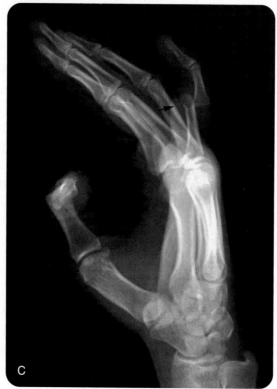

Figure 57.1 A: A second clinical picture of dorsal PIP dislocation presented at the beginning of the chapter. Note slight malrotation in supination. **B:** PA and lateral **(C)** radiographs of dorsal PIP dislocation, with evidence of small volar bony avulsion separated from the main body of the middle phalanx (*arrow*).

ligaments. A rotatory subluxation can be assessed by looking at the nails, as they should all lie in the same plane. A nail rotated out of the plane of the others signifies a rotational deformity.

Injuries at the distal interphalangeal (DIP) joint commonly result in rupture of the terminal slip of the extensor tendon ("mallet finger") (Fig. 57.3).[2] Less common but much more difficult to diagnose is rupture of the flexor profundus tendon at its attachment to the base of the distal phalanx. This may be easily confused with a sprained DIP joint, as both result in a swollen, stiff, painful joint. With an acutely injured joint, a patient can be coaxed into gently flexing the DIP joint if the examiner supports the middle phalanx. Even a slight amount of active flexion is evidence of an intact flexor mechanism.

The thumb, in addition to complete dislocations of interphalangeal, metacarpophalangeal (MCP), and carpometacarpal joints, is particularly susceptible to ligamentous injuries at the MCP joint. Most common is the "gamekeeper" or "skier" thumb, in which the ulnar collateral ligament is partially or completely ruptured. Occurring only 10% to 30% as frequently

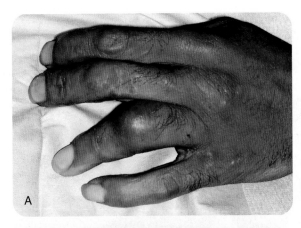

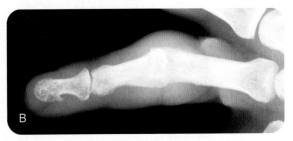

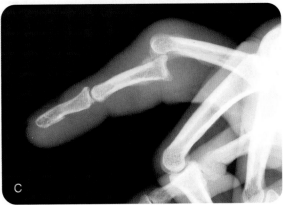

Figure 57.2 A: Volar PIP dislocation with more obvious pronation deformity. **B:** PA and lateral **(C)** radiographs of volar PIP dislocation. Rotational deformity can be appreciated on lateral by mismatch between the middle and proximal phalanges—perfect lateral of the base of the middle phalanx is not congruent with the oblique appearance of the proximal phalanx (two condyles of proximal phalanx are not perfectly superimposed).

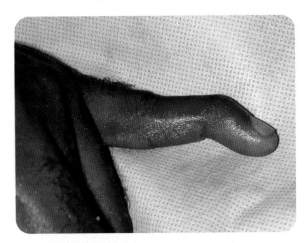

Figure 57.3 Mallet finger with rupture of terminal extensor tendon, causing droop at DIP joint.

NOT TO BE MISSED

- Open injuries
- Tendon injuries
- Unstable dislocations
- Complete ligament damage
- Fractures

are injuries to the radial collateral ligament.[1] Both may present with MCP tenderness, swelling, and stiffness as well as inability to generate forceful pinch.

A careful neurovascular exam should be documented prior to treatment (including the administration of any nerve blocks). The skin overlying the deformity must be evaluated for any disruption. Breaks in the skin should be assumed to communicate with the joint until proven otherwise.

Differential Diagnosis

Chronic dislocation
Septic joint
Inflammatory arthropathy
Charcot (neurogenic) joint
Flexor profundus rupture

Studies

Laboratory studies generally are not indicated; however, radiographs are extremely helpful. PA, lateral, and oblique views can determine the direction of subluxation or dislocation and assess for the presence of any associated fracture. It is important to obtain a lateral view of the individual affected finger so as not to obscure the dislocation by superimposition of

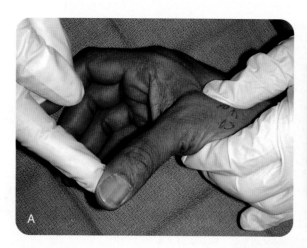
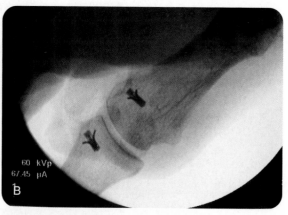

Figure 57.4 A: Significant laxity of the thumb MCP joint with stress testing due to complete rupture of the ulnar collateral ligament. **B:** Intraoperative radiograph of the thumb demonstrating correction of laxity. Two suture anchors have been placed in the bone to secure a tendon graft used to reconstruct a chronic deficiency of the collateral ligament.

other fingers. The head of the more proximal phalanx should fit symmetrically within the base of the more distal phalanx. If the joint space is not equal on both views, subluxation secondary to interposition of soft tissue structures within the joint should be considered. A rotational component may be detected in a volar PIP dislocation because the head of the proximal phalanx can "buttonhole" between the central slip and the lateral band of the extensor mechanism.[2] This can be observed on the lateral view, where the radial and ulnar aspects of each joint surface normally would be superimposed (Fig. 57.2C).

Common fractures to look for include avulsions of the volar plate at the base of the middle or distal phalanx. Larger fractures at this location make the injury a fracture dislocation, which may be unstable in extension. Avulsions of the extensor tendon at the dorsal base of the middle or distal phalanx should prompt careful testing of extensor function. Impacted fractures of the joint surface are best visualized on a true lateral view, allowing direct comparison of the radial and ulnar articular surfaces. In dorsal dislocations at the PIP joint, the middle phalanx is often hyperextended and deviated to the ulnar side. In a volar dislocation, rotation may be noticeable on the lateral view. Stress radiographs are occasionally helpful to test the integrity of supporting ligament, especially in MCP joint injuries of the thumb (Fig. 57.4A). Postreduction views should be obtained to rule out associated fractures and assess the adequacy of reduction.

Treatment

1. Attempt a reduction of dislocation with a gentle pull in the line of deformity. Check for ligament instability after reduction.

2. Irreducible dislocations require surgical intervention.

3. Splint for short periods and then buddy tape.

4. Permanent joint enlargement and some loss of motion are common.

Complete dislocations should be treated with early reduction, and a digital block using 1% lidocaine without epinephrine is frequently helpful. Reduction of dorsal dislocations is performed with accentuation of the deformity followed by flexion with slight longitudinal traction. Closed reductions should be done in a gentle manner and be limited to two or three attempts, as simple dislocations may be converted to complex ones with inappropriate or excessive reduction maneuvers.

Volar dislocations can be more problematic to treat. As mentioned, the proximal phalanx can "buttonhole" through a tear in the central slip of the extensor tendon. Reductions are done by hyperflexing the distal segment and then applying traction. This should be attempted only once.

After reducing the dislocation, the physical examination should be repeated, including palpating the point of maximum tenderness and performing a careful neurovascular exam. Postreduction stability should be assessed with full flexion–extension and gentle varus and valgus stress. The joint should stay reduced throughout the ROM. If instability or redislocation occurs with motion, an extension-block splint at an angle that preserves the reduction may be necessary (usually 30 degrees of flexion). If both active and passive ROM are impaired, there may be entrapment of a soft tissue structure in the joint.

Complex (irreducible) dislocations may occur secondary to soft tissue interposition or if the patient presents more than a few days from the time of injury. These require open reduction. If a dislocation is irreducible or unstable after reduction, referral to an orthopaedic or hand specialist is indicated. Other surgical indications include joints with significant collateral ligament laxity, complex fracture dislocations, volar dislocations accompanied by loss of complete extension, or chronically subluxed joints. Open dislocations require immediate incision and drainage, intravenous antibiotics, and tetanus prophylaxis.

Partial, stable collateral ligament injuries of the thumb MCP joint may be treated with a thumb spica splint or cast for 4 to 6 weeks. Severe laxity (>35 degrees joint opening during stress testing) or presence of a Stener lesion (mass in thumb index web space representing displacement of a completely torn ulnar collateral ligament) are usually indications for surgery (Fig. 57.4).

In general, splinting the finger in slight flexion after reduction for 7 to 10 days should promote proper healing, after which gentle, active ROM exercises can be performed.[3] The injured digit is often protected for 3 to 6 weeks after splinting with buddy taping to a neighboring uninjured digit (especially when a collateral ligament has been injured). Volar dislocations that are successfully reduced and stable can be splinted in full extension for 2 to 3 weeks, followed by buddy taping for 3 more weeks.

Patients should return for follow-up within a week to check for skin integrity and to confirm reduction in the splint. Repeat radiography is used to verify the reduction. The patient should perform gentle ROM exercises of any joint that does not require rigid immobilization. Ultimately, formal therapy can augment home exercises.

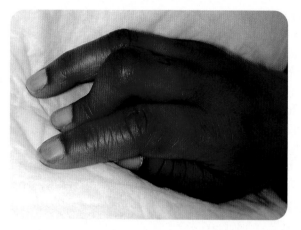

Figure 57.5 Chronic flexion deformity from rupture of the central slip of the extensor mechanism ("boutonniere deformity") after volar PIP dislocation.

Clinical Course

The prognosis is good in jammed fingers and simple dislocations, although patients should be informed that it may take as long as 12 months for pain and stiffness to completely resolve.[3] Slight loss of motion and permanent swelling are common and proportional to the energy of injury. The most common long-term complications are stiffness and flexion contractures (Fig. 57.5).[1] Permanent residual enlargement of the joint is not uncommonly seen, but chronic instability is rare.

Prognosis is poor in any dislocation that is incompletely reduced for more than a few days and for a dorsal fracture dislocation.[1] Delay in diagnosis and treatment may progressively worsen the prognosis, especially with concomitant injury to a tendon or ligament.

ICD9

834.00 Closed dislocation of finger, unspecified part
834.01 Closed dislocation of metacarpophalangeal (joint)
834.02 Closed dislocation of interphalangeal (joint), hand
834.10 Open dislocation of finger, unspecified part
834.11 Open dislocation of metacarpophalangeal (joint)
834.12 Open dislocation interphalangeal (joint), hand

References

1. Graham TJ, Mullen DJ. Athletic injuries of the adult hand. In: DeLee JC, Drez D, Miller MD, eds. *DeLee and Drez's Orthopaedic Sports Medicine*, 2nd ed. St. Louis, MO: Saunders; 2003:1388–1393.
2. Glickel SZ, Barron AO, Eaton RG. Dislocations and ligament injuries in the digits. In: Green DP, Hotchkiss RN, Pederson WC, eds. *Green's Operative Hand Surgery*, 4th ed. New York: Churchill Livingstone; 1999; 772–807.
3. Neviaser RJ. Dislocations and ligamentous injuries of the digits. In: Chapman MW, ed. *Operative Orthopaedics*, 2nd ed. Philadelphia: Lippincott Williams & Wilkins; 1993:1237–1250.

WHEN TO REFER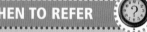

- Fracture dislocation
- Open dislocation
- Complex (irreducible) dislocation
- Complete collateral ligament injury of the thumb
- Chronic or recurrent dislocations
- Neurovascular compromise

58 Rheumatoid Arthritis of the Hand

Stephan G. Pill and David R. Steinberg

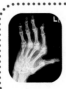 *A 55-year-old woman presents with a 3-month history of polyarticular arthralgias, worse at the metacarpophalangeal (MCP) and proximal interphalangeal (PIP) joints bilaterally.*

CLINICAL POINTS

- Carpometacarpal (CMC) and wrist joints are often affected.
- Symmetric involvement is characteristic.
- Disease progression may be rapid or slow.

PATIENT ASSESSMENT

1. Symmetrical swelling in the MCP joints
2. Can involve the proximal finger joints and the thumb later
3. Morning stiffness lasting more than 1 hour
4. Chronic inflammation leads to deformity of ulnar drift, swan neck, and boutonniere
5. Usually associated with carpal tunnel syndrome
6. X-rays show early notching in the periarticular area

Clinical Presentation

Rheumatoid arthritis (RA) usually manifests as an insidious onset of pain, stiffness, and swelling of multiple joints. The hands are commonly involved early in the course of disease, particularly the MCP and PIP joints. Involvement of thumb CMC and wrist joints are very common. The distal interphalangeal (DIP) joints may be involved later in the disease, but symptoms limited to these joints are more frequently associated with osteoarthritis. Although it may not be obvious initially, symmetric involvement is a characteristic feature of RA. Morning stiffness lasting more than 1 hour tends to be rather specific for RA, although many other inflammatory arthropathies can be associated with stiffness after prolonged periods of inactivity. The course of the disease is variable. In some cases, deterioration can occur rapidly; in others, deformity may progress slowly over many years (Fig. 58.1).

Physical Findings

Many early signs of the disease can be seen in the hands, such as symmetric effusions and swelling around the MCP and PIP joints (Fig. 58.2). Affected joints are tender to palpation and have restricted motion. In acute RA, the entire hand may be swollen, with pitting edema over the dorsum of the hand. Grip strength may be reduced and can be a useful marker of disease activity and progression. Extra-articular manifestations, including subcutaneous nodules, pulmonary nodules, vasculitis, pericarditis, or episcleritis, may be detected.

Later in the disease course, more characteristic joint deformities appear, including ulnar drift, swan neck, and boutonniere deformities. Ulnar drift occurs when the MCP joint becomes weakened, and elongation occurs of the MCP capsule and ligaments (Fig. 58.1). The resulting forces cause the extensor tendons to be displaced in an ulnar–palmar direction. Swan neck deformity refers to the deformity resulting from hyperextension of the PIP joint with flexion of the DIP joint (Fig. 58.3). The

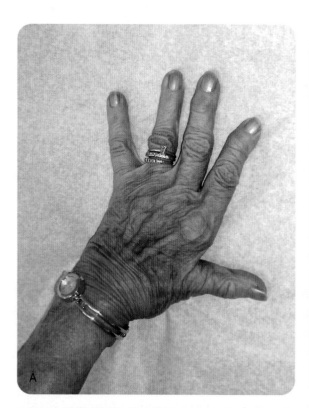 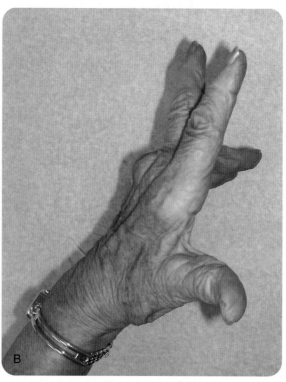

Figure 58.1 Clinical picture of typical rheumatoid hand deformities (refer to this patient's radiographs at of the beginning of the chapter). **A:** Dorsal and lateral **(B)** views demonstrate ulnar drift at the MCP joint, synovitis and early bony changes at the interphalangeal joints, thumb CMC disease, and wrist involvement including osteolysis of distal ulna.

volar plate at the PIP joint becomes stretched, and there is intrinsic muscle tightness, collateral ligament contracture, and DIP laxity. The boutonniere deformity begins with PIP synovitis, which leads to lengthening of the central extensor slip and triangular ligament. Volar displacement of the lateral bands leads to subsequent contracture of the transverse retinacular fibers and attenuation of the central slip and triangular ligament. The lateral bands become flexors of the PIP joint in this setting. This commonly affects the thumb in RA.

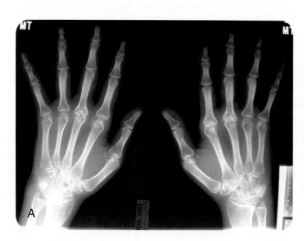 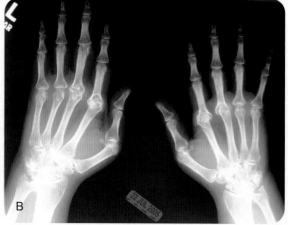

Figure 58.2 A, B: Radiographs of same patient 12 years apart demonstrate slows progression of bony destruction of the index and long MCP joints, joint space narrowing and subtle ulnar drift of the small and ring fingers, and progressive deterioration of the wrists.

Patients with RA will often present with loss of finger extension. This has multiple etiologies, which must be differentiated, as treatment is significantly different. Loss of extension at the MCP joint may be due to subluxation of the joint, volar subluxation of the extensor at the MCP joint due to attenuation of radial sagittal band, rupture of extensors over the distal ulna, or posterior interosseous nerve palsy secondary to nodules or synovitis over the radial head at the elbow.

Patients with RA may also present with carpal tunnel syndrome due to nerve compressions caused by synovial hypertrophy. This is manifested as paresthesia of the first three fingers and the radial side of the fourth finger and a positive Tinel or Phalen sign. Occasionally, tenosynovitis—infection of the tendon sheath—can mimic an acute flare of RA. Tenosynovitis may be detected by palpating the thickened extrinsic flexor tendons proximal to the MCP joint. Nodules may form along these tendon sheaths, resulting in catching or "triggering" when the patient attempts to extend the involved digit.

Differential Diagnosis

Psoriatic arthritis
Tophaceous gout
Pseudogout
Erosive inflammatory osteoarthritis
Reactive arthritis (originally described as Reiter syndrome)
Enteropathic arthritis
Systemic lupus erythematosus
Polymyositis/dermatomyositis
Scleroderma
Tenosynovitis

NOT TO BE MISSED

- Tenosynovitis
- Gout
- Tendon rupture
- Posterior interosseous nerve palsy

Studies

There are many laboratory markers for diagnosing and monitoring RA.[1] Rheumatoid factors and antibodies to citrulline-containing peptides (CCP) are helpful for diagnosis, while acute phase reactants are helpful in monitoring disease activity. In one cohort study, early determination of anti-CCP, IgA RF, anti-IL-1, ESR, CRP, and COMP predicted the development of joint damage in both the hands and feet.[2]

Plain radiographs are useful for diagnosing RA and determining the most appropriate therapeutic intervention. Erosions of cartilage and bone and periarticular decalcification are the cardinal features of RA. Early radiographs may appear normal until erosions of the cortex develop around the joint margins. Most erosions can be detected radiographically after the first 2 years of the disease. When ordering films, it is important to include oblique views of the hands to better visualize the periarticular joint surfaces.

MRI is a more sensitive technique than plain radiography for identifying bone erosions.[3] It can detect bone erosions earlier in the course of the disease and may also quantify the amount of hypertrophic synovial tissue, which tends to correlate with subsequent bone erosion. Ultrasonography is another alternative for estimating the degree of inflammation and volume of inflamed tissue.[3] However, MRI and ultrasonography are often not necessary and not yet widely accepted.

Treatment

1. Increasing use of disease-modifying antirheumatic drugs (DMARDs)
2. Splinting for persistent inflammation
3. Surgery for refractory synovitis or deformities

Managing RA is challenging. Patients are often given DMARDs as soon as the diagnosis is made in effort to prevent joint damage. Unfortunately, many of the DMARDs are associated with adverse or unacceptable side effects. Nonpharmacologic treatments serve as the foundation of therapy for every patient, along with activity modification, therapeutic exercise, and other general measures to prevent bone destruction and preserve function. The importance of an early therapy program cannot be overemphasized. Significant functional improvement and prevention of deformity can be obtained with resting and functional splints, adaptive aids, and various therapy modalities (Fig. 58.3).

Surgery is an option for those with functional abnormalities caused by proliferative synovitis, such as tendon rupture, or by bone and joint destruction. The primary goals of surgical treatment are pain relief, the restoration of function, and improved cosmesis. When considering surgical interventions, a few general principles are typically followed. First, in patients with involvement of multiple joints, the proximal joints are commonly addressed before distal ones, and lower extremity procedures are usually done before upper extremity surgery. Second, stabilizing procedures, such as arthrodesis, should be staged with mobilizing ones, such as arthroplasty, and not performed simultaneously.

Specific surgical interventions vary based on the severity and location of the disease. For problems related to the tendons or tendon sheaths, a tenosynovectomy may be selected for symptoms persisting for more than 4 to 6 months when medical management, splinting, and corticosteroid injections have been unsuccessful. In patients with severe synovitis, a synovectomy may be useful for pain relief, such as radiocarpal and distal radioulnar joint synovectomy for wrist synovitis. Partial arthrodeses of the radiolunate or scapholunate joints can prevent progression of carpal collapse in patients with intermediate disease. In patients with more severe disease, a total wrist arthrodesis can be performed. Wrist arthroplasty is a more motion-preserving alternative for patients with good bone stock, minimal deformity, and intact extensor tendons. Other surgical interventions include tenotomies and tendon transfers, which can improve cosmesis and function from various deformities, and carpal tunnel

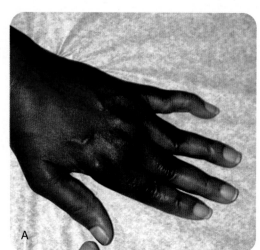
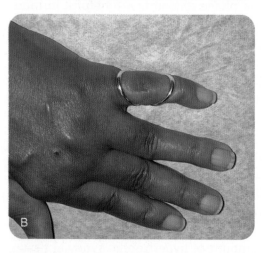

Figure 58.3 A: Mild swan neck deformity of the small finger corrected with a functional splint **(B)** that allows PIP flexion while preventing hyperextension.

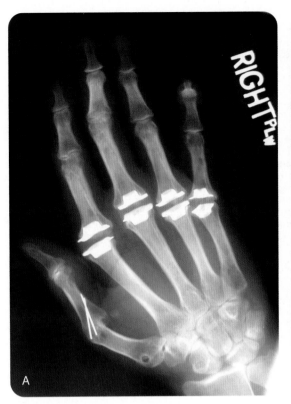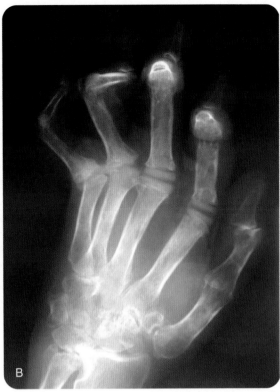

Figure 58.4 Successes and failures of treatment. **A:** Satisfactory correction of deformities with thumb MCP fusion and four MCP silicon arthroplasties (with metal grommets for additional support). **B:** Failed silicon arthroplasties at the ring and small finger MCP joints, with significant PIP and DIP zigzag deformities.

release in patients with compression of the median nerve. Silicon arthroplasties and extensor tendon reconstruction for MCP joint deformities remain popular. Early PIP deformities may be treated with soft tissue reconstruction; more severe deformities may require arthrodesis (preferred) or arthroplasty (Fig. 58.4).

Clinical Course

The long-term functional outlook is variable for patients who present early in the course of their illness and are treated appropriately. Use of effective DMARDs has been increasing, and this may be having a favorable effect on the severity of disability of patients with RA. The beneficial effects of DMARD treatment on function may be determined, at least in part, by the amount of joint damage that is present at the time such therapy is initiated. Early surgical consultation is advised for patients with functional impairments or pain from hand involvement who are not responding to medical intervention. The most gratifying results in reconstructive surgery for the rheumatoid hand can be obtained from MCP joint arthroplasty. An arc of 60 degrees of MCP joint motion, with a 10- to 15-degree extensor lag, has been reported. Ulnar drift may recur over many years (reported incidence ranges from 4%–43%). Results tend to deteriorate slowly over time.[2,4]

WHEN TO REFER

- Flexor or extensor tendon rupture[5]
- Nerve compression[5]
- Painful rheumatoid nodules[5]
- Persistent pain despite 6 months of medical therapy[5]
- Functional impairment[5]
- Unacceptable cosmetic deformities[5]

> *ICD9*
> *714.0 Rheumatoid arthritis*

References

1. Lindqvist E, Eberhardt K, Bendtzen K, et al. Prognostic laboratory markers of joint damage in rheumatoid arthritis. *Ann Rheum Dis* 2005;64:196–201.
2. Kirschenbaum D, Schneider L, Adams D. Arthroplasty of the metacarpophalangeal joints with use of silicone rubber implants in patients who have rheumatoid arthritis. *J Bone Joint Surg Am* 1993;75:3–12.
3. Backhaus M, Burmester GR, Sandrock D, et al. Prospective two year follow up study comparing novel and conventional imaging procedures in patients with arthritic finger joints. *Ann Rheum Dis* 2002;61: 895–904.
4. Stirrat C. Metacarpophalangeal joints in rheumatoid arthritis of the hand. *Hand Clin* 1996;12(3):515–529.
5. Steinberg DR. Management of the arthritic hand. In: Chapmann MW, ed. *Chapman's Orthopaedic Surgery*, 3rd ed. Philadelphia: Lippincott Williams & Wilkins; 2001:1943–1956.

59 Skin and Soft Tissue Injury

Jonas L. Matzon and David R. Steinberg

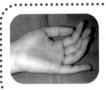

A 32-year-old right-hand dominant woman presents with a laceration of the left small finger after accidentally cutting herself with a kitchen knife.

CLINICAL POINTS

- Various types of accidents may result in injury.
- Injuries to the hand are the most common cause for emergency room visits.
- Injuries range in severity.
- A thorough history is necessary.

PATIENT ASSESSMENT

1. A great spectrum of problems may present, from minor lacerations to severe crushing.
2. For lacerations, check for nerve injury. For fractures, check for deformity.
3. X-rays required if there is a history of significant trauma.

Clinical Presentation

The human hand is of vital importance in interacting with surroundings, performing activities of daily living, and earning a living. Because of the hand's constant functional role, skin and soft tissue injuries to the hand are commonly encountered by primary care physicians, emergency medicine doctors, orthopaedic surgeons, and hand surgeons. Patients often present to the physician after domestic, recreational, or industrial accidents, and the clinical presentation varies greatly depending on the event. The first step in evaluating a patient with a skin or soft tissue injury to the hand is assessing the patient's current condition and determining how suitable it is for the resources available in the setting. Depending on the severity of the injury, the ABCDEs (airway, breathing, circulation, disability, and environment) should be performed, and the patient should be triaged to an appropriate facility. Once the patient is stable, a thorough history that includes the time, place, mechanism, and nature of injury should be obtained. Time elapsed since the injury must be known to assess possible ischemia time, risk of infection, and time period for repair. Place of injury is necessary information to determine likelihood of contamination. Mechanism of injury allows the practitioner to formulate an idea regarding the severity of tissue damage. Nature of the injury determines the amount of surrounding tissue that was concomitantly injured. Possible types include lacerations, crush injuries, burn injuries, and chemical injuries, and each of which has a different treatment algorithm.[1] Other key components of the history include dominant extremity, previous injuries to the extremity, preinjury functional capacity of the extremity, occupation, any pertinent past medical history such as immunosuppression, allergies, date of last tetanus shot, and time since the patient last ate or drank.

Physical Findings

The presentation of skin and soft tissue injuries of the hand vary greatly, depending on the nature and severity of the injury. When performing a physical examination, the first task is to thoroughly and completely inspect the hand. Special attention should be paid to the size and complexity of lacerations, any underlying exposed tendon, bone or neurovascular structure, any deformity that causes deviation from the normal resting posture of the hand, any areas that are actively bleeding or ischemic, any nail bed injury, and any obvious foreign bodies. Next, a full neurovascular examination evaluating the median/anterior interosseous, radial/posterior interosseous, ulnar, and digital nerves should be performed. Neuropathy should be assessed in relation to open wounds or areas of crush to determine whether there is a neuropraxia or neurotemesis. If active bleeding exists, pressure should be exerted over the area to tamponade the bleeding. Finally, isolated active and passive range of motion should be tested at all of the joints of the hand to assess tendon injury.

Different classification systems have been developed to better categorize injuries. Rank and colleagues[6] classified wounds as tidy or untidy. Tidy wounds incorporated simple cuts in the skin, a slicing injury with loss of soft tissue, a guillotine amputation, and a simple wound involving a tendon or nerve injury. Buchler and Hastings[3] developed a classification system that involved all of the relevant structural systems such as bones, joints, extrinsic extensors, extrinsic flexors, intrinsics, arteries, veins, skin, and nails. Injuries were classified as isolated if they involved only one relevant structural system or combined if they involved two or more systems.[3] Finally, Gustilo[4] proposed the widely accepted open fracture classification system. Type I fractures have a clean wound <1 cm, type II fractures have a 1- to 10-cm wound without extensive soft tissue damage, and type III fractures have either a wound >10 cm or extensive soft tissue damage. Type III injuries are further subdivided into IIIA fractures that have adequate soft tissue coverage; IIIB fractures that demonstrate periosteal stripping, bone exposure, and massive contamination; and IIIC fractures that have arterial injury requiring repair.[4]

In crush injuries to the hand, the physician should have a high index of suspicion for possible compartment syndrome (elevated intracompartmental pressures interfering with microcirculation to nerve and muscle). Early findings include a tense, swollen hand; pain out of proportion to other objective findings; and pain with passive motion of the digits. Immediate referral to a specialist and/or measurement of compartment pressures is indicated.

High-pressure injection injury is a relatively innocuous soft tissue injury that can have devastating consequences if missed. The patient presents with a tiny puncture wound, usually in the tip of a nondominant finger, that occurred after misfiring of a high-pressure paint, grease, or water gun (Fig. 59.1A) Two factors lead to significant soft tissue injury and necrosis: the introduction of a liquid under high pressure, causing a "minicompartment syndrome," and the local toxicity of the injected material (particularly grease and oil-based paint).

Laceration/crush injuries from a ring that is forcefully caught on a door ("ring avulsion injury") may cause only a small laceration or minimal surface wound but can lead to a dysvascular finger (Fig. 59.2). Careful

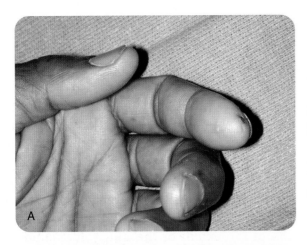

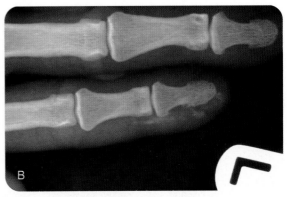

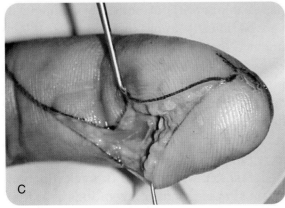

Figure 59.1 A: Small puncture wound at the tip of the index finger after a high-pressure paint injection. **B:** Radiograph demonstrating paint injected proximal to the distal interphalangeal (DIP) joint. **C:** Extensile exposure required to débride soft tissues and remove paint well proximal to the DIP joint.

NOT TO BE MISSED

- Nerve injuries
- Arterial injuries
- Nail bed injuries
- Flexor or extensor tendon injuries
- Open fractures
- Open joints
- High-pressure injection injuries
- Compartment syndrome of the hand

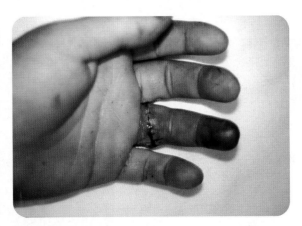

Figure 59.2 Ring avulsion injury. Small volar laceration does not indicate the more extensive, deeper soft tissue injury leading to disruption of both digital arteries and vascular compromise.

attention to the mechanism of injury will raise the physician's suspicion for this type of injury, which requires early consultation with a surgeon.

Studies

Radiographs of the hand are necessary to evaluate any underlying osseous injuries. PA and lateral views of the hand are usually sufficient, but occasionally, stress views are necessary to rule out ligamentous injuries. X-rays will often demonstrate depth of penetration of certain radiopaque agents after high-pressure injection injury (Fig. 59.1B). An arteriogram may be helpful if vascular injury is suspected but the degree or level of the injury is uncertain.

Laboratory values are generally not helpful in diagnosing skin or soft tissue injuries. Depending on the severity of the injury, a CBC may be useful in assessing blood loss, and preoperative labs are necessary when operative management is needed.

Treatment

1. Treatment depends on the nature and severity of the injury.

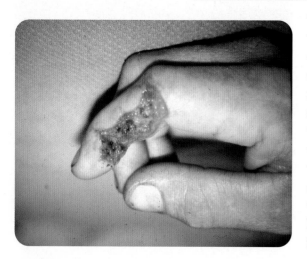

Figure 59.3 Large area of skin loss that eventually required a skin graft.

Treatment of skin and soft tissue injuries is based on the extent of the injury. All patients should receive adequate tetanus prophylaxis. Antibiotics may be given depending on wound contamination and whether there is an associated fracture. Subsequently, all wounds should be copiously irrigated with sterile saline and thoroughly debrided. This will allow definitive evaluation of the extent of the injury. If it is an isolated soft tissue injury without bone involvement, most wounds can be loosely approximated with 4.0 nylon suture under a local, digital, or wrist block (Chapter 72). Skin loss <1 cm in diameter can often heal by secondary intention with daily wet-to-dry dressing changes. Larger defects may require referral for skin grafting or a local flap (e.g., cross-finger flap) (Figs. 59.3, 59.4).

Flexor and extensor tendon lacerations involving >50% of the tendon require operative management, but this can be done in a primary delayed fashion within 2 to 3 weeks (patient should be referred earlier). Certain simple extensor lacerations over the hand can be repaired by the appropriate personnel in the emergency department. More

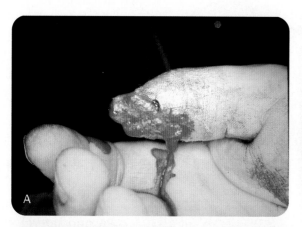

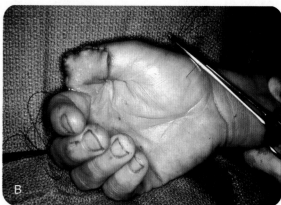

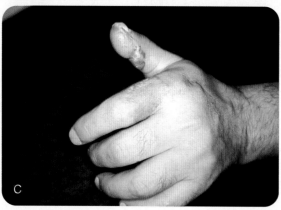

Figure 59.4 A: Extensive skin and soft tissue loss over the volar thumb. **B:** In order to restore a more functional soft tissue envelope over the distal phalanx of the thumb, a pedicled cross-finger flap from the dorsal index finger was harvested. **C:** The pedicle was inset after 3 weeks. This is the appearance of the new thumb pulp approximately 3 months later.

extensive extensor tendon injuries and those over the fingers often need to be addressed in the operating room.[5] Depending on the size of the nerve, the type of nerve transection, and the available resources, nerve lacerations can be managed with primary (within 24 hours) or delayed primary (within 2–3 weeks) repair. Sutures can be removed in 7 to 10 days and be replaced by an adhesive skin closure.

Nail injuries are extremely common and require special attention. Subungual hematomas on <50% of the nail surface are extremely painful and can be decompressed by using a heated paper clip or an 18-gauge needle. If the hematoma involves >50% of the nail surface, then the nail should be removed to allow for exploration of the nail bed. This can be done under digital block by using a freer elevator or fine scissors. Nail bed lacerations should be meticulously repaired with 6.0 chromic or plain gut. After repair, the nail or a nail substitute such as foil can be placed back in the nail fold to protect the nail bed during healing.[6,7]

If compartment syndrome is suspected or confirmed, immediate consultation is indicated. Once the diagnosis is made, urgent fasciotomy is required. Similarly, high-pressure injection injuries require urgent consultation with a specialist for possible débridement in the operating room (Fig. 59.1C).

Clinical Course

The clinical course depends on the severity and location of the injury.

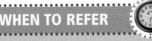

WHEN TO REFER

- Nerve injuries
- Arterial injuries
- Flexor or extensor tendon injuries
- Open fractures
- Open joints
- Severe soft tissue injuries

> *ICD9*
>
> *882.0 Open wound of hand except fingers alone, without mention of complication*
> *882.1 Open wound of hand except fingers alone, complicated*
> *883.0 Open wound of fingers, without mention of complication*
> *815.00 Closed fracture of metacarpal bone(s), site unspecified*
> *815.10 Open fracture of metacarpal bone(s), site unspecified*
> *927.3 Crushing injury of finger(s)*
> *944.10 Erythema due to burn (first degree) of unspecified site of hand*
> *944.11 Erythema due to burn (first degree) of single digit (finger [nail]) other than thumb*
> *944.12 Erythema due to burn (first degree) of thumb (nail)*
> *944.20 Blisters with epidermal loss due to burn (second degree) of unspecified site of hand*

References

1. Gupta, A, Shatford RA, Wolff TW, et al. Instructional course lectures, the American Academy of Orthopaedic Surgeons—treatment of the severely injured upper extremity. *J Bone Joint Surg Am* 1999;81:1628–1651.
2. Rank BK, Wakefield AR, Hueston JT. *Surgery of Repair as Applied to Hand Injuries*, 3rd ed. Edinburgh: Churchill Livingstone; 1968.
3. Buchler U, Hastings H. Combined injuries. In: Green DP, Hotchkiss RN, eds. *Operative Hand Surgery*, 3rd ed. New York: Churchill Livingstone; 1993:1563–1585.
4. Gustilo RB, Anderson JT. Prevention of infection in the treatment of one thousand and twenty-five open fractures of long bones: retrospective and prospective analyses. *J Bone Joint Surg Am* 1976;58:453–458.
5. Newport ML. Extensor tendon injuries in the hand. *J Am Acad Orthop Surg* 1997;5:59–66.
6. Fassler PR. Fingertip injuries: evaluation and treatment. *J Am Acad Orthop Surg* 1996;4:84–92.
7. Rozental TD, Steinberg DR. Skin and soft tissue defects. In: Beredjiklian PK, Bozentka DJ, eds. *Review of Hand Surgery*. Philadelphia: Elsevier; 2004:49–62.

SECTION 11　Hand

Common Pediatric Orthopaedic Problems

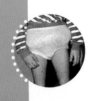

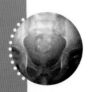

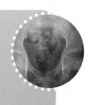

Chapter 64 ## Slipped Capital Femoral Epiphysis

David A. Spiegel and B. David Horn

Chapter 65 ## Septic Arthritis of the Hip

David A. Spiegel and B. David Horn

60 Intoeing

David A. Spiegel and B. David Horn

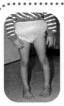
A five-year-old girl presents with a chief complaint of her feet pointing inward when she walks and runs. Her parents are concerned that she trips and falls frequently and that she tends to sit in a "W" position.

CLINICAL POINTS

- Deformity affects infants, toddlers, and children.
- The cause of deformity is inward rotation at the foot, lower leg, or hip.
- Bowing of the legs may occur.
- The deformity is a frequent concern of parents.
- Most fall within the range of normal variation, and improve with time
- Treatment is rarely required

PATIENT ASSESSMENT

1. Must examine the foot and the rotational profile.
2. Ask about the family history.

Clinical Presentation

Intoeing is a frequent cause for parental concern in infants, toddlers, and children. Most patients fall within a normal range of variation in rotational alignment, and while intrauterine position influences lower extremity alignment during infancy, genetic factors are likely to determine the alignment at skeletal maturity. The majority of these deformities improve with time, and there is little evidence to suggest any long-term morbidity in the vast majority of cases.

Intoeing results from inward rotation at the foot, lower leg, or hip, and more than one location may contribute to the deformity. The most common diagnosis in infants is metatarsus adductus, while medial tibial torsion is seen most frequently in toddlers. Medial tibial torsion may result in "apparent" bowing of the lower extremities. Parents observe that the child frequently trips and falls. In the older child and adolescent, excessive femoral anteversion (or medial femoral torsion) is most common. Medial femoral torsion becomes apparent at 3 to 5 years of age, and girls are affected more frequently than boys. Most torsional deformities improve with time, and a careful history and physical exam should identify the few patients who require further evaluation and/or treatment. Abnormal findings on the birth and/or developmental history may suggest a diagnosis of cerebral palsy. Families should be questioned regarding the presence of intoeing in other family members and/or any conditions that might be associated with rotational malalignment, including metabolic diseases, such as rickets, and the skeletal dysplasias.

Physical Findings

The primary care physician will recognize the internal rotation at the lower extremity. A rotational profile should be documented for all patients to determine both the location (foot, lower leg, or hip) and magnitude of the deformity.[1–4] This profile includes the foot progression angle (Fig. 60.1), the

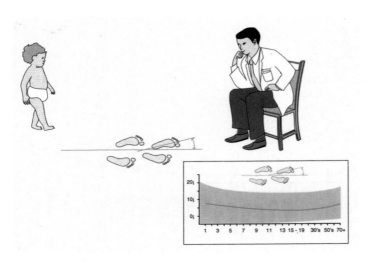

Figure 60.1 Foot progression angle. Normal variability in the angle between the axis of the foot and the line of progression. (From Staheli LT. *Practice of Pediatric Orthopaedics*. Philadelphia: Lippincott Williams & Wilkins; 2001:71.)

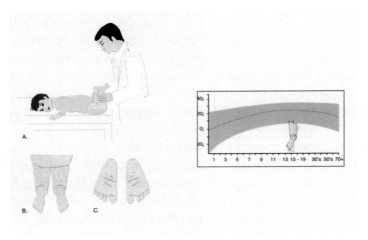

Figure 60.2 Rotational status of the lower leg and foot. The thigh–foot angle is measured in the prone position **(A, B)** and reflects rotation of both the lower leg (tibia/fibula) and the foot **(C)**. (From Staheli LT. *Practice of Pediatric Orthopaedics*. Philadelphia: Lippincott Williams & Wilkins; 2001:71.)

alignment of the foot, the thigh foot axis (Fig. 60.2) or transmalleolar axis, and the degree of femoral rotation (Fig. 60.3).[1–4] Findings on the rotational profile may be compared with the normative data of Staheli to determine where each child compares with the range of values for the population. Internal rotation may be identified at more than one location; for example, metatarsus adductus is commonly seen along with internal tibial torsion. Parents can then be counseled and reassured, and the few children who deviate significantly from mean values can be identified. Less than 1% of patients with such rotational deformities will ultimately require active treatment.

The foot progression angle represents the inward or outward rotation of the foot (degrees) relative to the direction of ambulation (Fig. 60.1). This quantifies the degree of intoeing but does not identify the location of the inward rotation.

Examination of the foot will reveal whether the lateral border is straight. A line bisecting the heel should normally go through the second web space, and the medial direction of the forefoot relative to the hindfoot is termed *metatarsus adductus* (Fig. 60.4).[5,6] The prognosis depends upon the degree of flexibility. If the forefoot can be abducted beyond neutral (a line bisecting the heel), the metatarsus adductus is flexible. If the forefoot can be brought just to neutral alignment (lateral board is straight), the foot is "partly flexible." If alignment cannot be brought to the neutral position, the deformity is "inflexible." Severe metatarsus adductus must be differentiated from two other conditions in which there is forefoot turning in, namely clubfoot and skewfoot. The hindfoot is turned in a clubfoot, while in the skewfoot the hindfoot is turned out.

The thigh–foot angle measures the rotational alignment of the lower leg (Fig. 60.2).[1–4] The examination is performed with the patient prone, and the knee is flexed to 90 degrees (Fig. 60.5).

Hip rotation is also measured with the patient prone and the knee flexed to 90 degrees. The degree of medial rotation is assessed by passively rotating the lower limb segment outward, away from the midline (Fig. 60.3). Femoral anteversion can be assessed clinically by rotating the hip medially until the greater trochanter is palpated at its most lateral position, and the angle between the lower limb segment and the vertical represents the degree of anteversion.[1–4] Normal anteversion is approximately 40 degrees in infants and 15 degrees in adults.

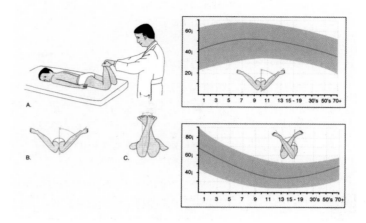

Figure 60.3 Assessment of hip rotation. The patient is placed in the prone position with the knee flexed 90 degrees **(A)**, and both medial **(B)** and lateral **(C)** rotation are measured as the angle between the lower limb and the vertical axis. (From Staheli LT. *Practice of Pediatric Orthopaedics*. Philadelphia: Lippincott Williams & Wilkins; 2001:71.)

Studies

Radiographs and/or other imaging studies are not required in the majority of children with intoeing, but they may be helpful in the presence of severe symptoms or marked abnormal physical findings in addition to the rotational profile. Weight-bearing AP and lateral radiographs of the foot should be obtained. A radiograph of the hip may be indicated in patients

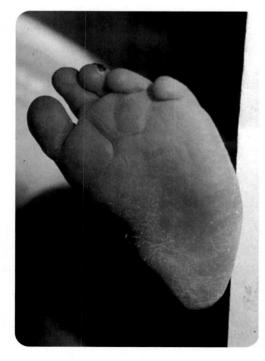

Figure 60.4 Metatarsus adductus is associated with an inward curvature of the lateral border of the foot. In this case, the heel bisector lies lateral to the fifth toe rather than through the second web space.

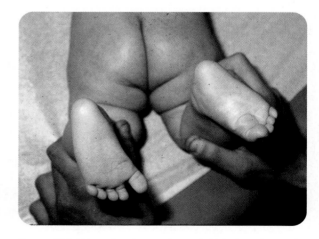

Figure 60.5 This patient has an internal thigh–foot axis on the left associated with an external axis on the right, ambulated with a "wind-swept" appearance.

with asymmetric rotation or in patients with known risk factors for hip dysplasia.

Treatment

1. Most rotational deformities correct spontaneously.
2. Tight, less flexible feet may require stretching.
3. The decision for surgery should be delayed until 12 years of age.

Active treatment is indicated in a minority of cases, and reassurance is usually all that is required.[1–4,7] Operative correction of rotational deformities of the tibia or the femur may be required in <1% of cases.[8–10]

Metatarsus adductus will resolve in approximately 90% of cases. As long as the deformity is flexible, symptoms are rare, and patients do well clinically over the long term.[11,12] Treatment is indicated when the deformity is not passively correctable and is ideally started within the first 8 months of life. For milder deformities, stretching exercises may be performed at home; however, there is no scientific evidence to support this. Serial casting followed by splinting may be considered when the deformity is more rigid.[13] Surgery is rarely required.

The treatment of tibial torsion is by observation in the majority of cases. Nonoperative measures such as stretching, bracing, or casting have not been shown to influence the natural history. As gradual improvement is expected and the rotational alignment of the tibial axis will not be established until 4 to 8 years of age, active treatment should be delayed at least until this time. Surgical treatment involves a tibial derotational osteotomy, which is usually performed distally.[9]

Femoral torsion usually becomes clinically evident at 4 to 6 years of age and improves until the early teenage years. Nonoperative measures such as physical therapy, braces, or twister cables have no influence on the natural history. In the rare case in which the torsion is severe and there are functional or cosmetic concerns, correction can be achieved by a derotational femoral osteotomy (proximal or distal). This should be delayed until at least 10 to 12 years of age.[10]

Clinical Course

The vast majority of children with rotational abnormalities like intoeing improve spontaneously. Persistent and symptomatic deformities may be corrected surgically, usually in late childhood or adolescence.

ICD9
754.53 Congenital bowing of tibia and fibula
736.89 Other acquired deformity of other parts of limb
755.69 Other congenital anomalies of lower limb, including pelvic girdle

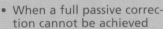

WHEN TO REFER

- When a full passive correction cannot be achieved
- When the deformity fails to resolve
- In cases of tibial torsion if there is any suspicion of an underlying neurologic diagnosis
- When the deformity is severe or fails to improve during the early childhood years
- In cases of patients with increased femoral anteversion when the deformity has not significantly improved or resolved by the late childhood years or when an underlying diagnosis is suspected

References

1. Lincoln TL, Suen PW. Common rotational variations in children. *J Am Acad Orthop Surg* 2003;11:312–320.
2. Staheli LT, Corbett M, Wyss C, et al. Lower-extremity rotational problems in children: normal values to guide management. *J Bone Joint Surg Am* 1985;67:39–47.
3. Staheli LT. Rotational problems in children. *J Bone Joint Surg Am* 1993;75:939–949.
4. Staheli LT. Rotational problems in children. *Instr Course Lect* 1994;43:199–209.
5. Bleck EE. Metatarsus adductus: classification and relationship to outcomes of treatment. *J Pediatr Orthop* 1983;3:2–9.
6. Smith JT, Bleck EE, Gamble JG, et al. Simple method of documenting metatarsus adductus. *J Pediatr Orthop* 1991;11:679–680.
7. Fabry G, Cheng LX, Molenaers G. Normal and abnormal torsional development in children. *Clin Orthop Rel Res* 1994;302:22–26.
8. Delgado ED, Schoeneker PL, Rich MM. Treatment of severe torsional malalignment syndrome. *J Pediatr Orthop* 1996;16:484–488.
9. Krengel WF III, Staheli LT. Tibial rotational osteotomy for idiopathic torsion: a comparison of the proximal and distal osteotomy levels. *Clin Orthop Rel Res* 1992;283:285–289.
10. Payne LZ, DeLuca PA. Intertrochanteric versus supracondylar osteotomy for severe femoral anteversion. *J Pediatr Orthop* 1994;14:39–44.
11. Farsetti P, Weistein SL, Ponseti IV. The long-term functional and radiographic outcomes of untreated and non-operatively treated metatarsus adductus. *J Bone Joint Surg Am* 1994;76:257–265.
12. Rushforth GF. The natural history of the hooked forefoot. *J Bone Joint Surg Br* 1978;60:530–532.
13. Katz K, David R, Soudry M. Below-knee plaster cast for the treatment of metatarsus adductus. *J Pediatr Ortho* 1999;19:49–50.

61 Bowed Legs

B. David Horn

A 3-year-old boy presents with bilateral bowed legs, which have been present since 1 year of age. The family reports that the bowing has worsened and that the child appears to have a limp.

Clinical Presentation

Angular deformities of the lower extremity in children are a common source of concern and anxiety for families. The majority of the time, these represent normal variations, are self-limiting, and correct with normal growth and development. Rarely, however, these can be secondary to localized growth disturbances or may be a manifestation of a systemic disease or disorder and require surgical or brace treatment.

The evaluation of the child with bowing of the lower extremity starts with a thorough history and physical examination. The history can be very useful in narrowing the differential diagnosis: sudden onset of the bowing suggests a traumatic or postinfectious cause. A gradual onset and progression is more consistent with a developmental condition or systemic disorder. The general health of the child should also be evaluated through the history, and a family history should also be obtained, as some patients with physiologic bowing, skeletal dysplasia, or rickets will have a positive family history for bowing.

CLINICAL POINTS

- Children are most often affected.
- This self-limiting condition generally resolves over time.
- History may be significant.

PATIENT ASSESSMENT

1. Physiologic bowing is a common problem and is frequently present from birth.

2. Very short and heavy children should be considered for Blount disease.

3. Progressive, unilateral deformity, associated with a thrust when walking, should be x-rayed to rule out structural abnormality.

Physical Findings

The physical examination should include evaluation of the child's height and weight. Height <5th percentile and weight >95th percentile are potential indicators of skeletal dysplasia or Blount disease.[1] The appearance of the limb in the frontal, sagittal, and axial planes should then be assessed. This should be done with the patella pointing forward in order to standardize assessment of the limb and remove the effect of hip rotation from the exam. A child with medial tibial torsion, for example, frequently has the appearance of tibia vara because the hip (and lower limb) is externally rotated to compensate for the medial tibial torsion. This pseudobowing is easily differentiated from tibia vara by examining the lower limb in a neutral position (i.e., with the patella forward), since the tibia has a normal alignment in pseudobowing. The location of the deformity should also be evaluated: a localized deformity suggests a localized growth disturbance such as Blount disease or posttraumatic deformity, whereas a generalized deformity suggests a systemic disease such as rickets or a metabolic disease. The child's gait should also be assessed. The presence of a lateral thrust of the affected knee in stance phase indicates significant tibia vara and is an indication for further evaluation.

NOT TO BE MISSED

- Physiologic bowing
- Blount disease
- Focal fibrocartilaginous dysplasia
- Rickets
- Skeletal dysplasia
- Anterolateral bowing (congenital pseudarthrosis of the tibia)
- Posterolateral bowing

Studies

Radiographs are not routinely indicated for bowing of the lower extremities in children <2 years of age. Indications for radiographs include age >24 months, stature <5th percentile, a lateral thrust while walking, and unilateral deformity. A standing radiograph should be obtained of each lower extremity in the AP and lateral projections. Care should be taken to obtain the radiographs with the patella pointed straight forward, as rotated images are difficult to interpret and can lead to misdiagnosis. If a systemic disorder is suspected, a skeletal survey may be ordered to image other bones that may be affected.[2]

The radiographs should be examined for physeal widening, irregularity, or deformity that may be signs of a systemic condition such as rickets or skeletal dysplasia. In young children, the tibial metaphyseal–diaphyseal angle can be measured on the AP radiograph.[3] This angle is formed by the intersection of a line drawn along the long axis of the tibia with a second line drawn along the proximal tibial metaphysis (Fig. 61.1). Metaphyseal–diaphyseal angles <10 degrees are normal, angles between 10 and 16 degrees are considered equivocal, while angles >16 degrees are considered indicative of Blount disease.[3] The distal femoral metaphyseal–diaphyseal angle (DFMDA) can also be measured, and the ratio of the DFMDA to the proximal tibial metaphyseal–diaphyseal angle (PTMDA) can then be calculated. A DFMDA/PTMDA ratio >1 (indicating that femur bow is equal to or greater than the tibial bow) is consistent with physiologic bowing.[4] More specialized imaging studies such as MRI may be obtained as a preoperative study or to further image an abnormal physis.

When rickets or metabolic bone disease are suspected, laboratory tests such as blood urea nitrogen, creatinine, calcium, and phosphorus can be obtained to further evaluate for any metabolic abnormalities.

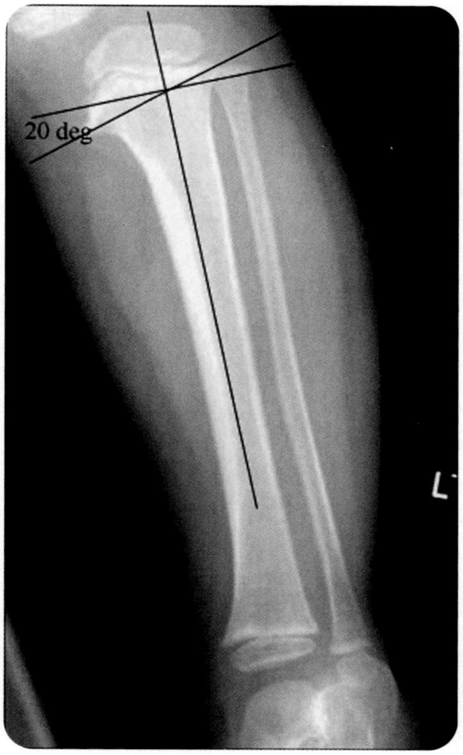

Figure 61.1 AP radiograph of a 30 month old with genu varum. The metaphyseal–diaphyseal angle is 20 degrees, indicating Blount disease.

Treatment

1. Most children with bowed legs correct spontaneously and require no treatment.
2. Complex causes for bowing require complex treatments.

Treatment and clinical course of lower extremity bowing depends on the diagnosis. The majority of patients seen for lower extremity

SECTION 12 Pediatric Orthopaedic Problems

bowing will have physiologic bowing. This typically is bilateral and involves both the femur and tibia. It is commonly seen in children who ambulate early, and there is often a history of bowlegs in the family. The natural history of physiologic bowing is benign, with spontaneous correction by 2 years of age. Braces, orthotics, special shoes, and the like have no role in the treatment of physiologic bowing. Children with physiologic bowing present after 24 months of age should have radiographs taken.

Infantile Blount disease represents the pathologic end of the spectrum of bowing and leads to progressive deformity that worsens with growth. Compressive forces from pre-existing physiologic bowing are believed to lead to a growth disturbance of the posteromedial aspect of the proximal tibial physis, which in turn causes bowing of the proximal tibia. In severe cases, this leads to deformity of the knee joint and permanent destructive changes in the proximal tibial physis. Infantile Blount disease has an onset between 1 to 4 years of age and is more common in obese children. Brace treatment may be effective for mild, unilateral disease; otherwise, surgery is indicated to correct the tibia vara of Blount disease.

Less common causes of bowlegs include focal fibrocartilaginous dysplasia, posteromedial bowing of the tibia, and anterolateral bowing of the tibia. Focal fibrocartilaginous dysplasia is a rare, unilateral growth disturbance of the proximal tibia or distal femur, where fibroblastic and cartilaginous tissue tethers the growth of the limb. Radiographs typically show an indentation in the medial cortex of the bone with growth of the affected bone into varus (Fig. 61.2). This condition often resolves spontaneously, so surgery is rarely needed.[5]

Posteromedial bowing of the tibia is a congenital, idiopathic, unilateral bowing of the tibia with the apex of the bow posteromedial. This is usually associated with shortening of the tibia and a calcaneovalgus foot. Both the foot deformity and bowing improves with growth, although shortening of the limb will persist and may require treatment. Anterolateral bowing (the apex of the bow is anterolateral) of the tibia is a pathologic condition that is a variant of and precursor to congenital pseudarthrosis of the tibia. Although the tibia may not be fractured at presentation, the bone may progress to fracture and subsequent pseudarthrosis. Anterolateral bowing of the tibia is associated with neurofibromatosis about 50% of the time, so all patients with this finding should have a thorough genetics evaluation.

Clinical Course

Most cases of physiologic tibial bowing in the infant correct spontaneously by the age of 2 years, and it is a benign condition. However, there are rare and challenging problems that present with progressive bowing, and these should be recognized and treated individually as noted previously.

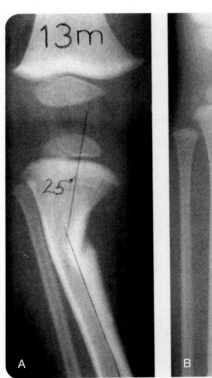
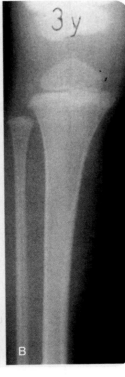

Figure 61.2 A: Radiographs of a 13 month old with focal fibrocartilaginous dysplasia of the tibia, with a follow-up radiograph **(B)** showing spontaneous resolution by the age of 3 years.

WHEN TO REFER

- Bowing in a child >2 years old or <5th percentile height
- Radiographs suspicious for skeletal or systemic disorders
- Posterolateral or antero-lateral bowing of the tibia

ICD9

736.42 Genu varum (acquired)
754.44 Congenital bowing of unspecified long bones of leg

References

1. Brooks WC, Gross RH. Genu varum in children: diagnosis and treatment. *J Am Acad Orthop Surg* 1995;3: 326–335.
2. Do TT. Clinical and radiographic evaluation of bowlegs. *Curr Opin Pediatr* 2001;13:42–46.
3. Levine AM, Drennan JC. Physiological bowing and tibia vara. The metaphyseal-diaphyseal angle in the measurement of bowleg deformities. *J Bone Joint Surg Am* 1982;64:1158–1163.
4. McCarthy JJ, Betz RR, Kim A, et al. Early radiographic differentiation of infantile tibia vara from phys-iologic bowing using the femoral-tibial ratio. *J Pediatr Orthop* 2001;21:545–548.
5. Jouve JL, Kohler R, Mubarak SJ, et al. Focal fibrocartilaginous dysplasia ("fibrous periosteal inclusion"): an additional series of eleven cases and literature review. *J Pediatr Orthop* 2007;27:75–84.

SECTION 12 Pediatric Orthopaedic Problems

62 Flatfoot

David A. Spiegel and B. David Horn

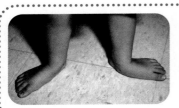

A healthy 6-year-old girl presents with mild, activity-related discomfort in the medial hind part of the foot.

Clinical Presentation

Flatfoot, or pes planovalgus, is a common finding in infants and children and is rarely a source of discomfort or functional problems. Flatfoot may best be described as a normal variant that is seen in up to 25% of the adult population.[1] There may be a positive family history, and flatfeet may be associated with generalized ligamentous laxity (familial) or with a connective tissue disease or syndrome. The longitudinal arch normally reaches its adult height by 10 years of age,[2,3] and there is some evidence to suggest that early shoe wear, especially shoes with a stiff sole, may be associated with flatfoot in later life.[4] Most flatfeet are flexible and usually cause no symptoms for the patient. Symptoms are more common when a flexible flatfoot is associated with a tendo Achilles contracture[5] or when range of motion is restricted (rigid flatfoot), as in a tarsal coalition.

Anatomically, flatfoot may be described as an alteration in the relationship between the bones of the hindfoot, with malalignment at the calcaneo-talo-navicular complex (Fig. 62.1).

The differential diagnosis for flatfoot depends on the age of the patient. In infants and toddlers, both a congenital vertical talus and a calcaneo-valgus foot may appear similar to a flexible flatfoot. During the childhood years, the most common diagnosis is a flexible flatfoot, with or without an associate tendo Achilles contracture. In older children and adolescents, the differential diagnosis includes rigid or structured forms of flatfoot such as tarsal coalition. Flatfoot, either flexible or structural, may also be associated with a variety of other diagnoses, including neurologic diseases (cerebral palsy), syndromes (Down), connective tissue disorders (Marfan, Ehler-Danlos), or inflammatory diseases such as juvenile rheumatoid arthritis.

CLINICAL POINTS

- This common finding in infants and children may occur in adults.
- A normal variant in most cases.
- The patient typically is asymptomatic.
- Pathology involves malalignment of the bones of the hindfoot.

Physical Findings

The musculoskeletal examination focuses on alignment and range of motion and should include an assessment of the degree of soft tissue laxity and a careful neurologic examination. An examination of the hips

1. No functional disability
2. Family history
3. Generalized ligament laxity
4. In infants, consider vertical talus
5. In childhood years, consider Achilles contracture
6. In adolescence, consider tarsal coalition
7. Obtain x-rays for rigid flatfeet

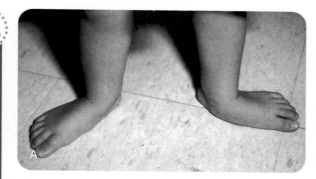

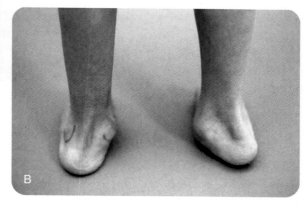

Figure 62.1 A, B: Clinical appearance of a flexible flatfoot. Note flattening of the longitudinal arch and abduction of the forefoot relative to the hindfoot **(A)**. Hindfoot valgus **(B)** is often a significant component of the deformity.

should be performed, especially in infants with a foot deformity. A flexible flatfoot will have a normal appearance in the nonweight-bearing position; however, the arch will flatten or disappear when the patient is standing (Fig 62.1). The skin over the medial hindfoot should be inspected for calluses or signs of irritation.

In infants, a calcaneovalgus foot may be confused with a flatfoot (Fig. 62.2). The calcaneovalgus foot will be everted and dorsiflexed, and the dorsum of the foot will often touch the lateral surface of the lower leg. The relationship between the midfoot and the hindfoot will be normal, and there is excessive dorsiflexion through the ankle.

The heel is in valgus, and the arch may be flattened. Passive inversion is mildly restricted.

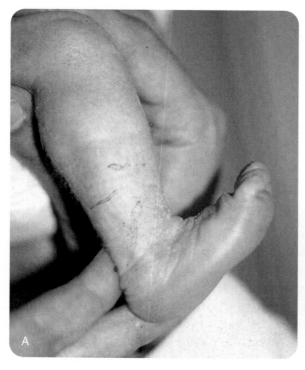

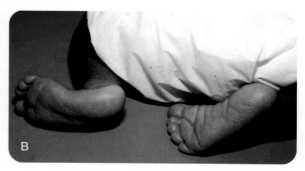

Figure 62.2 A, B: Calcaneovalgus foot.

SECTION 12 Pediatric Orthopaedic Problems

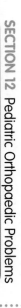

In the infant and toddler, congenital vertical talus should be ruled out. In the vertical talus, there is a convex border to the sole of the foot both with and without weight bearing. The deformity is usually rigid, and the dorsal midfoot subluxation cannot be corrected by plantar flexion. Congenital vertical talus is often bilateral and is commonly associated with a variety of underlying diagnoses, usually neuromuscular or syndromic. A comprehensive physical examination will often identify other abnormalities, and consideration should be given to a genetic or neurologic evaluation.

In late childhood and adolescence, tarsal coalition should be considered, especially when subtalar motion is restricted. This is a common cause of a painful flatfoot that involves bridging between the tarsal bones (fibrous, cartilaginous, or bony), most commonly the calcaneus and the navicular (calcaneonavicular), and the talus and the calcaneus (talocalcaneal).

Studies (Labs, X-rays)

Laboratory studies are not routinely indicated in the evaluation of a flatfoot, although inflammatory markers may be helpful in patients with stiffness and/or synovitis to rule out juvenile rheumatoid arthritis or other inflammatory disease. Radiographs are not routinely indicated in patients with bilateral flexible flatfoot and an otherwise normal examination.

When a congenital vertical talus is suspected with a convex sole, radiographs should be obtained (AP, lateral, and plantar flexion lateral).

In older children and adolescents in whom a tarsal coalition is suspected, weight-bearing AP and lateral radiographs should be obtained as well as an oblique view of the foot and a Harris view of the heel. As coalitions may be fibrous or cartilaginous, in many cases a CT scan is the best imaging modality to establish the diagnosis and to characterize the anatomy.

Treatment

1. Asymptomatic, flexible flatfeet do not require treatment.
2. Structural deformities associated with flatfeet may require surgical treatment.

The treatment depends on the age of the patient and the specific diagnosis. Asymptomatic flexible flatfeet do not require treatment, and there is no scientific evidence to suggest that shoe inserts or orthoses can influence the development of the longitudinal arch of the foot.[6] When asked about the best shoes for children, the importance of a flexible sole should be stressed rather than the brand name. For symptomatic flexible flatfoot, a medial arch support may be sufficient; in severe cases, particularly those associated with connective tissue diseases or laxity syndromes, an orthotic such as a UCBL (University of California Biomechanics Laboratory) may be required to control the hindfoot.

NOT TO BE MISSED

- Flexible flatfoot
- Flexible flatfoot with a tight tendo Achilles
- Calcaneovalgus foot
- Congenital vertical talus
- Tarsal coalition
- Flatfoot associated with other diagnoses (neurologic, syndromic, connective tissue disorder)

Operative treatment can be considered for the rare case in which a flexible flatfoot, with or without an associated tendo Achilles contracture, remains symptomatic despite these measures. The most common procedure recommended currently is a calcaneal lengthening osteotomy, which realigns the hindfoot bones.[7–9]

Patients diagnosed with a tarsal coalition are only treated if symptoms are present. Nonoperative measures include activity modification or restriction, nonnarcotic analgesics, range-of-motion exercises, and short-term immobilization (short leg cast or CAM Walker). Patients with persistent symptoms and/or functional deficits may benefit from excision of the fibrous, cartilaginous, or osseous coalition.

A congenital vertical talus is first treated by serial casting; however, the majority of cases are quite rigid, and surgery is required to restore the anatomic relationships.

Clinical Course

Children with flexible flatfeet do not require specific treatment. They are generally asymptomatic and function well with the flatfoot. Occasionally, medial arch supports will be beneficial.

> ### ICD9
> 734 Flat foot

WHEN TO REFER ⊙

- Most flexible flatfeet in normal infants and children do not require referral.

- In the infant and toddler age groups, patients with a convex border to the sole in whom a vertical talus is suspected should be referred.

- Calcaneovalgus feet (toe out) should be referred if the deformity does not resolve in the first few weeks after birth.

- During the childhood years, flatfeet associated with a tight heel cord, or any symptomatic flatfeet, should be referred.

- In older children and adolescents, the presence of pain, stiffness, or functional impairment should prompt referral.

References

1. Harris RI, Beath T. *Army Foot Survey: An Investigation of Foot Alignment in Canadian Soldiers*, Vol. 1. Ottawa: National Research Council of Canada; 1947.
2. Gould N, Moreland M, Alvarez R, et al. Development of the child's arch. *Foot Ankle* 1989;9:241–245.
3. Staheli LT, Chew DE, Corbett M. The longitudinal arch: a survey of eight hundred and eighty two feet in normal children and adults. *J Bone Joint Surg Am* 1987;69:426–428.
4. Sachithanandam V, Joseph B. The influence of footwear on the prevalence of flatfoot: a survey of 1846 skeletally mature patients. *J Bone Joint Surg Br* 1995;77:254–257.
5. Harris RI, Beath T. Hypermobile flatfoot with short Achilles tendon. *J Bone Joint Surg Am* 1948;30:116.
6. Wenger DR, Mauldin D, Speck G, et al. Corrective shoes and inserts as treatment for flexible flatfoot in infants and children. *J Bone Joint Surg Am* 1989;71:800–810.
7. Mosca VS. Calcaneal lengthening for valgus deformity of the hindfoot: results in children who had severe, symptomatic flatfoot and skewfoot. *J Bone Joint Surg Am* 1995;77:500–512.
8. Mosca VS. Flexible flatfoot and skewfoot. *Instr Course Lect* 1996;45:347–354.
9. Sangoreazan BJ, Mosca V, Hansen ST Jr. Effect of calcaneal lengthening on relationships among the hindfoot, midfoot, and forefoot. *Foot Ankle* 1993;14:136–141.

SECTION 12 Pediatric Orthopaedic Problems

CHAPTER 63 Perthes Disease

David A. Spiegel and B. David Horn

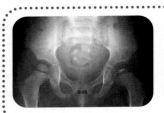

A six-year-old boy presents with an intermittent left-sided limp associated with occasional pain in the left knee.

Clinical Presentation

Perthes disease may be best described as idiopathic osteonecrosis of the femoral head in children. While the etiology remains unknown, the pathophysiology involves a loss of blood supply (segmental or total) to the capital femoral epiphysis. The disease is most common in boys from 4 to 8 years of age and is bilateral in 10% to 12% of cases. Up to 3% of patients have had a history of transient synovitis of the hip, and approximately 90% will have a decrease in bone age (mean of 21 months). Short stature is exhibited in 90% of patients, and approximately one third have been diagnosed with attention deficit hyperactivity disorder. While several reports have implicated thrombophilia, more recent studies find no evidence of a heritable coagulopathy. The condition has been associated with exposure to secondhand smoke. Although there is a positive family history in 1% to 20% of patients, there is no evidence that Perthes disease is inherited.

Patients present with the insidious onset of a limp, and pain is often experienced in the groin, thigh, or knee. The pain usually occurs with activity and is relieved by rest. Fever is typically absent.

Physical Findings

On physical examination, there is a decrease in range of abduction and medial rotation of the hip, and there may be discomfort or guarding at the extremes of rotation. Muscle spasm may also be observed, and atrophy of the gluteal muscles is a common physical finding. During ambulation, patients tend to shift the body weight over the involved hip during stance phase. The Trendelenburg test should also be performed. The patient is observed from behind and is asked to lift the opposite leg off the ground. Normally, the gluteal muscles on the stance side will contract and maintain the contralateral hemipelvis in an elevated position. In the presence of gluteal weakness (or pain), the contralateral hemipelvis will drop down. Patients should be tested for 10 seconds.

CLINICAL POINTS

- The disease is most common in young boys (4–8 years of age).
- Short stature is characteristic of most patients.
- Rest relieves the pain that occurs with activity.

Studies

LABORATORY

Laboratory studies are commonly performed in children who present with a limp, including a CBC with a differential, ESR, and CRP. Additional studies such as Lyme titer, RH, antistreptolysin O titer, and ANA may also be considered.

IMAGING

Plain films are usually all that is required to make the diagnosis of Perthes disease. AP and frog-leg lateral views should be obtained, and additional studies may be necessary when other diagnoses are suspected. Plain radiographs help to determine the extent of physeal involvement and to follow patients through the course of their disease.

The radiographic findings evolve over 2 to 5 years, as described by Waldenstrom. The earliest findings (initial stage) include a decrease in the size of the ossific nucleus relative to the contralateral side and an increase in the medial joint space (Fig. 63.1A). Next is the fragmentation stage, in which there are areas of both radiolucency and radiodensity within the capital femoral epiphysis, generally during the first 6 to 9 months (Fig. 63.1B–E). A subchondral fracture ("crescent sign") may be identified on the frog lateral. Following collapse of the capital femoral epiphysis, the disease progresses to the reossification stage, in which healing of the femoral head occurs. Areas of increased radiodensity are seen in regions that were radiolucent, along with changes in the shape of the femoral head, neck, and acetabulum. In the fourth stage (residual deformity), permanent changes in morphology are seen. In cases of bilateral disease, each hip is typically at a different stage of the disease.

Several patterns of residual deformity may be observed. The radiographic outcome depends on the degree of involvement of the capital femoral epiphysis and the presence of physeal involvement. Coxa magna (enlarged femoral head) is common, and there may be flattening of the femoral head. Disturbance of proximal femoral physeal growth may result in shortening (coxa breva) and widening of the femoral neck. The growth cartilage of the greater trochanter is spared, resulting in a relative overgrowth of the trochanter in relation to the femoral head, and may disturb hip abductor mechanics, resulting in a lurch during ambulation. Asymmetric physeal arrest may result in valgus angulation of the proximal femur and a more horizontal physis. Osteochondral lesions may also be seen, especially in older patients.

Changes on the acetabular side of the joint may also be observed. Younger patients (<4–6 years old) have the capacity for acetabular remodeling, and the shape of the acetabulum changes to accommodate

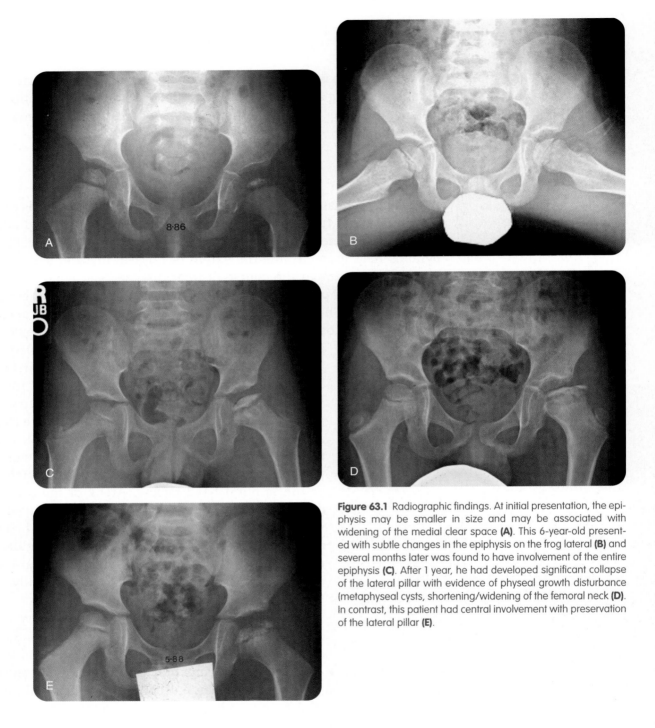

Figure 63.1 Radiographic findings. At initial presentation, the epiphysis may be smaller in size and may be associated with widening of the medial clear space **(A)**. This 6-year-old presented with subtle changes in the epiphysis on the frog lateral **(B)** and several months later was found to have involvement of the entire epiphysis **(C)**. After 1 year, he had developed significant collapse of the lateral pillar with evidence of physeal growth disturbance (metaphyseal cysts, shortening/widening of the femoral neck **(D)**. In contrast, this patient had central involvement with preservation of the lateral pillar **(E)**.

changes in femoral head morphology. As such, younger patients have a higher likelihood of achieving a congruous relationship between the femoral head and the acetabulum at healing. Stulberg and colleagues presented a five-part classification of deformity that was correlated with long-term outcome and can be summarized as follows. The best outcome is seen when the femoral head is spherical at healing and a congruous relationship is preserved. An intermediate prognosis is likely when the head is aspherical but the acetabulum has remodeled such that congruity is maintained.

When changes consistent with Perthes disease are identified in both hips, an AP radiograph of the wrists and the knees in addition to a lateral view of the spine should be obtained to rule out a skeletal dysplasia. In patients presenting with the typical symptoms of Perthes disease who have a normal radiograph, additional imaging studies may help to make the diagnosis. A three-phase bone scan can be helpful as well as an MRI study.

RADIOGRAPHIC CLASSIFICATION

Three classification schemes have been popularized in the literature.[1-4] The lateral pillar classification focuses on the height of the lateral portion of the epiphysis, or pillar.[2,3] In group A, there is no involvement of the lateral portion of the epiphysis (Fig. 63.1E). In group B, more than 50% of the height of the lateral pillar is maintained, while in group C <50% of the height of the lateral pillar is maintained (Fig. 63.1C,D). Involvement of the lateral portion of the epiphysis is important when establishing the prognosis, as those with significant lateral pillar involvement have a greater severity of the disease and are more likely to heal with greater deformity and incongruence.

Treatment

1. Restore and maintain range of motion
2. Symptomatic relief by rest (bedrest or use of crutches and analgesics)
3. Goal is to achieve containment of the femoral head
4. Brace treatment (nonsurgical containment) is rarely practiced in North America
5. Indications and techniques for surgical containment remain controversial

The treatment of Perthes disease is one of the most controversial topics in pediatric orthopaedics. While the general principles are well established, the indications for reconstructive surgery for containment of the femoral head remain under investigation. The first priority is to restore or maintain an adequate range of motion. Symptomatic relief may be provided by activity restriction, including periods of bed rest and/or limited weight bearing, mild analgesics (usually NSAIDs), and gentle range-of-motion exercises. A home traction program may help in selected cases, and physical therapy may be indicated to maintain or enhance joint range of motion. For patients who have developed a soft tissue contracture despite these measures, surgical release of the adductors, and occasionally the hip flexors, may be necessary to regain the range of motion. The release is commonly followed by up to 6 weeks in long leg casts with the knees extended and the hips abducted.

In addition to preservation of motion, containment of the diseased femoral head within the acetabulum theoretically affords the greatest chance of retaining a congruous joint at healing, especially in patients

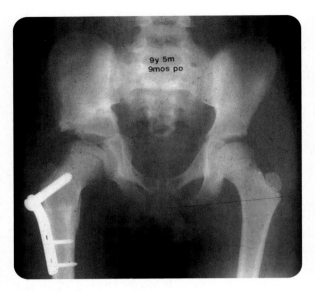

Figure 63.2 Examples of surgical containment. In patients requiring a greater degree of realignment to contain the anterolateral epiphysis under the acetabulum, a combined osteotomy (varus femoral osteotomy and redirectional pelvic osteotomy) may be recommended.

who are felt to have a poor prognosis. Containment may be achieved with or without surgery.[5–7]

Clinical Course

The long-term concern in patients with Perthes disease is premature osteoarthritis of the hip, and a worse prognosis is expected in patients >8 years of age who have involvement of >50% of the epiphysis.[1,7–10]

Patients with an incongruent articulation at the time of healing may develop arthritis as early as the third or fourth decade of life. When the femoral head is aspheric but the joint is congruent, the onset of degenerative changes may be delayed until the fifth or sixth decade of life. Prognostic factors include the age at the onset of disease, the degree of involvement of the epiphysis, the amount of growth disturbance, the deformity of the femoral head, and joint congruity at healing (Fig. 63.2).

ICD9

732.1 Juvenile osteochondrosis of hip and pelvis

References

1. Cattarall A. The natural history of Perthes disease. *J Bone Joint Surg Br* 1971;53:37–53.
2. Herring JA, Kim HT, Browne R. Legg-Calve-Perthes disease. Part I. Classification of radiographs with use of the modified lateral pillar and Stulberg classifications. *J Bone Joint Surg Am* 2004;86:2103–2120.
3. Herring JA, Neustadt JB, Williams JA, et al. The lateral pillar classification of Legg-Calve-Perthes disease. *J Pediatr Orthop* 1992;12:143–150.
4. Salter RB, Thompson GH. Legg-Calve-Perthes disease: the prognostic significance of the subchondral fracture and a two-group classification of femoral head involvement. *J Bone Joint Surg Am* 1984;66:479–489.
5. Herring JA, Kim HT, Browne R. Legg-Calve-Perthes disease. Part II. Prospective multicenter study of the effect of treatment on outcome. *J Bone Joint Surg Am* 2004;86:2121–2134.
6. Meehan PL, Angel D, Nelson IM. The Scottish Rite abduction orthosis for the treatment of Legg-Perthes disease: a radiographic analysis. *J Bone Joint Surg Am* 1992;74:2–12.
7. Weinstein SL. Legg-Calve-Perthes syndrome. In: Morrissey RT, Weinstein SL, eds. *Lovell and Winter's Pediatric Orthopaedics*, Vol. 2, 6th ed. Philadelphia: Lippincott Williams & Wilkins; 2006:1039–1083.
8. Stulberg SD, Cooperman DR, Wallenstein R. The natural history of Legg-Calve-Perthes disease. *J Bone Joint Surg Am* 1981;63:1095–1108.
9. Weinstein SL. Long term followup of pediatric orthopaedic conditions: natural history and outcomes of treatment. *J Bone Joint Surg Am* 2000;82:980–990.
10. Yrjonen T. Prognosis in Perthes disease after noncontainment treatment: 106 hips followed for 28-47 years. *Acta Orthop Scand* 1992;63:523–526.

WHEN TO REFER

- Most children with a limp that lasts more than several days are referred for orthopaedic evaluation.

64 Slipped Capital Femoral Epiphysis

David A. Spiegel and B. David Horn

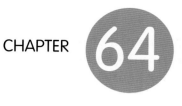

A 13-year-old boy presents with a 6-month history of progressively worsening pain in the left knee and thigh that has a caused a limp.

Clinical Presentation

Slipped capital femoral epiphysis represents a progressive displacement of the upper portion of the femur relative to the capital femoral epiphysis. In the majority of cases, the epiphysis maintains a normal position with respect to the acetabulum, and there is displacement of the proximal femur (anterior, proximal, external) relative to the epiphysis and the acetabulum.

The disorder is seen most frequently in adolescent boys, and blacks are affected more frequently than whites and Hispanics. Most patients are obese and are noted to ambulate with an externally rotated gait. Slipped epiphysis most commonly occurs in boys from 13 to 15 years of age and in girls from 11 to 13 years of age. Bilateral involvement is seen in approximately 25% to 50% of patients.

The etiology of this condition remains unknown and is likely multifactorial. Both anatomic and biomechanical abnormalities may render the physis more susceptible to shear stresses, including retroversion of the hip, weakening of the perichondrial ring (in association with the adolescent growth spurt), and a greater inclination of the proximal femoral physis. As more than 50% of patients will be above the 95th percentile for weight, mechanical factors are also felt to play an important role. While endocrinologic abnormalities have been suspected and slipped capital femoral epiphysis may be seen in association with endocrinopathies and metabolic disorders, the vast majority of patients will have a normal endocrinologic evaluation. An underlying endocrinopathy should be suspected when the diagnosis is made in a thin patient or when the age is atypical for a slipped epiphysis (<10 years of age or >16 years of age). Underlying diagnoses associated with a slipped epiphysis include hypothyroidism, growth hormone deficiency (with or without replacement therapy), panhypopituitarism, and renal disease (secondary hypoparathyroidism). Patients who have received pelvic irradiation are also susceptible.

Patients commonly present with pain in the groin, but the discomfort may also be referred to the thigh or the knee, and 15% may present with

CLINICAL PRESENTATION

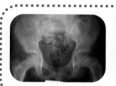

- The condition most commonly occurs in adolescent boys.
- When affected, girls are often younger than boys.
- Pain in the groin, thigh, or knee.
- Etiology may involve several factors.

knee pain alone.[1] The pain is dull in character, worsened by activity, and progressive in nature. A small subset of patients will present with the acute onset of severe pain, often following a minor injury.

There have been two schemes used to classify slipped capital femoral epiphysis. The first is a temporal classification, including *acute* (<3 weeks duration of symptoms), *chronic* (>3 weeks duration), and *acute on chronic* (recent exacerbation of symptoms that have been present for weeks to months). The clinical classification of *stable* versus *unstable* is perhaps more useful, as it more accurately defines the prognosis. A patient has an unstable slip if he or she is unable to bear weight (with or without crutches) and a stable slip if able to bear weight (with or without crutches).[2] Patients with an unstable slip (approximately 5%) have a much higher risk of avascular necrosis (up to 47%), which is usually associated with a poor outcome due to premature joint degeneration.[2] The clinical presentation of patients with an unstable slipped epiphysis is similar to that of a physeal fracture.

The long-term outcome relates to the degree of displacement at the time of stabilization (or at closure of the physis) and whether or not complications such as chondrolysis or avascular necrosis occur.

Physical Findings

Patients are usually obese and ambulate with an externally rotated gait. Those who are able to ambulate will shift their body weight over the involved hip (or hips) during stance phase, and the degree of external rotation is greater on the affected side in those with unilateral involvement. On bench examination, while absolute motion may not be decreased, the range of motion is reoriented. There is a decrease in flexion and internal rotation relative to the normal side. The extremity will roll into external rotation with progressive flexion of the hip, and there is often discomfort at the extremes of motion, especially internal rotation. Both hips should always be assessed, as 20% of patients will present with bilateral disease. Patients with an unstable slip, in addition to the inability to bear weight, may present with the limb held in flexion, abduction, and external rotation and may resist any attempts to move the extremity.

Studies

Laboratory studies are typically not indicated in the evaluation of slipped epiphysis. Most cases of slipped capital femoral epiphysis can be diagnosed by using plain radiographs alone. The earliest finding is widening and irregularity of the physis, and this is occasionally termed a *preslip*. On the AP radiograph, a line drawn parallel to the superior femoral neck (Klein line) should intersect the lateral portion of the capital femoral epiphysis (Fig. 64.1A). A slipped epiphysis is suspected when this finding is not observed. The degree of displacement is best appreciated on the lateral view (ideally, a true lateral), and there will be a prominence of the anterior femoral neck at the junction of the epiphysis

PATIENT ASSESSMENT

1. Obesity common
2. Bilateral involvement in 25% to 60%
3. Painful limp
4. Pain in groin, anterior thigh, or knee
5. Modest limitation of flexion and internal rotation
6. X-rays demonstrate slipped epiphysis
7. First sign is widening of the physis
8. Later can note displacement of head

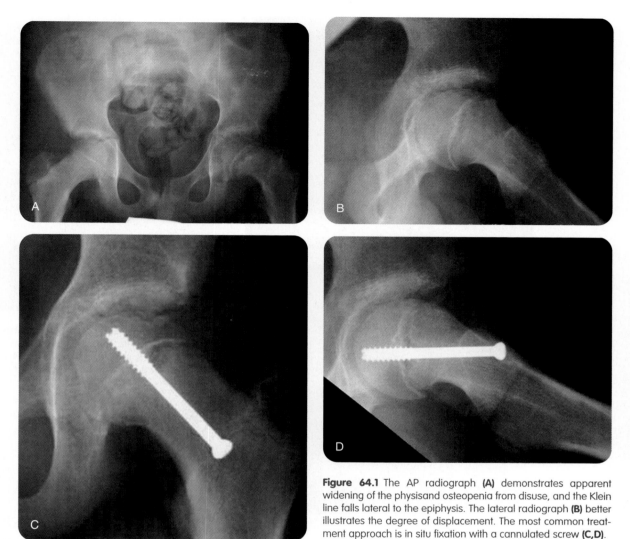

Figure 64.1 The AP radiograph **(A)** demonstrates apparent widening of the physisand osteopenia from disuse, and the Klein line falls lateral to the epiphysis. The lateral radiograph **(B)** better illustrates the degree of displacement. The most common treatment approach is in situ fixation with a cannulated screw **(C,D)**.

SECTION 12 Pediatric Orthopaedic Problems

NOT TO BE MISSED

- Overuse injuries of the muscles around the hip or knee
- Perthes disease
- Infection
- Tumor

and the neck. This prominence may become smoother over time due to metaphyseal remodeling (Fig. 64.2). Other imaging modalities are not routinely indicated.

Treatment

1. Prevent progression of deformity with pin stabilization.

The goals of treatment are to prevent progression of the deformity through stabilization of the epiphysis, avoid complications of the disease process and/or treatment (avascular necrosis, chondrolysis), and maximize function.

The most common treatment of a stable slipped epiphysis is in situ fixation with a single cannulated screw. Routine implant removal is not required.

An unstable slipped capital femoral epiphysis is usually treated as an emergency, and patients are admitted for stabilization. Controversial topics include the timing of intervention, the need for decompression of the

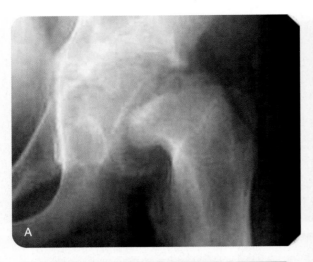

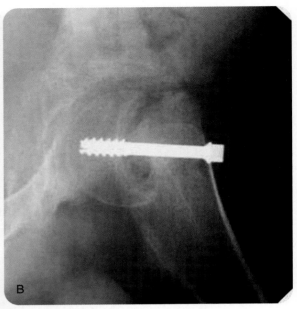

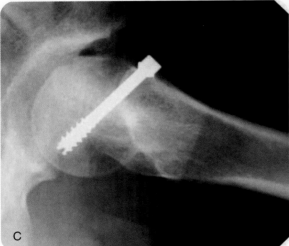

Figure 64.2 Severe slipped capital femoral epiphysis. The AP radiograph demonstrates the initial deformity **(A)**, and the epiphysis was stabilized in situ with a single screw **(B)**. At physeal closure **(C)**, there was some remodeling of the prominence along the anterior femoral neck.

joint, the role of manipulative reduction,[3,4] and the type of fixation. Many authors liken the unstable slipped epiphysis to a displaced proximal femoral physeal fracture and recommend emergent stabilization with or without decompression of the joint capsule by aspiration or arthrotomy.

Complications of the disease and its treatment include chondrolysis and avascular necrosis,[3–8] both of which may occur with or without treatment. Avascular necrosis is most commonly seen in association with unstable slipped capital femoral epiphysis, and evidence from pretreatment bone scanning suggests that the loss of blood supply is often present at the time of diagnosis. Patients present with pain in the hip, often after several months, and radiographically there is a progressive collapse of the femoral head (Fig. 64.3). Chondrolysis represents a progressive thinning or degeneration of the articular surface, and while the etiology remains unknown, an immunologic mechanism is suspected.[5] Clinical findings include pain and a decrease

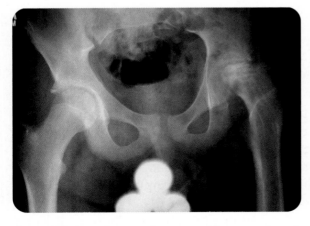

Figure 64.3 Avascular necrosis may result in progressive collapse of a significant portion of the femoral head, predisposing to early degenerative joint disease.

in the range of motion, and radiographically there is a decrease in the joint space to <3 mm. There may be partial reconstitution of the joint space once the acute phase of the disease resolves. The treatment includes rest or activity modification, NSAIDs, and physical therapy.

As between 20% and 61% of patients will ultimately be diagnosed with bilateral disease, the role of prophylactic pinning of the contralateral hip has been debated.[3,9,10] A common approach has been to counsel patients and their families regarding this possibility and asking them to seek immediate medical attention if any discomfort or limp is experienced. Further study will be required to resolve this issue. Prophylactic fixation is recommended for patients with an underlying endocrinologic or metabolic disease and in juvenile patients (<10 years of age).

WHEN TO REFER

- Limping children or adolescents, refer for x-rays and possible orthopaedic evaluation.
- Children or adolescents with pain in the groin, thigh, or knee should have an examination of the knee and hip, radiographs, and referral if SCFE diagnosis made or if symptoms do not resolve.

Clinical Course

The clinical course of patients with slipped epiphysis depends on the degree of slip and when it was diagnosed and treated. With a minimal slip and early pin fixation, the prognosis is excellent. With severe slips or progressive deformity from delayed diagnosis, the patients will initially do reasonably well as young adults but will be predisposed to early arthritis.[3,11,12] It is important to recognize this disease process early.

ICD-9
732.2 Nontraumatic slipped upper femoral epiphysis

References

1. Matava MJ, Patton CM, Luhmann S, et al. Knee pain as the initial symptom of slipped capital femoral epiphysis: an analysis of initial presentation and treatment. *J Pediatr Orthop* 1999;19:455–460.
2. Loder RT, Richards BS, Shapiro PS, et al. Acute slipped capital femoral epiphysis: the importance of physeal stability. *J Bone Joint Surg Am* 1993;75:1134–1140.
3. Loder RT. Controversies in slipped capital femoral epiphysis. *Orthop Clin North Am* 2006;37:211–221.
4. Peterson MD, Weiner DS, Green NE, et al. Acute slipped capital femoral epiphysis: the value and safety of urgent manipulative reduction. *J Pediatr Orthop* 1997;17:648–654.
5. Lubicky JP. Chondrolysis and avascular necrosis: complications of slipped capital femoral epiphysis. *J Pediatr Orthop* 1996;5:162–167.
6. Rattey T, Piehl F, Wright JG. Acute slipped capital femoral epiphysis. Review of outcomes and rates of avascular necrosis. *J Bone Joint Surg Am* 1996;78:398–402.
7. Rhoad RC, Davidson RS, Heyman S, et al. Pretreatment bone scan in SCFE: a predictor of ischemia and avascular necrosis. *J Pediatr Orthop* 1999;19:164–168.
8. Tomakova KP, Stanton RP, Mason DE. Factors influencing the development of osteonecrosis in patients treated for slipped capital femoral epiphysis. *J Bone Joint Surg Am* 2003;85:798–801.
9. Kocher MS, Bishop JA, Hresko MT, et al. Prophylactic pinning of the contralateral hip after unilateral slipped capital femoral epiphysis. *J Bone Joint Surg Am* 2004;86:2658–2665.
10. Stasikelis PJ, Sullivan CM, Phillips WA, et al. Slipped capital femoral epiphysis: prediction of contralateral involvement. *J Bone Joint Surg Am* 1996;78:1149–1155.
11. Carney BT, Weinstein SL, Noble J. Long term followup of slipped capital femoral epiphysis. *J Bone Joint Surg Am* 1991;73:667–674.
12. Leunig M, Casillas MM, Hamlet M, et al. Slipped capital femoral epiphysis. Early mechanical damage to the acetabular cartilage by a prominant femoral metaphysis. *Acta Orthop Scand* 2000;71:370–375.

SECTION 12 Pediatric Orthopaedic Problems

CHAPTER 65 Septic Arthritis of the Hip

David A. Spiegel and B. David Horn

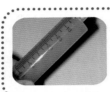

A 2-year-old boy presents with a 1-day history of left hip pain, refusal to bear weight on the left side, and a temperature of 39°C.

CLINICAL POINTS

- Infection may be due to bacteria in the blood or to the spread of osteomyelitis.

- Resulting inflammation leads to destruction of the hip if untreated.

- Surgical emergency if diagnosed.

Clinical Presentation

Septic arthritis of the hip is a common musculoskeletal infection in children. This is primarily due to a delay in diagnosis secondary to vague presenting symptoms, a large differential diagnosis, and the young age of patients. Prompt diagnosis, surgical intervention, and intravenous antibiotics are the mainstays of treatment for hip sepsis and are vital in preventing complications.

Most patients with septic arthritis of the hip are infected from a hematogenous route. Transient bacteremia may result in organisms settling in the subsynovial layer of the hip. This tissue is unique in that it does not contain a basement membrane, so bacteria can easily gain access into the hip joint itself. A second route of infection in children with septic arthritis of the hip is from osteomyelitis in the adjacent proximal femoral metaphysis. The metaphysis is intra-articular in the proximal femur, radial neck, proximal humerus, and distal fibula. Osteomyelitis in these regions can therefore easily expand beyond the bone and into the joint. Children <18 to 24 months of age also have blood vessels that transverse the physis and these transphyseal vessels may be a route of infection into the hip joint.

Regardless of the exact mechanism of introduction, intra-articular bacteria multiply rapidly. The resultant infection incites an inflammatory response, and polymorphonuclear cells migrate into the joint. This inflammatory response, as well as production of plasma proteins inside of the joint, causes a tense hip effusion.

Destruction of the hip joint can be caused by several mechanisms. First, the cells of the synovium and polymorphonuclear leukocytes directly produce proteolytic enzymes, which attack the hyaline cartilage. Second, the infection triggers a monocyte-mediated inflammatory cascade, which leads to the release of various proteases by synovial and cartilage cells within the joint. These proteases also damage the hyaline articular cartilage. Third, a tense hip effusion can tamponade the blood vessels supplying the femoral head, leading to avascular necrosis of the femoral head.

The diagnosis of hip sepsis is also made difficult by the fact that there are a large number of conditions that cause hip pain in children. The differential diagnosis of hip pain in children includes transient synovitis, juvenile rheumatoid arthritis, Lyme disease, pyogenic abscess of the psoas muscle, pelvic osteomyelitis, Legg-Calve-Perthes disease, leukemia, and other neoplasms.

Physical Findings

Children with septic arthritis in the hip have an acute clinical illness and may appear toxic. Although children with hip sepsis are typically febrile, neonates and infants may be afebrile. There may also be a history of a prodromal infection, such as streptococcal pharyngitis or otitis media. Antibiotics given for these conditions may also mask the early presentation of septic hip. In infants, an early clinical sign may be irritability during diaper changes. Infants and toddlers may exhibit general irritability and have a decreased appetite. They may also cease to crawl or ambulate. Older children may complain of pain in the groin, thigh, or knee (hip pain may be referred to the thigh or knee).

Patients with a septic hip will frequently hold the hip in abduction, flexion, and external rotation. This position maximizes the volume of the hip joint, which helps to accommodate the joint effusion that is invariably present. Any motion of the hip usually produces intense pain, and patients will guard against any attempted motion of the hip. Palpation of the hip and pelvis may reveal tenderness over the anterior hip joint as well as regions of bony tenderness that may be more consistent with pelvic or femoral osteomyelitis.

Studies (Labs, X-rays)

The laboratory and radiographic evaluation of patients with suspected septic arthritis of the hip should include a WBC count, ESR, CRP, blood cultures, and urine and throat cultures (if clinically indicated). Radiographic studies should include an AP view of the pelvis and a lateral radiograph of the involved hip. An ultrasound of the hip is often useful to determine the presence of a hip effusion and to guide aspiration of the hip, if needed.

The WBC count is elevated 40% to 60% of the time in hip sepsis. An increased WBC count is seen more frequently in older children, and the count may be normal in neonates. The ESR, a nonspecific indicator of inflammation, is elevated about 90% of the time. The ESR reflects fibrinogen production by the liver, so it is an indirect marker of inflammation, which is why the ESR often is increased 24 to 48 hours after the onset of infection. Although an elevated ESR is helpful, it is a nonspecific marker and may be normal in neonates, sickle cell disease, or early presentation of hip sepsis. The CRP is an acute-phase reactant. It is directly synthesized by the liver and rises rapidly in response to infection. It will be elevated 6 to 8 hours after onset of infection and is useful in tracking response to

---

PATIENT ASSESSMENT

1. Early findings may be nonspecific; irritability, cease to crawl, groin pain, or bear weight
2. Usually febrile
3. Any motion of the hip is painful

NOT TO BE MISSED

- Transient synovitis of the hip
- Juvenile rheumatoid arthritis
- Lyme disease
- Pelvic osteomyelitis
- Psoas muscle abscess
- Legg-Calve-Perthes disease
- Leukemia and other neoplasm

treatment. Blood cultures yield positive results 40% to 50% of the time and should be obtained prior to initiating antibiotic treatment, as a positive blood culture is very useful in guiding antibiotic treatment.

The hip joint should be radiographically evaluated for joint space widening, subluxation, or dislocation. Radiographs should also be scrutinized for periosteal reaction or lucency that may be suggestive of osteomyelitis or neoplasm.

Ultrasound is valuable for confirming the presence of a hip effusion. Distention of the hip capsule by 2 mm or more when compared with the opposite side is diagnostic for a hip effusion. However, the character or quantity of the joint fluid as seen on ultrasound has not been proven to be reliable in differentiating septic arthritis from other causes of a hip effusion. Ultrasound can also be used to guide a subsequent hip aspiration (either by marking the entry site or to provide real-time guidance for the aspiration).

Hip aspiration is frequently confirmatory for septic arthritis and should be performed if the diagnosis is uncertain. A large-gauge needle should be used, and if the aspiration is not performed under ultrasound guidance, an arthrogram should be performed in order to confirm intra-articular placement of the needle. Joint fluid should then be sent for cytologic and chemical studies, including a WBC count with differential, Gram stain, aerobic and anaerobic cultures, and synovial glucose level (along with a serum glucose level). A WBC count >50,000 cells/mL and a differential of >90% polymorphonuclear cells are considered diagnostic for septic arthritis. A synovial fluid glucose level 40 mg/dL less than the serum level (or a synovial fluid/serum glucose ratio of <0.5) is also suggestive of septic arthritis. Positive Gram stain or positive synovial fluid cultures are diagnostic for hip sepsis. Gram stain is positive about 30% to 40% of the time, while synovial fluid cultures will be positive 50% to 70% of the time.

Differentiating between septic arthritis and transient synovitis of the hip may be particularly challenging. In general, individuals with transient synovitis will have a less acute clinical course than those with septic arthritis, including decreased pain, greater hip motion, and ability to bear weight (albeit with a limp). Several studies have tried to further separate these two conditions on the basis of clinical and laboratory factors. Kocher and colleagues identified four variables—temperature >38°C, inability to bear weight on the affected hip, ESR >40 mm hour, and serum WBC count >12,000/mL—that they hypothesized would help to predict the presence of septic arthritis. They found that if one of these predictors were present, the probability of septic arthritis was 3%. If two predictors were present, the probability of a septic hip was 40%, with three predictors, the probability was 93.1%; and with all four predictors present, the probability of septic arthritis was 99.6%.[1] Although helpful, this approach has not been consistently validated with subsequent prospective studies.[2,3] These factors (along with CRP >2.0 mg/dL), however, are still useful in differentiating a septic hip from transient synovitis but should be used in conjunction with sound clinical judgment. In equivocal cases, hip aspiration should be performed to help further establish the diagnosis.

Treatment

1. Urgent hip arthrotomy
2. Intravenous antibiotics specific for the organism

Hip arthrotomy should be performed as urgently as possible. An irrigation and debridement of the hip evacuates the bacteria and the inflammatory residue, which left undrained can rapidly degrade articular cartilage. An arthrotomy also decompresses the hip joint and helps to prevent tamponade of the blood vessels supplying the femoral head, which may help to prevent avascular necrosis of the hip and allows for débridement and drainage of any concomitant proximal femoral osteomyelitis.

Intravenous antibiotics should be started after all initial cultures are obtained (including synovial fluid from hip arthrocentesis). The results from the Gram stain should be used to guide initial antibiotic treatment. If the Gram stain is negative, then antibiotics should be selected based on the patient's age, immunization status, and local epidemiology. Neonates are most commonly infected with group B β-hemolytic streptococci, *Staphylococcus aureus*, and gram-negative bacilli. Treatment in this age group, therefore, typically would consist of ceftriaxone or cefotaxime and oxacillin. Children from 1 month to 3 years of age typically have *S. aureus*, *Streptococcus pneumoniae*, and *Streptococcus pyogenes* as causative organisms, so antibiotics in this age group should include nafcillin, oxacillin, cefotaxime, or ceftriaxone. Historically, *Haemophilus influenzae B* was a major cause of hip sepsis in children. Since immunization against this organism began in 1992, the incidence of infections caused by *H. influenzae B* has declined dramatically. Children who are not immunized for *H. influenzae B* or with an unknown immunization status should be started on an antibiotic that is effective against *H. influenzae B* (typically cefuroxime). Septic arthritis in children >3 years of age are usually caused by *S. aureus*, *S. pneumoniae*, or *S. pyogenes*.[4] In this age group, oxacillin or cefazolin are typically recommended as an initial antibiotic. It is important to bear in mind, however, that there appears to be an increasing number of osteoarticular infections caused by community-acquired methicillin-resistant *S. aureus* (MRSA). In areas with a large presence of MRSA, strong consideration should be given to using clindamycin (or another antibiotic effective against MRSA) as initial treatment for septic arthritis of the hip.

The duration of intravenous antibiotics is controversial. Generally, 2 to 6 weeks of total antibiotic treatment is needed, with longer duration used for more virulent organisms. At least 1 to 2 weeks of intravenous antibiotics should generally be given, and conversion to oral antibiotics can be considered after that point.

Clinical Course

Most patients will make a complete recovery with prompt diagnosis and treatment. Risk factors for a proper prognosis following hip sepsis include patient age <6 months, >4-day delay in treatment, infection with

SECTION 12 Pediatric Orthopaedic Problems

WHEN TO REFER

- Inability to bear weight, hip irritability, and fever in a child should be investigated further for possible septic arthritis of the hip.

S. *aureus*, and concomitant osteomyelitis of the proximal femur.[4] Rapid diagnosis and prompt treatment are therefore vital to prevent complications from this devastating infection.

ICD9

711.05 Pyogenic arthritis involving pelvic region and thigh

References

1. Kocher MS, Zurakowski D, Kasser JR. Differentiating between septic arthritis and transient synovitis of the hip in children: an evidence-based clinical prediction algorithm. *J Bone Joint Surg Am* 1999;81:1662–1670.
2. Caird MS, Flynn JM, Leung YL, et al. Factors distinguishing septic arthritis from transient synovitis of the hip in children. A prospective study. *J Bone Joint Surg Am* 2006;88:1251–1257.
3. Luhmann SJ, Jones A, Schootman M, et al. Differentiation between septic arthritis and transient synovitis of the hip in children with clinical prediction algorithms. *J Bone Joint Surg Am* 2004;86:956–962.
4. Sucato DJ, Schwend RM, Gillespie R. Septic arthritis of the hip in children. *J Am Acad Orthop Surg* 1997;5:249–260.

General Medical Problems

Chapter 70

The Use of Nonsteroidal Anti-inflammatory Drugs

Marc L. Cohen and Joan M. Von Feldt

Chapter 71

The Use of Corticosteroid Preparations: Intra-articular and Soft Tissue Injections

Jennifer Kwan-Morley and

Joan M. Von Feldt

CHAPTER 66 Osteoporosis

Ankur A. Karnik and Joan M. Von Feldt

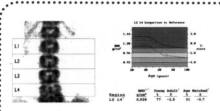

A 65-year-old woman is concerned that she is becoming short. She believes that she has lost about 2 or 3 inches in height. She feels well but has had several episodes of mid back pain, each lasting a few weeks; the last one occurred suddenly as she was attempting to open a window.

CLINICAL POINTS

- The condition is most likely to affect elderly women.
- Vertebral fractures are the most common clinical feature.
- Pain and loss of height may occur.
- Physical disability may be severe in affected individuals.

Clinical Presentation

Osteoporosis is the most common bone disease as well as the most common and eminently preventable risk factor for fracture. In the United States, there are 1.5 million osteoporotic fractures per year, with a direct annual cost of approximately $14 billion in 1995.[1] Approximately one half are vertebral fractures, and one fifth each are hip, wrist, and other fractures.[2] Unlike osteomalacia, osteoporosis is asymptomatic until a fracture occurs. Pain and other subtle symptoms are related to fractures and consequent to deformity.

Hip fractures affect 15% of women and 5% of men by age 80. The 1-year mortality is 20% for those <70 years of age, 30% for those between 70 and 79, and 40% for those >80. Survivors often have severe physical and social limitations; only 50% are able to ambulate independently, and 13% can climb stairs.[3]

Vertebral fractures are the most common clinical manifestations of osteoporosis. About two thirds are asymptomatic and are discovered as an incidental finding on chest or abdominal radiographs. In women who have a vertebral fracture, approximately 19% will have another fracture in the next year. Fractures typically occur during routine activities such as lifting or bending and can cause acute pain. This pain is replaced by a chronic pain that may persist for a long time or eventually subside. Successive fractures can lead to thoracic kyphosis with height loss and a "dowager's hump."[1] Abdominal contents are compressed into less vertebral space, which results in a protuberant belly; patients complain of weight gain that is apparent rather than real. Patients may have early satiety or constipation as well as pain in their neck muscles, as they have to constantly extend their neck. Finally, kyphosis can also lead to dyspnea and a restrictive defect on pulmonary function testing. De Smet and colleagues[4] found that solitary wedge fractures did not occur above the seventh thoracic vertebra in a study of 87 osteoporotic women. They

343

therefore suggested that if a solitary vertebral fracture is found above seventh vertebra, a cause other than osteoporosis must be considered.

Physical Findings

A recent meta-analysis reported that certain physical exam findings in patients who do not meet screening recommendations suggest the presence of osteoporosis or spinal fracture and warrant further workup:

Table 66.1	**Screening Guidelines for Osteoporosis using Bone Mineral Density Testing**
AGENCY	**RECOMMENDATION**
U.S. Preventive Services Task Force (2002)	• Routine screening of women age 65 years and older (grade B recommendation). Begin screening at age 60 for women at increased risk for osteoporotic fractures[a] (grade B recommendation). • No recommendation for or against routine screening in postmenopausal women <60 years old or in women aged 60 to 64 who are not at increased risk for osteoporotic fractures (grade C recommendation).
National Institutes of Health Consensus Statement (2000)	• BMD testing should be considered in patients receiving glucocorticoid therapy for 2 or more months and for patients with other conditions that place them at high risk for osteoporotic fracture. • Individual decisions regarding screening can be based on the preliminary evidence that the risk for fracture increases with age and with an increased number of additional risk factors.[b] • BMD testing should be considered when it would help the patient decide whether to receive treatment to prevent osteoporotic fracture.
National Osteoporosis Foundation (1999)	• All women aged 65 and older, regardless of additional risk factors. • Younger postmenopausal women with one or more risk factors for osteoporosis (other than being white, postmenopausal, and female).[c] • Postmenopausal women who present with fractures (to confirm diagnosis and determine disease severity).

[a] Lower body weight (<70 kg) is the single best predictor of low BMD. No current use of estrogen is another risk factor. Less evidence supports smoking, weight loss, family history, decreased physical activity, alcohol or caffeine use, or low calcium and vitamin D intake as risk factors. At any given age, black women on average have higher BMD than white women and so are thus likely to benefit from screening.

[b] Predictors of low bone mass include female gender, increased age, estrogen deficiency, white race, low weight and body mass index, family history of osteoporosis, smoking, and history of prior fracture. Late menarche, early menopause, and low endogenous estrogen levels are also associated with low BMD in several studies.

[c] Major risk factors for osteoporosis and related fractures in white postmenopausal women include personal history of fracture as an adult, history of fragility fracture in a first-degree relative, low body weight (<~127 lb), current smoking, and use of oral corticosteroid therapy for more than 3 months.

PATIENT ASSESSMENT

1. Presentation varies from asymptomatic to presentation with back deformity and fracture.

2. History should include a family history and risk factors (Table 66.1).

3. Physical exam may show kyphotic skeletal deformity.

4. Diagnosis may be suggested by osteopenia on plane radiographs and confirmed by dual-energy x-ray absorptiometry (DEXA).

- Secondary causes of osteoporosis include endocrine, rheumatologic, gastrointestinal, renal, and oncologic disease as well as nutritional deficiency and pharmacotherapy.

- Other causes of atraumatic compression fractures include osteomalacia, tumor, osteonecrosis, infection, and metabolic disorders.

- A solitary vertebral fracture above seventh vertebra is unlikely to be due to osteoporosis,

(a) presence of a wall-occiput gap (inability to touch occiput to wall with back and heels to wall), (b) weight <51 kg, (c) rib–pelvis distance (<2 fingerbreadths from the inferior margin of ribs to superior surface of pelvis at the midaxillary line), (d) <20 teeth, and (e) self-reported humped back.[1]

Studies

At this time, universal screening for all postmenopausal women for low bone mineral density (BMD) is not recommended. Although numerous risk factors have been identified, it is not clear which women merit screening. National practice guidelines on postmenopausal osteoporosis screening have been created by the U.S. Preventive Services Task Force, the National Institutes of Health, and the National Osteoporosis Foundation; these are summarized in Table 66.1. All of these organizations support an individualized approach rather than universal screening.

DUAL-ENERGY X-RAY ABSORPTIOMETRY SCAN

DEXA, the preferred screening test, uses dual-energy photon beams to measure bone mineral content (BMC) and bone area (BA) of the L1-4 vertebrae and hip. BMD is calculated by dividing BMC by BA. A T-score, used for diagnosis of osteoporosis, compares patient BMD with a sex- and ethnicity-matched young adult. Z-scores compare patient values to age-, sex-, and ethnicity-matched peers. DEXA is the most accurate method for detecting low BMD, is predictive of fracture risk, and is the method by which the World Health Organization defines osteoporosis.[3] The 10-year risk of a fragility fracture in a postmenopausal woman with a T-score ≤ -2.5 is 5% at age 50 but 20% at age 65; absolute risk increases with additional risk factors such as previous fragility fractures. Although it is a good predictive tool of fractures on a population level, it is only modestly successful on an individual basis. Of those women >65 years of age, 7% with normal BMDs will suffer a fracture; of those with severe osteoporosis (T-score <4), less than half will ultimately experience a fracture. Furthermore, osteoarthritis, aortic arteriosclerosis, and intervertebral disk chondrocalcinosis may artifactually increase measured spinal BMD.[5] Ironically, aortic calcification is associated with lower BMD of the femur and an independent predictor of hip fracture. Finally, peripheral densitometry, which measures radius, heel, and hand BMD, does not show good T-score correlations with those of central DEXA scans.[5]

QUANTITATIVE COMPUTED TOMOGRAPHY

Another imaging option is quantitative CT, which separately analyzes trabecular and cortical bone. While it can detect early vertebral bone loss quite sensitively, it has not been validated, is more costly, and has more radiation exposure than DEXA.[5]

BIOCHEMICAL MARKERS

Biochemical markers (BCMs) for bone formation and resorption, while not meant for screening, are indicated for patients with low Z-scores and may be helpful when secondary causes of bone fragility and loss are suspected[5] (Table 66.2). Additionally, because these markers change in

Table 66.2 Biochemical Markers and Other Laboratory Tests for Primary and Secondary Osteoporosis

CONDITION	TEST	ASSOCIATION
Primary osteoporosis	Osteocalcin Bone-specific alkaline phosphatase Carboxyterminal and aminoterminal propeptides of type I collagen	Bone formation
	Serum skeletal acid phosphatase Urinary excretion of calcium, hydroxyproline, and collagen cross links (deoxypyridinoline and peptide-bound alpha-1 to alpha-2 N-telopeptide cross links and C-telopeptide cross link with an isomerized bond between the aspartate and the glycine)	Bone resorption
Secondary osteoporosis	25-Hydroxyvitamin D PTH, calcium TSH, free T4 Serum testosterone, LH, FSH, GnRH, sperm count LFTs, ANA, antimitochondrial antibodies	Vitamin D deficiency Hyperparathyroidism Hyperthyroidism Hypogonadism Liver disease (primarily primary biliary cirrhosis)
	Vitamin B$_{12}$ Serum homocysteine ANA, RF, ESR	Pernicious anemia Homocytinuria Rheumatic disease (e.g., lupus, rheumatoid arthritis, psoriatic arthritis)

PTH, parathyroid hormone; TSH, thyroid-stimulating hormone; LH, luteinizing hormone; FSH, follicle-stimulating hormone; GnRH, gonadotropin-releasing hormone; LFTs, liver function tests; ANA, antinuclear antibodies; RF, rheumatoid factor; ESR, erythrocyte sedimentation rate.

response to treatment more quickly than does BMD, they may have a role in monitoring response to therapy.[3] Derangements are associated with increased fracture risk, but there is significant variability.[5]

Treatment

1. Adequate dietary calcium and vitamin D
2. Weight-bearing exercise
3. Calcium and vitamin D supplements
4. Bisphosphonates
5. Estrogens
6. Synthetic parathyroid hormone

To be of practical use, a discussion of the approach to management should be based on the stage of the disease. Decision making should take into consideration certain caveats: (a) treatment can reduce the risk of fractures in postmenopausal women by 50%, but some women have fractures despite treatment; (b) a substantial number of fractures occur in women who have

T-scores >-2.5; (c) in some cases, there is substantial discrepancy between the spine and hip T-scores; (d) changes in lifestyle and the use of pharmacologic treatment are lifelong commitments, so cost, compliance with medication regimen, and safety must be considered in the decisions on therapy.[6]

Regardless of BMD, postmenopausal women should be counseled on their risk for osteoporosis and encouraged to do weight-bearing exercise, consume adequate calcium (1,000–1,500 mg) and vitamin D (400–800 IU), abstain from smoking, and avoid excess alcohol.[3] Pharmacologic options are generally divided into antiresorptive agents (bisphosphonates, estrogens, selective estrogen-receptor modulators, calcitonin, strontium), and anabolic agents (sodium fluoride, synthetic parathyroid hormone). A summary of available agents, formulations, cost, and side effects is presented in Table 66.3.

CALCIUM AND VITAMIN D

A study of over 36,000 healthy postmenopausal women showed a small benefit to hip BMD with supplementation of 1,000 mg of elemental calcium and 400 IU of vitamin D but no benefit to fracture risk. However, a recent meta-analysis of 12 randomized clinical trials showed a 26% reduction of hip fractures and 23% reduction of nonvertebral fractures with 700 to 800 IU/day of vitamin D; no benefit was shown with 400 IU/day.[7] Those who use these supplements may be at higher risk for kidney stones. 25-Hydroxyvitamin D levels correlate with BMD and are useful in identifying individuals at risk as well as guiding endpoints to treatment.[5]

ANTIRESORPTIVE AGENTS

Bisphosphonates are the most widely used antiresorptive agents that are considered by many to be first-line therapy for postmenopausal osteoporosis. They have strong affinity for hydroxyapatite crystals in bone and are powerful inhibitors of bone resorption via their actions on osteoclasts and possibly osteoblasts.[6] Currently, there are four FDA-approved bisphosphonates for the prevention and treatment of postmenopausal osteoporosis: alendronate, risedronate, ibandronate, and zolendronate.

Alendronate has been shown to decrease incidence of vertebral, hip, and other fractures. Alendronate reduces vertebral fractures in osteopenic and osteoporotic women as well as in those with established vertebral fractures.[6] Duration of optimal treatment is unknown. In one study, women who stopped alendronate after 5 years had a lower BMD and more bone turnover than those who continued it; however, both groups had higher values than at baseline.[8]

Risedronate reduces vertebral and nonvertebral fractures in postmenopausal osteoporotic women. It also reduces the incidence of new fractures by 40% in women with prior fragility fractures. While there is evidence that alendronate produces more gains in BMD and greater reductions in BCM than risedronate, the significance on fracture risk is not well studied.[6]

Ibandronate, which comes in monthly or daily formulations, was approved in 2005 for the prevention and treatment of osteoporosis. The BONE study is the only major study published so far that shows >50%

Table 66.3 Medications Approved by the Food and Drug Administration for the Treatment or Prevention of Postmenopausal Osteoporosis[a]

DRUG	METHOD OF ADMINISTRATION AND DOSE	REDUCTION IN RISK OF FRACTURE	SIDE EFFECT	FDA APPROVAL
Bisphosphonates	Oral		Esophagitis, myalgias	For treatment and prevention[b]
Alendronate	35–70 mg weekly, 5–10 mg daily (oral)	Vertebral, nonvertebral, and hip fracture		
Risedronate	30–35 mg weekly, 5 mg daily (oral)	Vertebral, nonvertebral, and hip fracture		
Ibandronate	150 mg monthly, 2.5 mg daily (oral)	Vertebral fracture	First dose[c]	
Zolendronate	5 mg yearly (intravenous)	Vertebral, nonvertebral, and hip fracture	Atrial fibrillation	
SERM	Oral			For treatment and prevention
Raloxifene	60 mg daily	Vertebral fracture only	Hot flashes, nausea, DVT, leg cramps	
Anabolic agents PTH (3–34) teriparatide	Subcutaneous, daily 20 μg	Vertebral and nonvertebral fracture	Hypercalcemia, nausea, leg cramps	Approved for treatment only: generally used for severe osteoporsis
Calcitonin[d]	Subcutaneous or nasal, 100–200 IU	Vertebral fracture only	Nasal stuffiness, nausea	Approved for treatment only
Estrogens	Oral or transdermal		Risk of DVT, risk of cardiovascular disease, breast cancer	Approved for prevention only
Conjugated equine estrogens	Oral, 0.30–1.25 mg daily	Vertebral, nonvertebral and hip fracture (at dose of 0.625 mg daily)		
17β-estrodiol[e]	Oral, 0.025–0.10 mg, or transdermal twice weekly	No data from randomized, controlled trials		For prevention only
	Ultra low dose (0.014 mg/d, given weekly)	No data available		

SERM, selective estrogen-receptor modulator; DVT, deep vein thrombosis; PTH, parathyroid hormone.

[a] All agents approved for treatment have demonstrated efficacy in reducing fractures, as determined in randomized, placebo-controlled trials with fractures as the primary end point.

[b] There has been limited post marketing experience with ibandronate for prevention.

[c] There may be .a response to the first dose at 150 mg consisting of myalgias, joint aches, and low-grade fever, which is similar to a response to the first intervenous administration of bisphosphonates containing nitrogen.

[d] The use of calcitonin is not generally recommended.

[e] A reduction in the risk of hip fracture has not been established for 17β-estradiol in a randomized, controlled trial.

Adapted from Rosen CJ. Postmenopausal osteoporosis. *N Engl J Med* 2005;353:594–603.

reduction in vertebral fractures after 3 years of treatment in postmenopausal women with prior fractures.[9]

Once yearly intravenous zolendronate was approved in 2007 for the treatment of postmenopausal osteoporosis. It significantly reduces the risk of vertebral, hip, and other fractures.[10]

Pamidronate is used in the treatment of malignant hypercalcemia, multiple myeloma, and skeletal metastases. It is currently not approved for the treatment of osteoporosis. Studies have been small and have focused on BMD as an end point, although one study did find a benefit on vertebral fracture risk compared with placebo.[3]

The benefits of antiresorptive therapy on fracture reduction may be greater than predicted by improvements in BMD; even women who lose up to 4% of BMD while on bisphosphonates have a reduced vertebral fracture risk.[11] However, increase in BMD does correlate well with reduction in rate of vertebral and nonvertebral fractures.[12]

Selective estrogen-receptor modulators such as raloxifene slow bone resorption by osteoclasts. Raloxifene is the only nonbisphosphonate antiresorptive agent that is FDA-approved for the prevention and treatment of osteoporosis. It increases BMD and decreases vertebral fractures by 40% in women with osteoporosis; it has not yet been demonstrated to have an effect on nonvertebral fractures.[13]

Calcitonin is an inhibitor of bone resorption by decreasing osteoclast formation and attachment. Nasal and subcutaneous formulations are approved for the treatment and prevention of postmenopausal osteoporosis. The PROOF trial, the only major study of this compound, showed a 33% reduction in vertebral fractures and 36% in nonvertebral fractures with 100 IU/day compared with placebo; however, due to the large dropout rate, lack of blinding, and lack of dose-response effect, the results are in question.[6] A meta-analysis including other studies suggests a benefit from 250 IU/day only on vertebral fractures.[14]

Estrogen is FDA-approved for the prevention (not treatment) of osteoporosis. Estrogen's principle effect on bone is to inhibit resorption; it also affects calcium balance and cytokine signaling to osteoclasts. The Women's Health Initiate Trial demonstrated a 33% risk reduction in hip fractures with those treated with conjugated estrogens (with or without a progestin).[6] While one meta-analysis showed nonsignificant benefits on vertebral and nonvertebral risk, another showed a 27% risk reduction of nonvertebral fractures.[15] Estrogen therapy may not have as long-lasting effects as bisphosphonates after discontinuation;[6] how this affects fracture risk is unknown.

Strontium ranelate is a trace element with anabolic and antiresorptive activity. In vitro, it increases collagen and noncollagen protein synthesis, enhances preosteoblast differentiation, and inhibits osteoclast differentiation and function. In one study of postmenopausal women with osteoporosis and previous fracture, there was a 41% relative risk reduction of vertebral fractures in those treated with 2 g of strontium. Another study demonstrated a 19% risk reduction of nonvertebral fractures in postmenopausal women with osteoporosis or other risk factors for fracture.[16]

ANABOLIC AGENTS

Sodium fluoride stimulates osteoblast proliferation and new bone formation. There are no large trials investigating its use, and those that exist give conflicting information. Whereas three studies using 20 to 50 mg/day of sodium fluoride found significant risk reduction in vertebral fractures in postmenopausal women with osteoporosis or prior fracture,[17] two studies using 60 to 75 mg/day had showed increased numbers of nonvertebral and vertebral fractures in those treated with fluoride.[18] Interestingly, there may be a dose-related effect, as these later two studies used higher quantities of fluoride.

Parathyroid hormone (PTH 1-34) stimulates osteoblast production and bone formation. Teriparatide is a portion of human PTH approved for the treatment of osteoporosis in postmenopausal women or men with a high risk for fracture. A large, randomized, controlled trial showed a relative risk reduction of >60% for vertebral and around 40% for nonvertebral fractures in postmenopausal women with prior fractures treated with 20 to 40 μg of subcutaneous PTH 1-34. There is a black box warning on PTH 1-34, as rats treated with extremely large doses (30–60 times the FDA-approved dose) developed osteosarcoma. For this reason, the current recommendation is to limit its use to 2 years.[6]

COMBINATION THERAPY

There have been several trials evaluating combination treatment, usually alendronate and another modality. They are mostly small, however, and they overwhelmingly use BMD rather than fractures as their outcome measure. Alendronate may not be synergistic with PTH in increasing BMD when started simultaneously but may be of benefit when daily or cyclic PTH is added to an existing alendronate regimen. It also appears that gains made in BMD after 1 year of PTH therapy are lost unless followed by antiresorptive therapy.[6] Finally, hormone replacement therapy (HRT) in combination with alendronate has longer-lasting effects on BMD after withdrawal of treatment than does treatment with HRT alone.[12] One possible explanation for the lack of synergy between PTH and antiresorptive treatments is that antiresorptive agents reduce bone turnover and bone formation, thus limiting the number of mature osteoblasts for PTH to act on. An alternative is to use PTH for a maximum of 2 years and then use antiresorptive agents to maintain and possibly enhance the gains made in BMD.

TREATMENT IN MEN

Men age 50 and older have a 13% lifetime risk for fracture. The morbidity and mortality following a fracture is greater in men than it is in women.[19] For men with osteoporosis, 30% to 60% of cases are associated with secondary causes, most commonly hypogonadism, glucocorticoid therapy, and alcohol abuse.[2] Currently, there are no guidelines on osteoporosis screening in men. Workup should be based on history of prior fractures, presence of risk factors, or clinical suspicion. Although alendronate and teriparatide are the only FDA-approved drugs for osteoporosis in men, other drugs have been shown to increase BMD in men, including androgens, raloxifene, and combination therapy.

Clinical Course

Prior fractures are the most important risk for future fractures independent of mineral density. Apart from prior fragility fractures, silent fractures (seen radiographically) causing more than 2 cm of height loss and traumatic

- Evaluation or treatment of secondary causes of fractures

- Those who have failed treatment

- Those with multiple fractures causing spinal instability or severe kyphosis affecting breathing

- Any fracture that needs surgical repair

fractures should prompt further inquiry. Other risks for fragility fractures include factors that increase fall risk; inflammatory disorders of the musculoskeletal, gastrointestinal, and pulmonary systems; glucocorticoids; discontinuation of HRT in postmenopausal women; hypogonadism from drugs, anorexia, or athleticism; and neurologic disorders that cause immobilization.[5] Failure of therapy should be considered if the patient is compliant; has had sufficient time for treatment (>1 year); and secondary causes such as hypercalciuria, vitamin D deficiency, and malignancy are ruled out. In this circumstance, it may be appropriate to try an anabolic agent such as PTH, although there is no solid evidence to drive such a decision.

ICD9

733.00 Osteoporosis, unspecified
733.01 Senile osteoporosis
733.02 Idiopathic osteoporosis
733.03 Disuse osteoporosis
733.09 Other osteoporosis

References

1. Green AD, Colon-Emeric CS, Bastian L, et al. Does this woman have osteoporosis? *JAMA* 2004; 292:2890–2900.
2. Mauck KF, Clarke BL. Diagnosis, screening, prevention, and treatment of osteoporosis. *Mayo Clin Proc* 2006;81:662–672.
3. Wei GS, Jackson JL, Hatzigeorgiou C, Tofferi JK. Osteoporosis management in the new millennium. *Prim Care* 2003;30:711–741.
4. De Smet AA, Robinson RG, Johnson BE, Lukert BP. Spinal compression fractures in osteoporotic women: patterns and relationship to hyperkyphosis. *Radiology* 1988;166:497–500.
5. Raisz LG. Clinical practice. Screening for osteoporosis. *N Engl J Med* 2005;353:164–171.
6. Rosen CJ. Postmenopausal osteoporosis. *N Engl J Med* 2005;353:594–603.
7. Bischoff-Ferrari HA, Willett WC, Wong JB, et al. Fracture prevention with vitamin D supplementation. *JAMA* 2005;293:2257–2264.
8. Ensrud KE, Barrett-Connor EL, Schwartz A, et al. Randomized trial of effect of alendronate continuation versus discontinuation in women with low BMD: results from the Fracture Intervention Trial longterm extension. *J Bone Miner Res* 2004;19:1259–1269.
9. Chesnut III CH, Skag A, Christiansen C, et al. Effects of oral ibandronate administered daily or intermittently on fracture risk in postmenopausal osteoporosis. *J Bone Miner Res* 2004;19:1241–1249.
10. Black DM, Delmas PD, Eastell R, et al. Once-yearly zoledronic acid for treatment of postmenopausal osteoporosis. *N Engl J Med* 2007;356:1809–1822.
11. Cummings SR, Karpf DB, Harris F, et al. Improvement in spine bone density and reduction in risk of vertebral fractures during treatment with antiresorptive drugs. *Am J Med* 2002;112:281–289.
12. Greenspan SL, Resnick NM, Parker RA. Combination therapy with hormone replacement and alendronate for prevention of bone loss in elderly women. *JAMA* 2003;289:2525–2533.
13. Riggs BL, Hartmann LC. Selective estrogen-receptor modulators-mechanisms of action and application to clinical practice. *N Engl J Med* 2003;348:618–629.
14. Cranney A, Tugwell P, Zytaruk N, et al. Meta-analyses of therapies for postmenopausal osteoporosis. VI. Meta-analysis of calcitonin for the treatment of postmenopausal osteoporosis. *Endocr Rev* 2002;23:540–551.
15. Torgerson DJ, Bell-Syer SE. Hormone replacement therapy and prevention of nonvertebral fractures: A meta-analysis of randomized trials. *JAMA* 2001;285:2891–2897.
16. Reginster JY, Seeman E, De Vernejoul MC, et al. Strontium ranelate reduces the risk of nonvertebral fractures in postmenopausal women with osteoporosis: treatment of Peripheral Osteoporosis (TROPOS) study. *J Clin Endocrinol Metab* 2005;90:2816–2822.
17. Rubin CD, Pak CY, Adams-Huet B, et al. Sustained-release sodium fluoride in the treatment of the elderly with established osteoporosis. *Arch Intern Med* 2001;161:2325–2333.
18. Gutteridge DH, Stewart GO, Prince RL, et al. A randomized trial of sodium fluoride (60 mg) +/− estrogen in postmenopausal osteoporotic vertebral fractures: increased vertebral fractures and peripheral bone loss with sodium fluoride; concurrent estrogen prevents peripheral loss, but not vertebral fractures. *Osteoporos Int* 2002;13:158–170.
19. Amin S. Male Osteoporosis: epidemiology and pathophysiology. *Curr Osteoporos Rep* 2003;1:71–77.

CHAPTER 67 Crystal-induced Arthritis

Jennifer Kwan-Morley and Joan M. Von Feldt

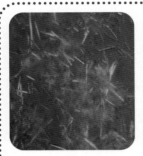

A 45-year-old overweight man comes to clinic for the evaluation of an exquisitely tender first toe, which started abruptly in the middle of the night. He has a history of hypertension, hyperlipidemia, and kidney stones and states that he had spent the prior evening with his friends having several rounds of beer. He then awoke in the middle of the night with severe, 10/10, pain in his toe, not relieved by acetaminophen and only minimally relieved by ibuprofen. He could not bear weight on his foot and noted that "even the pressure of the sheet on my toe was painful."

CLINICAL POINTS

- The condition is more common in men but is also found in postmenopausal women.

- Monoarticular arthritis of the first metatarsal joint can be the first presenting sign.

- Abrupt onset of pain, with inflammation, is characteristic.

GOUT
Clinical Presentation

Gout is one of the oldest known types of arthritis. The association between gout and uric acid has been known for centuries, but it was only after the biochemistry of uric acid was elucidated in the 1960s that better treatment and prevention of gout became available. Today, it is one of the most successfully treated forms of arthritis.

Gout is predominantly a disease of adult men, with its peak incidence in the fifth decade of life. The prevalence of self-reported gout in the United States was estimated to be 13.6 per 1,000 men and 6.4 per 1,000 women in 1986. However, the rates of gout in women significantly increase as they enter into menopause and afterwards approach similar rates as men.[1]

The classic presentation of gout is a monoarticular arthritis of the first metatarsal joint, known as *podagra*. However, gout can present as a monoarticular arthritis of almost any joint or can have a polyarticular presentation (Fig. 67.1). Joints predominantly involved include the metatarsalphalangeal (MTP) joints, ankles, knees, small joints of the hands, wrists, and elbows. An attack is usually abrupt in onset, often occurring in the middle of the night, and rapidly progresses to inflammation of the joint and surrounding tissues. In fact, the skin surrounding a gouty joint can appear so inflamed that it is often mistaken for an overlying cellulitis. Patients will often describe exquisite tenderness such that sheets touching the skin above the joint is painful, inability to ambulate or bear weight, and an abrupt onset of the pain. A typical gout flare can last from several days to a week but can be significantly shortened with treatment at the onset of an attack.

Physical Findings

In the initial attack of gout, there are often no physical findings that are associated with gout except for the inflammatory arthritis. Tophi are usually not present during the first presentation of gout and generally develop after 10 years of intercritical gout. Subcutaneous gouty tophi can be found almost anywhere but most commonly are found on the fingers, toes, ears, knees, olecranon bursa, Achilles tendons, and pressure points along extensor surfaces. A history of uric acid nephrolithiasis could be helpful in the diagnosis of gout.

PATIENT ASSESSMENT

1. Acute monoarticular arthritis
2. Surrounding inflammatory response; marked tenderness
3. Polyarticular arthritis less common, but can occur
4. Resolves in days to a week
5. Tophi over extensor surfaces
6. Serum uric acid >7 mg/dl
7. Birefringent synovial fluid analysis—crystals

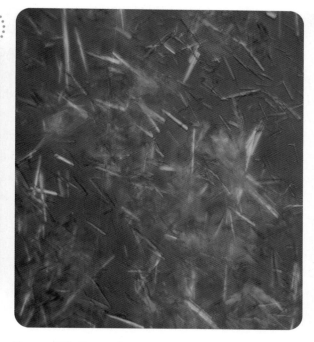

Figure 67.1 Monosodium urate crystals under polarized microscopy. Note the long needle-shaped crystals and the difference in color of the crystals at 90-degree angles. Monosodium urate crystals are strongly negatively birefrigent under polarized light. (Picture courtesy of H. Ralph Schumacher, M.D.)

NOT TO BE MISSED

Patterns of Arthritis in Common Conditions

Monoarthritis

- Crystal-induced arthritis
- Infectious arthritis
- Lyme arthritis
- Monoarticular presentation of a systemic disease (e.g., rheumatoid arthritis, systemic lupus erythematosus)
- Psoriatic
- Reactive arthritis
- Fracture
- Malignancy

Podagra Is Not Always Gout. Consider:

- Infection
- Trauma/Fracture
- Malignancy
- Systemic disease
- Foreign body

Polyarthritis

- Crystal induced arthritis
- Inflammatory osteoarthritis
- Spondyloarthropathies including psoriatic arthritis
- Rheumatoid arthritis
- Systemic autoimmune disease
- Systemic lupus erythematosus
- Palindromic rheumatism
- Sarcoidosis
- Whipple disease
- Malignancy

PATHOGENESIS

Uric acid is the normal end product of degradation of purine compounds. In humans, gout is a consequence of a lack of the enzyme uricase, which oxidizes uric acid to the soluble allantoin. Uric acid is derived from both ingestion of purines as well as the endogenous synthesis of purine nucleotides. The major route of uric acid disposal is renal excretion, which accounts for approximately two thirds of urate loss.

Traditionally, patients with gout have been subcategorized into two major categories: uric acid overproducers and underexcretors.[2] Both increased uric acid production as well as decreased uric acid renal secretion contributes substantially to hyperuricemia. To distinguish the two categories, 24-hour urine collections are calculated for uric acid concentrations. A person is classified as an uric acid overproducer if there is >750 mg of uric acid. If there is <750 mg of uric acid, then the patient is classified as an underexcretor. Table 67.1 lists the most common causes of overproduction and underexcretion.

The course of gout tends to pass through three distinct stages (Table 67.2): asymptomatic hyperuricemia, acute intermittent gout, and chronic

Table 67.1 Causes of Uric Acid Overproduction/Underexcretion

URIC ACID OVERPRODUCERS	URIC ACID UNDEREXCRETORS
Primary	*Primary*
Idiopathic	Idiopathic
Inherited enzyme abnormalities	
Secondary	*Secondary*
Dietary intake	Renal insufficiency[a]
Malignancy, hemolytic disease	Medications
Alcohol abuse	Dehydration
Hypertension	
Insulin resistance	

[a]Most common cause of hyperuricemia.

tophaceous gout.[3] Asymptomatic hyperuricemia is defined physiologically as a level above the normal soluble concentration of monosodium urate crystals in body fluid, which is 6.8 mg/dL. In adult men, the level of uric acid is reached during puberty, whereas in women, the levels are lower but approximate the levels in men after menopause. The second stage starts with the initial attack of gout. After resolution of an acute attack, there can be periods of quiescence with long intervals between attacks (intercritical gout). Over time, these intervals can become shorter or more joints may be involved until development into chronic tophaceous gout. This usually develops after years of intermittent gout, usually 10 years or more. The involved joints become persistently uncomfortable and swollen, and very often, clinically evident tophi are detected.

Studies

LABORATORY AND RADIOLOGIC FEATURES

Elevated serum uric acid is commonly seen in gout patients, but as reported previously, asymptomatic hyperuricemia can precede true gout attacks by decades. In order to have a definitive diagnosis of gout, aspiration of synovial fluid and microscopy with polarized light showing bright, negatively birefringent needle-shaped crystals must be performed.[4]

Table 67.2 Stages of Gout

Asymptomatic hyperuricemia

Acute gout

Chronic tophaceous gout

Often, early in the course, there are no specific radiologic features of gout, except for possible soft tissue swelling around the joint. However, in long-standing gout, and in particular tophaceous gout, erosions may be present. These erosions are usually distinguishable from other inflammatory arthrides in that the gouty erosion often has an "overhanging edge" with preserved joint space until very late in the disease.

Treatment and Clinical Course

1. Colchicine or NSAIDs
2. Corticosteroids
3. Xanthine oxidase inhibitors (allopurinol) as preventive treatment

PHARMACOLOGIC

Acute

Colchicine can be used in acute attacks of gout as well as for prevention of gout. It impairs granulocyte chemotaxis and phagocytosis and thus prevents the inflammatory reaction. When taken at the very start of a gouty attack, it usually provides relief within 24 hours. The usual dose of Colchicine in patients without renal insuffiency is a 0.6 mg tablet by mouth every hour until relief or nausea, vomiting, abdominal pain, or diarrhea. Many patients find this regimen difficult to manage, and often Colchicine is given 0.6 mg by mouth two or three times daily for the first few days and then tapered to daily when symptoms improve, and then it is stopped. In renal insufficiency, the dose should be significantly decreased. The dosage should be halved for patients with a glomerular filtration rate <50 to 60 mL/minute, and a typical dose is 0.6 mg by mouth every other day. The main side effects of Colchicine are gastrointestinal symptoms (nausea, diarrhea, abdominal pain), and excessive doses can cause bone marrow toxicity.

NSAIDs do not prevent the gouty attack but diminish the inflammation and pain associated with a gout flare. The classic treatment is indomethacin 25 to 50 mg by mouth two or three times daily during an acute attack, but any NSAID can be used. Caution should be used in patients with renal insufficiency.

Both oral and intra-articular corticosteroids are of benefit in the acute gouty attack. Intra-articular corticosteroids are usually given if the gouty flare is limited to fewer than three joints. Corticosteroids can be exceedingly useful in those with renal insufficiency, those who cannot tolerate the gastrointestinal side effects of Colchicine, or in those with a contraindication to oral medications. Caution should be used in diabetic patients due to the systemic effect of corticosteroids and associated hyperglycemia.

Preventative

Allopurinol is a xanthine oxidase inhibitor that directly reduces the production of uric acid. It is the mainstay in the treatment of gout and can be used in overproducers and underexcretors of uric acid. It is indicated in patients with urate overproduction, tophus formation, nephrolithiasis, and increasing attacks of gout (usually more than three attacks/year). Gastrointestinal upset, rash, and headache are the most common side effects and are rare. The usual starting dose is 100 mg/day and is titrated up based on the serum uric acid. The dose is stabilized once the goal of the serum uric acid of <6 mg/dL is achieved. The dose should be adjusted appropriately in those with renal insufficiency. It is not recommended to start allopurinol during acute flares, as fluctuations in the serum uric acid levels can worsen gout. Allopurinol is generally started 2 to 4 weeks after the resolution of an acute attack. It is important to note that a rare but serious toxicity known as *allopurinol hypersensitivity syndrome* can occur, characterized by fever, rash and which should prompt the patient to seek immediate medical attention.

Probenecid is a drug that promotes the excretion of uric acid in the urine and is thus most beneficial in uric acid underexcretors. Caution should be used in overproducers, as it can precipitate uric acid nephrolithiasis. Initial doses start at 500 mg/day and can be increased to a maximum of 1 gm twice a day. Side effects include rash, gastrointestinal upset, and nephrolithiasis and are rare. It is contraindicated in patients with uric acid nephrolithiasis, in those with a glomerular filtration rate <50 to 60 mL/minute, and in those who are unable to drink at least 2 L of fluid a day.

The use of dietary modification is controversial and is not consistently recommended by all practitioners. A low purine diet is often recommended, with avoidance of foods high in purine such as organ meats (kidney, liver, sweetbreads), sardines/anchovies, shellfish (scallops, shrimp), and beer and alcohol. In addition, plenty of fluids are recommended to prevent dehydration, which can precipitate gout flares.

For adjuvant therapies, there are two medications that have known uricosuric effects. Losartan is an angiotensin II receptor antagonist that promotes uric acid secretion in the urine. This is an effect specific to losartan and not a class effect. Another medication with similar uric acid–lowering properties is fenofibrate, which is used in the treatment of hypercholesterolemia. Both reduce serum uric acid by 10 to 15% and can be used as adjunctive therapy.

Newer therapies include the use of Febuxostat and uricase. Febuxostat is a nonpurine inhibitor of xanthine oxidase that is an even more selective inhibitor than allopurinol. As of this writing, it is not available in the United States. It is a completely different molecule than allopurinol and thus can be used in patients with allopurinol hypersensitivity syndrome. In addition, it is not dependent on renal function and therefore can be used in chronic renal insufficiency with less difficulty.[5] Current studies are under way looking at uricase in chronic gout, and in particular in chronic tophaceous gout, as its dramatic lowering of serum uric acid can lead to relatively rapid resolution of tophi.[6]

WHEN TO REFER

- Suspected genetic disorder presenting as asymptomatic hyperuricemia in a young patient
- Joint aspiration required for diagnosis (e.g., rule out infection)
- Hyperuricemia or gout heralding systemic disorder (malignancy, chronic kidney disease, etc.)
- Gouty arthritis not responding to medical therapy
- Complications of tophi (spinal or neural compression, parenchymal organ involvement, etc.)

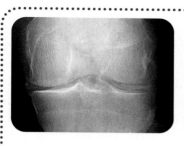

An 85-year-old woman with a history of general osteoarthritis and primary hyperparathyroidism, status post parathyroid resection with resultant hypothyroidism and generalized osteoarthritis, is hospitalized for an acute left hip fracture that occurred after a fall in her nursing home. She was admitted to the orthopedic surgery service, and a successful ORIF procedure was performed without complications. However, on postoperative day 2, she notices a relatively abrupt onset of pain and swelling of her right knee. She also notes warmth, swelling, and erythema of the knee and is unable to participate in physical therapy because of the pain.

CALCIUM PYROPHOSPHATE DIHYDRATE
Clinical Presentation

Pseudogout is the deposition of calcium pyrophosphate dihydrate (CPPD) crystals in the synovial fluid. It is similar to gout flares in that it can cause similar symptoms, although the mechanism of disease is markedly different. Whereas gout is caused by the deposition of uric acid in the synovium because of increased serum uric acid, pseudogout is caused by CPPD deposition. Pseudogout, like gout, is a self-limited attack that can present in almost any joint, although classically the knees are affected. It is often precipitated by trauma, surgery, and acute illness. Chondrocalcinosis refers to the presence of calcium-containing crystals in cartilage, which can be detected on plain radiographs. This is most often due to CPPD deposition but can also represent other calcium-containing crystals such as calcium hydroxyapatite, basic calcium phosphate, or others. Chondrocalcinosis shows an increasing prevalence with age. However, not all chondrocalcinosis is symptomatic, and it is often discovered only after a first pseudogout attack. Several clinical associations have been made with CPPD arthritis (Table 67.3). There are familial, autosomal dominant patterns of CPPD arthritis, but the largest associations with CPPD arthritis are due to age and other secondary causes. Those associations include hyperparathyroidism, hemochromatosis, hypothyroidism, hypomagnesemia, and hypophosphatemia (the 5 H's) as well as amyloidosis. In a patient <55 years old documented to have CPPD in synovial fluid or with severe recurrent attacks, evaluation should include calcium, iron/TIBC ratio, magnesium, phosphorus, alkaline phosphatase, parathyroid hormone, and thyroid stimulation hormone for completeness.

Table 67.3 Clinical Associations with Gout
Renal insufficiency
Hypertension
Obesity
Hyperlipidemia
Transplantation
Familial gout

PATIENT ASSESSMENT

1. Monoarticular or poly-articular acute arthritis
2. Synovial analysis—crystals
3. Joint x-rays
4. Consider secondary causes

Physical Findings

The physical findings of CPPD mimic those of gout, particularly when the presentation is monoarticular. The single joint most often involved in CPPD is the knee, while in gout it is the MTP joint. Upper extremity involvement, particularly the wrist in elderly patients, is common. The findings of monoarthritis are otherwise similar to those of gout and include intense inflammation with redness, warmth, and swelling. Less commonly, patients will have multiple joints involved, occasionally mimicking rheumatoid arthritis, or osteoarthritis. Other physical findings of CPPD are those of the associated underlying illness (see above).

Studies

Confirmation of CPPD arthritis is done by identification of the classic weakly positive birefringent rhomboid-shaped crystals under polarized light. Plain radiographs showing chondrocalcinosis in the affected joint also is helpful diagnostically (Fig. 67.2). Figure 67.3 shows CPPD crystals under polarized microscopy.

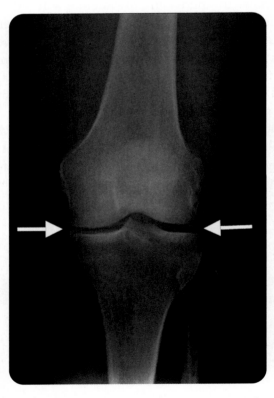

Figure 67.2 Plain radiograph of the left knee. Note the chondrocalcinosis in the medial and lateral compartments of the knee. Note also the mild osteoarthritis with evidence of medial joint space narrowing and osteophyte formation.

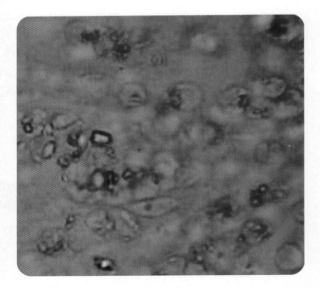

Figure 67.3 CPPD crystals under polarized microscopy. Note the rhomboid-shaped crystals, which are weakly positively birefringent under polarized light. Note also the presence of intracellular as well as extracellular crystals. (Picture courtesy of H. Ralph Schumacher, M.D.)

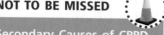
Treatment and Clinical Course

1. Colcichine or NSAIDs
2. Intra-articular or oral corticosteroids

Unlike gout, there is no easy way to extract CPPD crystals from cartilage. Acute attacks can be treated with NSAIDs in those with normal renal function and without other contraindications. Colchicine can be effective if treated early but has less effect than on gout. Intra-articular corticosteroid injection can be beneficial once the absence of infection is confirmed. Oral or parenteral corticosteroids may be necessary in a polyarticular episode.

ICD9

274.9 Gout, unspecified

References

1. Hochberg MC, Thomas J, Thomas DJ, et al. Racial differences in the incidence of gout: the role of hypertension. *Arthritis Rheum.* 1995;38:628–632.
2. Choi HK, Mount DB, Reginato AM. Pathogenesis of gout. *Ann Intern Med.* 2005;143:499–516.
3. Schumacher HR. Monosodium urate crystal deposition arthropathy part I: review of the stages and diagnosis of gout. *Adv Stud Med.* 2005;5(3):133–138.
4. Underwood M. Diagnosis and management of gout. *BMJ.* 2006;332;1315–1319.
5. Schumacher HR. Febuxostat: a non-purine, selective inhibitor of xanthine oxidase for the management of hyperuricaemia in patients with gout. *Expert Opin Investig Drugs.* 2005;14(7):893–903.
6. Terkeltaub R, Businsku DA, Becker MA. Recent developments in our understanding of the renal basis of hyperuricemia and the development of novel antihyperuricemic therapeutics. *Arthritis Res Ther.* 2006;8(Suppl 1):S4.

SECTION 13 General Medical Problems

Joan M. Von Feldt

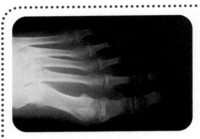

A 44-year-old woman presents with joint pain and fatigue of 3 months duration. She works as a third-grade teacher and has had difficulty getting to school on time because of morning pain and fatigue. She normally works out at the gym three mornings a week but lately feels too tired to do so. She complains of foot pain, which she attributes to standing on her feet in the classroom and poor shoe wear. On direct questioning, she notes 45 minutes of morning stiffness and pain primarily in her feet and wrists.

Rheumatoid arthritis (RA) is the most common autoimmune rheumatic disease, affecting 1% to 2% of the population.[1] It affects women more than men in a ratio of 5:1, with a peak age of onset between 30 and 55 years of age. Untreated, it can cause deformity, significant disability. and premature death.[2,3] Although there is no cure for RA, there has been an explosion of new treatments and combination therapies available to treat the condition, and many patients can achieve near remission with aggressive therapeutic regimens.

The characteristic findings in RA include inflammatory arthritis that is destructive to joints. This destruction is measured as erosions and joint space narrowing. The destructive arthritis is also accompanied by muscle atrophy, and inflammation of the tendon sheaths that can lead to tendon rupture. Structural damage to the joints and supporting ligaments and tendons are usually irreversible. The degree of damage is closely linked to inflammation, and hence to disease activity. Extra-articular manifestations can be present as well. RA, like other systemic inflammatory conditions, is associated with premature mortality, usually attributed to cardiovascular events.[4] Therefore, early recognition of the disease and aggressive intervention are warranted.

Clinical Presentation

The typical presentation of RA is a young woman with morning stiffness of multiple joints of the hands, wrists, and feet, although almost any joint can be involved. Morning stiffness is usually more prominent than pain.[5] Frequently, women present with chronic foot pain, which they incorrectly attribute to poor shoe wear. Subcutaneous nodules (rheumatoid nodules) can be present on extensor surfaces, although they can be found in lung

CLINICAL POINTS

- The condition is most common autoimmune rheumatic disease.

- Women are affected more often than men.

- Inflammatory arthritis that destroys joints is characteristic.

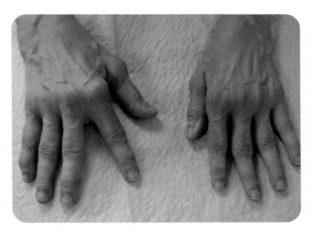

Figure 68.1 Patient with moderate RA. Note swelling of the MCP and PIP joints and right wrist, with accompanying hyperextension of the PIP joints, especially of the third and fourth fingers of left hand and the third finger of the right hand. Interosseous muscle atrophy of the dorsum of the hand is present. The dominant hand is more affected, which frequently occurs.

and other tissues as well. On examination, the involved joints are usually swollen, painful on range of motion, and tender, but the findings are usually more subtle than, for example, an inflamed joint affected by gout (Fig. 68.1).

The ACR criteria for the diagnosis of RA is summarized below. Patients should be considered to have the diagnosis of RA if they have the presence of four of these criteria for at least 6 weeks.

- Morning stiffness for at least 1 hour
- Swelling of three or more joints
- Swelling of wrist, metacarpophalangeal (MCP), or proximal interphalangeal (PIP) joints
- Symmetric joint swelling
- Hand x-ray changes typical of RA that must include erosions or unequivocal bony decalcification
- Rheumatoid subcutaneous nodules
- Rheumatoid factor

More frequent extra-articular features of RA include anemia, serositis (pleuropericarditis), scleritis, and secondary Sjögren syndrome (dry eyes and dry mouth). Less commonly, splenomegaly, vasculitis, neuropathy, interstitial lung disease, and renal disease may occur during the course of the disease and can be life threatening. Neck pain should raise concern because of possible involvement of the atlantoaxial joint of the cervical spine and subsequent neck instability. Prompt imaging and referral should occur with the development of neurologic findings.

Physical Findings

The physical findings of RA reflect the form of clinical presentation, which most often is a symmetrical polyarthritis with inflammation; swelling and warmth of the MCP and interphalangeal joints of the fingers, wrists and metatarsophalangeal (MTP) joints of the toes; along with symmetrical involvement of the elbows, shoulders, ankles, and knees. Patients typically manifest tenderness and limitation of motion in involved joints as well as other signs of inflammation. The degree of structural damage varies greatly among patients but generally follows chronicity and disease severity. In established, chronic RA, ulnar deviation, swan neck deformity of the fingers, and other physical evidence of joint destruction and tendon dislocation are found. Extra-articular features of RA include anemia, subcutaneous nodules, and dry mucous membranes from secondary Sjogren (Felty syndrome). Patients with extra-articular findings usually also have a more severe coarse.

Studies

LABORATORY

Although the rheumatoid factor (RF) is positive in 80% of patients within 2 years of disease onset, the RF can be negative at initial presentation.

PATIENT ASSESSMENT

- Pain and morning stiffness greater than one hour
- Polyarticular, symmetric arthritis
- Radiologic abnormalities
- Laboratory evidence of RA

SECTION 13   General Medical Problems

Anti-CCP antibodies have been shown to be more sensitive in early disease and therefore should be checked when the illness is suspected. The sensitivity and specificity of anti-CCP antibodies for RA is dependent on the characteristics of the assay kit employed.[6] Acute-phase reactants that measure systemic inflammation such as ESR and CRP may be elevated. For ESR, if the blood is not processed properly (cold specimen, tilted tube), pregnancy and certain drugs (dextran) can cause a false increase, and alternatively, hyperglycemia, leukocytosis, clotted blood, and other drugs (quinine) can cause a false decrease.

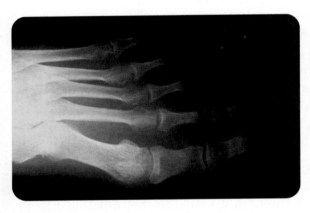

Figure 68.2 Radiograph of a patient with early RA. Note marginal erosion of the third and fifth MTP joints.

RADIOGRAPHIC EVALUATION

Joint erosions can be seen very early with sensitive imaging such as MRI or musculoskeletal ultrasound, but even on x-rays, erosions of the MCP, PIP, or MTP joints can be seen within 3 months of disease onset.[7] Radiographic findings include marginal erosions and joint space narrowing, most easily appreciated in the small joints of the hands, wrists (especially the ulnar–carpal joint), and feet (Fig. 68.2). The presence of RF, anti-CCP Ab, rheumatoid nodules, ≥20 joints involved, and early erosions are all associated with a poorer prognosis.

Treatment and Clinical Course

1. Disease-modifying antirheumatic drugs (DMARDs) such as methotrexate (MTX)
2. NSAIDs and/or prednisone
3. Biological therapy

Patients with the diagnosis of RA should be promptly referred to a rheumatologist for evaluation and treatment. There has been an evolution of therapeutic strategy in the past decade as more effective therapy has been studied. Spontaneous remission is rare, and prompt aggressive therapy is warranted. The ACR guidelines for the management of RA were updated in 2002[8] (Fig. 68.3). Methotrexate (MTX) is the standard of care for initial management. However, other agents can be utilized if there is a contraindication to MTX. MTX is one of the disease modifying antirheumatic drugs (DMARD) used to treat RA. MTX has a low-toxicity profile in most patients, although liver function tests (LFT) and a complete blood count (CBC) should be monitored regularly.[8] Patients with liver disease are at increased risk of MTX toxicity, and therefore, patients should be screened for hepatitis B and C prior to starting MTX. Patients with a history of heavy alcohol intake and diabetes also have a risk of increased liver toxicity from MTX, and alcohol is contraindicated while on MTX. The dose of MTX is usually 15 to 20 mg, taken once a week, and is usually well tolerated. Folic acid supplementation is recommended while on MTX, since it decreases other side effects such as mucositis.

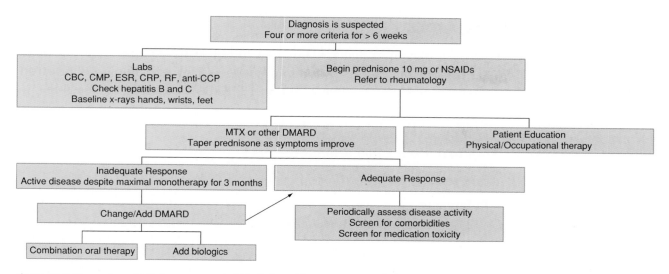

Figure 68.3 Diagnosis and initial management of RA. (Adapted from American College of Rheumatology Subcommittee on Rheumatoid Arthritis Guidelines. Guidelines for the management of rheumatoid arthritis: 2002 update. *Arthritis Rheum* 2002;46:328–346.)

Other alternatives to MTX include sulfasalazine in doses up to 3 g/day and leflunomide 10 to 20 mg/day.[9,10] The advantage of sulfasalazine is that it does not have any liver toxicity and is nonimmunosuppressive. Leflunomide has similar toxicity to MTX. Leflunomide, MTX, and sulfasalazine have all demonstrated efficacy in decreasing bone erosions and joint space narrowing in RA.

For early symptomatic relief while DMARDs take effect (which can be 4–6 weeks), NSAIDs and/or prednisone can be helpful. There is data suggesting that prednisone may delay bone erosions and joint space narrowing, although its myriad side effects usually has the rheumatologist weaning the dose as quickly as possible. NSAIDs can also be associated with many side effects (Chapter 70).

If initial therapy with MTX (or other DMARD) has less than a good response at 3 months, combination therapy with MTX and other oral DMARDs, or the new biologics can be considered.[11] Most rheumatologists would add a TNF inhibitor as the second line of therapy, but many considerations are given, including; cost, availability of prescription drug insurance coverage, and toxicity profiles of the DMARDs alone or in combination, special patient considerations such as upcoming pregnancy, lactation, risk of liver disease, renal function, and convenience.[12] Some biologic agents (such as abatacept, infliximab, and rituximab) require infusion in a practitioner's office, whereas other agents are subcutaneous injections that the patient can self-administer (adalimumab or etanercept).

In patients with unacceptable levels of pain, loss of range of motion, or limitation of function due to structural damage of the joint, surgical procedures should be considered and are discussed elsewhere in this text (Fig. 68.4).

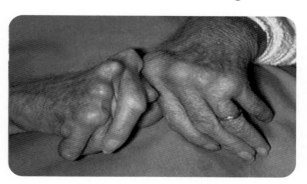

Figure 68.4 Patient with severe RA. Note swelling, subluxation, and ulnar deviation of the MCP joints leading to a clawlike hand.

WHEN TO REFER

- All patients with RA should be referred to a rheumatologist.

Summary

RA is a disabling disease, but new therapeutic agents offer the hope of remission (on therapy). Patients suspected of RA should be referred to rheumatologists and instituted on DMARDs as quickly as possible.

ICD9

714.0 Rheumatoid arthritis

References

1. Lawrence RC, Helmick CG, Arnett FC, et al. Estimates of the prevalence of arthritis and selected musculoskeletal disorders in the United States. *Arthritis Rheum* 1998;41(5):778–799.
2. Wolfe F, Hawley DJ. The longterm outcomes of rheumatoid arthritis: work disability: a prospective 18 year study of 823 patients. *J Rheumatol* 1998;25(11):2108–2117.
3. Maradit-Kremers H, Nicola PJ, Crowson CS, et al. Cardiovascular death in rheumatoid arthritis: a population-based study. *Arthritis Rheum* 2005;52(3):722–732.
4. Choi HK, Hernan MA, Seeger JD, et al. Methotrexate and mortality in patients with rheumatoid arthritis: a prospective study. *Lancet* 2002;359(9313):1173–1177.
5. Lineker S, Badley E, Charles C, et al. Defining morning stiffness in rheumatoid arthritis. *J Rheumatol* 1999;26(5):1052–1057.
6. van Gaalen FA, Linn-Rasker SP, van Venrooij WJ, et al. Autoantibodies to cyclic citrullinated peptides predict progression to rheumatoid arthritis in patients with undifferentiated arthritis: a prospective cohort study. *Arthritis Rheum* 2004;50(3):709–715.
7. van der Heijde DM. Joint erosions and patients with early rheumatoid arthritis. *Br J Rheumatol* 1995;34(Suppl 2):74–78.
8. American College of Rheumatology Subcommittee on Rheumatoid Arthritis Guidelines. Guidelines for the management of rheumatoid arthritis: 2002 update. *Arthritis Rheum* 2002;46:328–346.
9. Strand V, Cohen S, Schiff M, et al. Treatment of active rheumatoid arthritis with leflunomide compared with placebo and methotrexate. Leflunomide Rheumatoid Arthritis Investigators Group. *Arch Intern Med* 1999;159(21):2542–2550.
10. Smolen JS, Kalden JR, Scott DL, et al. Efficacy and safety of leflunomide compared with placebo and sulphasalazine in active rheumatoid arthritis: a double-blind, randomised, multicentre trial. European Leflunomide Study Group. *Lancet* 1999;353(9149):259–266.
11. O'Dell JR. Therapeutic strategies for rheumatoid arthritis. *N Engl J Med* 2004;350(25):2591–2602.
12. Messori A, Santarlasci B, Vaiani M. New drugs for rheumatoid arthritis. *N Engl J Med* 2004;351(9):937–938.

CHAPTER 69 Fibromyalgia and Regional Pain Syndromes

Joan M. Von Feldt, Jonathan Dunham, and Lan X. Chen

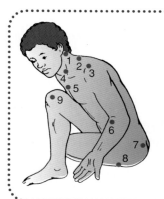

A 35-year-old woman presents with 3 years of worsening fatigue and diffuse pain. She has a 7-year-old and a 4-year-old at home and relates her symptoms beginning shortly after the birth of her second child. Her pain is "all over" but mainly in her upper back/neck, lower back, hips, and knees.

Fibromyalgia is a common cause of chronic musculoskeletal pain. It is one of a group of soft tissue pain disorders that affect muscles and soft tissues such as tendons and ligaments. Fibromyalgia is *not* associated with tissue inflammation, and the etiology of the pain is not known.

Fibromyalgia is likely the most common cause of generalized, musculoskeletal pain in women between 20 and 55 years of age, with a prevalence of 2%.[1] It is usually associated with a sleep disturbance and nonrestorative sleep. The precise pathophysiologic mechanism of fibromyalgia is unclear. However, some aberrancy in central nervous system function is likely. In fact, patients with fibromyalgia have higher levels of substance P, a neurotransmitter involved in pain transmission, in their cerebrospinal fluid.[2] The exact trigger of fibromyalgia is unknown, but it is possible that some psychosocial stressor may be important.

Clinical Presentation and Physical Findings

CLINICAL POINTS

- The condition is probably the most common cause of generalized musculoskeletal pain in women.
- Pain may be widespread and diffuse.
- Associated fatigue is usually present.

The major criteria for the diagnosis of fibromyalgia includes (a) widespread musculoskeletal pain and (b) excess tenderness in at least 11 of 18 tender points, in association with nonrestorative sleep. Tender points are predefined anatomic sites in the muscles of the upper and lower back and extremities that are excessively tender on manual palpation (Fig. 69.1). Excessive tenderness is defined as eliciting pain when the examiner applies a digital force of 4 kg/cm^2 to a fibromyalgia tender point or enough pressure to result in blanching of the fingernail of the examiner. Although most patients give a history of frequent waking throughout the night, some patients do not recall a poor sleep pattern but awaken in the

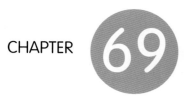

night, some patients do not recall a poor sleep pattern but awaken in the

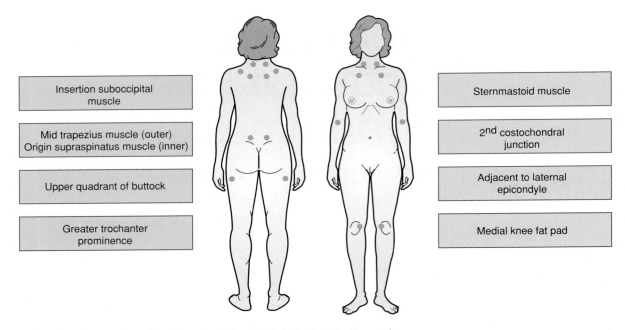

Insertion suboccipital muscle		Sternmastoid muscle
Mid trapezius muscle (outer) Origin supraspinatus muscle (inner)		2nd costochondral junction
Upper quadrant of buttock		Adjacent to laternal epicondyle
Greater trochanter prominence		Medial knee fat pad

Figure 69.1 Nine paired tender points adapted from 1990 ACR criteria for fibromyalgia.

morning with nonrestorative sleep. This is due to a sleep arousal disorder, with disruption of deep sleep, or EEG-measured alpha wave intrusion on delta wave sleep, which is frequently found in patients with fibromyalgia.[3]

Patients with fibromyalgia frequently have accompanying fatigue, and their fatigue is disproportionate to amount of time resting and sleeping. They describe moderate or severe fatigue with lack of energy and decreased exercise endurance. Often, the fatigue is more of a problem and more troubling than the pain. Since they feel fatigued, patients usually will exercise less, exacerbating the poor sleep.

Fibromyalgia is a diagnosis of exclusion, and systemic conditions need to be considered in evaluating a patient with diffuse pain. Additionally, since a sleep disturbance can coexist with many rheumatic disorders and many rheumatic and systemic illnesses present with generalized arthralgias, myalgias, and fatigue, rheumatic conditions need to be carefully considered in a patient with diffuse pain. Also, fibromyalgia can coexist in patients with rheumatic disorders. For example, 25% of patients with systemic lupus erythematosus can have coexistent fibromyalgia.[4]

In evaluating a patient with diffuse pain, some practitioners find it helpful to provide an anatomic figure and ask the patient to identify areas of pain. The more diffuse the pain, the more likely it is to be fibromyalgia. A patient with polyarticular arthritis, such as rheumatoid arthritis, will identify the articulations as painful but will rarely point to muscles or the back.

The initial approach to a patient with complaints suggestive of fibromyalgia is a thorough history and physical examination. Sleep apnea and restless leg syndrome or nocturnal myoclonus may interfere with sleep and promote symptoms of fibromyalgia.[5] Thus, a careful sleep

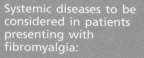

PATIENT ASSESSMENT

1. Noninflammatory areas of pain and tenderness

2. Associated syndromes of regional pain, fatigue, and sleep disorders

3. Negative laboratory evaluation

NOT TO BE MISSED

Systemic diseases to be considered in patients presenting with fibromyalgia:

- Hypothyroidism and other endocrine disorders (e.g., diabetes, Addison disease, growth hormone deficiency)

- Chronic hepatitis B and C infections

- Sleep disorders such as sleep apnea and restless leg syndrome

- Rheumatoid arthritis, systemic lupus erythematosus, Sjögren syndrome, polymyalgia rheumatica, and other autoimmune diseases

- Medications (especially lipid-lowering drugs, antiviral agents)

- Vitamin D deficiency

- Celiac disease

- Malignancy

history should be obtained in patients with fibromyalgia symptoms. Also, a psychiatric history may be important to look for concomitant mood disorders, as these are prevalent in patients with fibromyalgia. Careful examination of the joints and muscles and testing for tender points is very important.

Studies

Baseline blood tests should be limited to a CBC, ESR, standard blood chemistries, thyroid function tests, and CPK—especially since many patients are on statins. With certain risk factors, it would be suggested to check HIV and hepatitis serologies. These tests are all usually normal in patients with fibromyalgia, and any abnormalities might suggest the presence of an alternative diagnosis. Patients with possible sleep apnea or nocturnal myoclonus should be referred to a sleep clinic for further evaluation and treatment.

REGIONAL PAIN SYNDROMES (MYOFASCIAL PAIN SYNDROMES)

Regional pain syndrome, or myofascial pain syndrome, sometimes termed *muscle strain* or *repetitive strain syndrome*, overlaps considerably with fibromyalgia. People with myofascial pain syndrome complain of pain in one anatomic region, such as the right side of the neck and shoulder, with tenderness being confined to that area.

Myofascial pain is a relatively common problem in patients with soft tissue disorders.[6] The pain of myofascial pain disorder is of a deep, aching quality, occasionally accompanied by a sensation of burning or stinging. The pain is defined by the presence of trigger points that are found in a taut band in the muscle. A characteristic referral pain pattern is frequently elicited when pressure is applied to a trigger point. By contrast, tender points, as seen in fibromyalgia, are soft tissue sites that are excessively tender on manual palpation.

In evaluating a person with a regionalized pain syndrome, it is important to determine the patient's activities, including hobbies, and work description and habits, such as carrying a heavy briefcase. Occasionally, a severe enough regionalized pain syndrome could lead to nonrestorative sleep, and symptoms of diffuse pain could develop.

Treatment and Clinical Course

1. Pain control
2. Restoration of normal sleep patterns
3. Management of coexisting mood disorders

Treatment of fibromyalgia and regional pain syndromes is dependent on the degree of symptoms and interferences with usual activities of daily living. Although regional pain syndromes may be treated locally, there is occasionally a need for a more global approach. For fibromyalgia, optimal treatment involves a multidisciplinary approach by using pharmacologic and nonpharmacologic treatment. Treatment should be individualized for the patient. Pharmacologic treatment should address issues of pain control, sleep disturbance, fatigue, and any underlying coexisting mood disorder. Nonpharmacologic treatment should include patient education, a regular exercise and stretching program, stress coping mechanisms, and cognitive behavioral therapy. All of these are essential to improving functional capacity and quality of life.

Although only partly beneficial in most patients, tricyclic antidepressants, selective serotonin reuptake inhibitors, NSAIDs, and nonopioid analgesics are frequently initially used, alone or in combination. Opioid analgesics should be avoided. The use of antiepileptic drugs and antispasticity agents have been supported by anecdotal data and a few clinical trials.[7,8]

Included in the evaluation and treatment of patients with fibromyalgia should be a proper assessment of the cause of the nonrestorative sleep, an important component of the fibromyalgia syndrome. If patients have restless legs syndrome or sleep apnea, the focus of treatment should be on the underlying sleep disorder. In patients without sleep apnea, behavioral approaches to improve sleep hygiene help the disturbances in circadian sleep–wake rhythms. Other secondary causes of fibromyalgia should also be ruled out, such as hypothyroidism, autoimmune disease, chronic hepatitis B or C infection, vitamin D deficiency, and celiac diseases.

Exercise is a critical component of treatment for fibromyalgia, and the authors have never seen lasting improvement in patients with fibromyalgia without patients participating in at least modest cardiovascular exercise. Perhaps because of its beneficial effect on sleep, exercise can improve the pain and fatigue in fibromylagia. Traditional hypnotic agents, while helpful in initiating and maintaining sleep and reducing daytime tiredness, do not provide restorative sleep or reduce pain. Tricyclic drugs such as amitriptyline and cyclobenzaprine may provide long-term benefit for improving sleep but may not have a continuing benefit beyond 1 month for reducing pain. The use of a biologic agent that facilitates sleep-related neuroendocrine functions (e.g., growth hormone) is reported to improve symptoms, but the need for injection and high cost restrict its use.[9] Since fibromyalgia is not an inflammatory condition, medications used in inflammatory rheumatologic conditions such as steroids, biologic agents, or other immunosuppressant agents have *no* role in the treatment of fibromyalgia.

Local therapy for fibromyalgia and regional pain syndromes can be an alternative for both patients and their health care provider. Local measures can be perceived as going directly to the source of pain and in general offer less risk compared with systemic delivery. The hands-on approach of some these local therapies is also often an important part of a therapeutic relationship.

An alternative and attractive approach to pain control is to apply drugs locally to the site of origin of the pain. Other advantages of topical application are lack of drug interactions and the ease of use. Topical application of NSAIDs offers the advantage of local, concentrated drug delivery to affected tissues with a reduced incidence of systemic adverse effects, such as peptic ulcer disease and gastrointestinal hemorrhage. Topical tolmetin as Tolectin gel 5%, acetylsalicylic acid, salicylic acid, indomethacin, and diclofenac hydroxyethylpyrrolidine patch have all been used in small studies and have demonstrated efficacy.

Topical application leads to relatively high NSAID concentrations in the dermis. Concentrations achieved in the muscle tissue below the site of application are variable but are at least equivalent to that obtained with oral administration.[10] NSAIDs applied topically over joints do reach the synovial fluid, but the extent and mechanism (topical penetration vs. distribution via the systemic circulation) remain to be determined.

Local anesthetics have long been used to abolish pain temporarily by blocking nerve conduction, but local anesthetics, such as lidocaine patch or gel, are now used as an effective treatment for many chronic pain conditions.[11]

Massage is a popular remedy for fibromyalgia and regional pain syndromes. The possible physiologic benefits of massage include stimulation of nonnociceptive nerve endings, which contributes to the release of endorphins, increases serotonin levels, and the reflex responses can cause the reduction of blood pressure.[12,13] The "language" of human touch may provide these patients with a feeling of relaxation, warmth, and renewed vitality, which can counteract the stresses and pressures experienced in everyday life.

Transcutaneous electrical nerve stimulation (TENS) is a noninvasive therapeutic modality widely used in clinical practice for pain relief by electrically stimulating peripheral nerves via skin surface electrodes. Clinical studies demonstrate a wide range of success rates with TENS varying from 25% to 95%.[14] Systematic reviews on TENS in the treatment of chronic pain with placebo and control groups have reported inconclusive results. Anecdotally, the authors have used it in some patients with modest success.[15]

Many reports of success with acupuncture for fibromyalgia have fueled a cottage industry. A recent meta-analysis included five randomized, controlled trials; three trials suggested positive but mostly short-lived effects, and two yielded negative results. There was no significant difference between the quality of the negative and the positive trials. Although the authors concluded that effective symptomatic treatment for fibromyalgia is not supported by the results from rigorous clinical trials, acupuncture is still used for the treatment of fibromyalgia and may be beneficial as an adjunct to therapy.[16]

In conclusion, fibromyalgia and regional pain syndromes are common causes of musculoskeletal pain and present to the primary care physician frequently. Careful evaluation with a good history and physical examination and limited laboratory studies can obviate many expensive evaluations. Treatment should be individualized to the patient.

WHEN TO REFER

- Depression refractory to standard therapy
- Suspected sleep apnea
- Therapy involving other health professionals, including physical therapy, nutritional therapy, and counseling

ICD9

729.0 Rheumatism, unspecified and fibrositis
729.1 Myalgia and myositis, unspecified

SECTION 13 General Medical Problems

References

1. Lawrence RC, Helmick CG, Arnett FC, et al. Estimates of the prevalence of arthritis and selected musculoskeletal disorders in the United States. *Arthritis Rheum* 1998;41(5):778–799.
2. Russell IJ, Orr MD, Littman B. Elevated cerebrospinal fluid levels of substance P in patients with the fibromyalgia syndrome. *Arthritis Rheum* 1994;37(11):1593–1601.
3. Moldofsky H. Management of sleep disorders in fibromyalgia. *Rheum Dis Clin North Am* 2002;28(2): 353–365.
4. Middleton GD, McFarlin JE, Lipsky PE. The prevalence and clinical impact of fibromyalgia in systemic lupus erythematosus. *Arthritis Rheum* 1994;37(8):1181–1188.
5. Shah MA, Feinberg S, Krishnan E. Sleep-disordered breathing among women with fibromyalgia syndrome. *J Clin Rheumatol* 2006;12(6):277–281.
6. Walker-Bone K, Palmer KT, Reading I, et al. Prevalence and impact of musculoskeletal disorders of the upper limb in the general population. *Arthritis Rheum* 2004;51(4):642–651.
7. Baker K, Barkhuizen A. Pharmacologic treatment of fibromyalgia. *Curr Psychiatry Rep* 2006;8(6):464–469.
8. Barkhuizen A. Rational and targeted pharmacologic treatment of fibromyalgia. *Rheum Dis Clin North Am* 2002;28(2):261–290.
9. Geenen R, Jacobs JW, Bijlsma JW. Evaluation and management of endocrine dysfunction in fibromyalgia. *Rheum Dis Clin North Am* 2002;28(2):389–404.
10. Heyneman CA, Lawless-Liday C, Wall GC. Oral versus topical NSAIDs in rheumatic diseases: a comparison. *Drugs* 2000;60(3):555–574.
11. Galer BS, Rowbotham MC, Perander J, et al. Topical lidocaine patch relieves postherpetic neuralgia more effectively than a vehicle topical patch: results of an enriched enrollment study. *Pain* 1999;80(3): 533–538.
12. Ironson G, Field T, Scafidi F, et al. Massage therapy is associated with enhancement of the immune system's cytotoxic capacity. *Int J Neurosci* 2002;84:205–217.
13. Field T, Diego M, Cullen C, et al. Fibromyalgia pain and substance P decreases and sleep improves after massage therapy. *J Clin Rheumatol* 2002;8(2):72–76.
14. Offenbacher M, Stucki G. Physical therapy in the treatment of fibromyalgia. *Scand J Rheumatol Suppl* 2000;113:78–85.
15. Carroll D, Moore RA, McQuay HJ, et al. Transcutaneous electrical nerve stimulation (TENS) for chronic pain. *Cochrane Database Syst Rev* 2001;(3):CD003222.
16. Mayhew E, Ernst E. Acupuncture for fibromyalgia—a systematic review of randomized clinical trials. *Rheumatology (Oxford)* 2006;46:801–804.

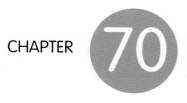

The Use of Nonsteroidal Anti-inflammatory Drugs

Marc L. Cohen and Joan M. Von Feldt

NSAIDs are available in variable dosages and forms, both over the counter and by prescription, and are used for both acute and chronic indications by a worldwide market of over 60 million people. Some NSAIDs (ibuprofen, naproxen, aspirin) are among the most popular over-the-counter medications sold in the United States.[1] Point prevalence for prescription NSAID use among the elderly has exceeded 10%, with close to 40% of patients receiving at least a short-term course of NSAID treatment each year.[2]

The mechanism believed to be responsible for the majority of effects of NSAIDs involves inhibition of the cyclooxygenase enzyme (COX). This enzyme has two isoforms: COX-1 and COX-2. The COX-1 enzyme is expressed constitutively in most tissues and helps to maintain the integrity of gastric and duodenal mucosa. It also modulates renal plasma flow (particularly in patients who are dehydrated or have significant congestive heart failure, cirrhosis, or kidney disease). The COX-2 enzyme is an "inducible enzyme" whose expression is increased during inflammatory states. It also modulates glomerular blood flow and helps to mediate renal electrolyte and water balance.[3,4] At high doses of NSAIDs used for anti-inflammatory effects, it is hypothesized that they may also operate via other non-COX–dependent mechanisms.[5]

Pharmacokinetics

NSAIDs are almost completely absorbed,[6] metabolized primarily in the liver (most via p450 CYP 2C9), and excreted in the urine. They have widely varying half-lives, the longest serum half-life belonging to piroxicam (average 57 hours) (Table 70.1). They generally have no first-pass metabolism; however, some (sulindac, nabumetone) have been designed as "pro-drugs" and are changed to their active form on first-pass metabolism.[4] All NSAIDs, except piroxicam and salicylates, are >98% albumin bound; thus, in the setting of hypoalbuminemia, the clinician should consider starting an NSAID at a lower-than-usual dose.[6]

KEY POINTS

- In the setting of hypoalbuminemia, the clinician should consider starting an NSAID at a lower-than-usual dose.

- If a patient fails one NSAID, a trial with an NSAID from another class is appropriate.

- COX-2–selective NSAIDs have shown approximately 10-fold inhibition of COX-2 compared with COX-1 in vitro, although this specificity is diminished at higher anti-inflammatory doses.

Table 70.1 Duration of Action of Various Nonsteroidal Anti-inflammatory Drugs

SHORT ACTING (usually dosed q2–q6h)	MEDIUM ACTING (usually dosed two or three times daily)	LONG ACTING (usually dosed once or twice daily)
Fenoprofen	Diclofenac	Celecoxib
Ibuprofen	Diflunisal	Meloxicam
Ketoprofen	Etodolac	Nabumetone
Meclofenamate	Sulindac	Naproxen
		Oxaprozin
		Piroxicam

Although there are some specific exceptions, no major differences in efficacy between specific NSAIDs have been shown for most diseases. Thus, the choice of NSAID should generally be made based on differences in side effect profiles, dosing regimen preferences, and availability/cost. Interestingly, despite an inability to find differentials in response between large populations or specific disease states, there seems to be wide variability in individual response to various NSAIDs.[6] For this reason, it is generally recommended that if a patient fails one NSAID, a trial with an NSAID from another class is appropriate.[4]

Aspirin (acetylsalicylic acid), one of the earliest NSAIDs, is a very effective inhibitor of the COX enzyme and does so irreversibly via alkylation. It is available under a wide range of names and variable doses. Because of its effective, irreversible effect on the COX enzyme and thus on platelet aggregation, it is commonly used as a cardioprotective agent. It is available in regular, buffered, and enteric-coated forms. The nonacetylated salicylates are approximately 100 times less effective than aspirin as COX inhibitors yet are as effective as aspirin clinically at decreasing pain, joint tenderness, and joint swelling (suggesting that they may work via some mechanisms apart from COX inhibition)[6] (Table 70.2).

The nonsalicylate NSAIDs are a large grouping of agents. The propionic acids are the most widely used, with several forms (ibuprofen, naproxen, ketoprofen) available in over-the-counter dosage forms. Some NSAIDs (oxaprozin, meloxicam, etodolac, nabumetone [a naphthylalkanone]) are referred to as *COX-2–selective* NSAIDs. These have shown approximately 10-fold inhibition of COX-2 compared with COX-1 in vitro, although this specificity is diminished at higher anti-inflammatory doses. These agents have been associated with less ulcer risk when used at their lower doses than earlier-generation NSAIDs. Most recently, COX-2–specific NSAIDs (celecoxib, rofecoxib, valdecoxib) were developed. These agents are at least 300 times more effective at inhibiting COX-2 than COX-1 and have no measurable effect on COX-1–mediated events at therapeutic doses. The hope that these agents would have a much more favorable risk–benefit ratio compared with previous agents has been squelched recently by debate among scholars and the lay press over potential cardiac risk associated with these drugs.[3,4]

Table 70.2 Examples of Available Nonsteroidal Anti-inflammatory Drugs

GENERIC NAME	TRADE NAMES
Salicylates/Carboxylic Acids	
Acetylated	
Aspirin (regular, buffered, & enteric coated)	Anacin, Aspergum, Bayer, BC Powder, Bufferin, Ecotrin
Nonacetylated	
Choline salicylate	Arthropan
Magnesium salicylate	Doan's Pills, Mobigesic
Choline + magnesium salicylates	Tricosal, Trisilate
Sodium salicylate	*Generic only*
Salsalate	Amigesic, Salsatab
Diflunisal	Dolobid
Nonsalicylate Nonsteroidal Anti-inflammatory Drugs	
Proprionic Acids	
Ibuprofen	Advil, Excedrin IB, Midol IB, Motrin IB, Nuprin
Naproxen sodium	Aleve, Anaprox, Anaprox DS
Naproxen	Naprosyn, Naprapac (naproxen + lansoprazole copackaged)
Fenoprofen	Nalfon
Flurbiprofen	Ansaid
Ketoprofen	Orudis
Oxaprozin	Daypro
Indolacetic Acids	
Indomethacin	Indocin
Sulindac	Clinoril
Etodolac	Lodine
Pyrrolacetic Acids	
Ketorolac	Toradol
Tolmetin	Tolectin
Phenylacetic Acids	
Diclofenac potassium	Cataflam
Diclofenac sodium	Voltaren (delayed release), Voltaren XR (extended release)
Diclofenac + misoprostol	Arthrotec
Anthranilic Acids	
Mefenamic acid	Ponstel
Meclofenamate	Meclomen
Enolic Acids	
Meloxicam	Mobic
Phenylbutazone	Butazolidin
Piroxicam	Feldene
Naphthylalkanones	
Nabumetone	Relafen
Cyclooxygenase-2–specific Inhibitors	
Celecoxib	Celebrex
Rofecoxib	Vioxx (*withdrawn from market*)
Valdecoxib	Bextra (*withdrawn from market*)
Lumiracoxib	Prexige (*not available in U.S. market*)
Etoricoxib	Arcoxia (*in development*)

Indications for Use

NSAIDs are used widely for their analgesic, antipyretic, and anti-inflammatory effects. Aspirin is effective in these roles but has not proved more effective than equal doses of acetaminophen, which in most circumstances has a more favorable risk–benefit ratio. NSAIDs, however, have been shown to be excellent analgesics as a class and in certain settings have been found to provide analgesia equal to starting doses of narcotics. Unlike narcotics, however, NSAIDs do have a ceiling dose above which no additional analgesia is obtained. Higher doses may be useful when used for anti-inflammatory purposes.[7]

Given their ability to both blunt the inflammatory response and control pain, NSAIDs are commonly used in the setting of acute athletic injury. Recently, their use has been the subject of some debate, as inflammation may be necessary for proper healing in certain injuries. Prostaglandins play a major role in bone formation and resorption and are critical to bone repair. Prospective studies in animals have suggested that NSAIDs have a negative effect on bone fracture healing, and most human studies, while retrospective, have raised concerns about delayed healing or nonunion. No study has examined NSAID effects on athletic stress fractures. Long-term NSAID use may also interfere with muscle repair and regeneration. Currently, NSAIDs are thought to be beneficial in the acute setting of injury to either muscle or ligament, as they aid in pain and inflammation control and generally allow faster return to activity. This is particularly true for soreness related to eccentric muscle injury. NSAID courses should generally be limited to 3 to 7 days for these injuries. NSAIDs may also be useful for decreasing inflammation associated with tendinitis or transiently for analgesia associated with tendinopathy. However, except for transient use for analgesia, many experts discourage their use in chronic muscle injury or in acute fracture, particularly completed fractures or stress fractures at risk for nonunion.[8]

NSAIDs are also a large part of the armamentarium for treatment of rheumatologic joint diseases. NSAIDs have been shown to be helpful in the management of osteoarthritis (OA), with no difference in efficacy between specific NSAIDs.[9–11] The effect of NSAIDs over acetaminophen (4 g/day) for OA was modest in head-to-head trials, and results of a crossover trial suggest that acetaminophen may actually be less effective if given after a course of an NSAID.[12] Thus, acetaminophen should be used as first-line treatment for OA before NSAIDs. There has also been some debate as to whether chronic NSAID use may accelerate joint failure.[5] While immune-modulating agents are more often being used today, NSAIDs have been shown to provide significant improvement in ACR 20 criteria in rheumatoid arthritis (RA).[5,13,14]

Drug–Drug Interactions

NSAIDs have been described as the "best recognized cause of iatrogenic pathology"[1] and in fact are estimated to be related to as many as 16,500 deaths in the United States per year. At one point in the late 1980s, one fourth of adverse drug reactions reported to the Committee on Safety of Medicine in the United Kingdom were due to NSAIDs.[5]

Given the common usage of NSAIDs, issues surrounding their interaction with other medications are a frequent occurrence. One particularly interesting issue raised recently in the literature involves the interaction of aspirin and other NSAIDs. Recent data suggests that some NSAIDs when used in combination with aspirin may in fact inhibit the cardioprotective effects of aspirin. A 2001 study[15] found that when ibuprofen was taken before aspirin, aspirin's ability to inhibit thromboxane formation was prevented. It is thought this results from ibuprofen competitively inhibiting aspirin's ability to bind and irreversibly inactivate platelet COX-1. Naproxen's effects are still debated. Naproxen interferes with aspirin's ability to permanently inhibit COX; however, the simultaneous administration of naproxen and aspirin still results in effective inhibition of the COX enzyme, likely due to the long half-life of naproxen. However, it remains unclear as to whether twice daily naproxen provides clinically effective cardioprotection.[16]

Given the available data, in patients on cardioprotective doses of aspirin, acetaminophen should be chosen before an NSAID, if appropriate. If the benefit to treatment with an NSAID is deemed significant enough to warrant its use over other options, a nonenteric-coated aspirin should be taken in the morning at least 2 hours prior to the first dose of an NSAID. NSAIDs with short to medium half-lives requiring multiple daily dosing should be avoided, and the treatment should be limited to the shortest possible course. Delayed-release diclofenac preparations may be one of the safest NSAIDs to use in combination with aspirin from a cardiac standpoint based on current studies. If used in combination, aspirin should ideally be taken at least 6 to 8 hours after the last dose of ibuprofen or 36 to 48 hours after naproxen.[16]

Given NSAID effects on platelets and the risk of bleeding, it is important to carefully consider options before beginning an NSAID in a patient taking warfarin. NSAIDs can prolong prothrombin time in patients taking concomitant warfarin (rarely), and INR should be carefully followed when NSAIDs are added to a regimen including warfarin.[6] The relative risk (RR) of presenting with hemorrhage among anticoagulant users is 4.3 for those not using NSAIDs and 12.7 for those who do.[2] All NSAIDs, with the exception of nonacetylated salicylates, inhibit platelet aggregation.[6] For this reason, patients should be told to stop aspirin 1 to 2 weeks prior to surgery, while other NSAIDs can be stopped several half-lives before surgery. Nonacetylated salicylates may be good choices for patients in whom inhibiting platelet activity is a concern.

Providers should also be aware that NSAIDs can inhibit metabolism of phenytoin, valproic acid, and oral hypoglycemic agents; inhibit excretion of lithium and methotrexate; and interfere with binding of any protein-bound medications.[5,6] All of these interactions may affect levels of medications, which are often tightly monitored. Dosage of the NSAID itself may need to be adjusted when used in combination with probenecid, which may reduce metabolism and renal clearance of NSAIDs; barbiturates, which may affect NSAID clearance; and antacids, cholestyramine, metoclopramide, and caffeine, which may affect the rate and degree of NSAID absorption.[5]

Adverse Effects

Gastrointestinal side effects are the most common adverse events related to the use of NSAIDs. While dyspepsia is most common, NSAID-induced ulceration and associated morbidity and mortality is the most significant. The FDA reports an overall risk of 2% to 4% per year for NSAID-induced gastric ulcer development and its complications.[4] Users of NSAIDs are at an approximate three times greater risk for developing serious adverse GI events than nonusers. Risk appears to be equal among men and women.[17] Multiple risk factors for the development of these complications have been identified and include prior history of a gastrointestinal event (RR 4.76), age >60 (RR 5.52), concurrent use of corticosteroids (RR 4.4), concurrent use of anticoagulants (RR 12.7), and dosage >2 times normal (RR 10.1) (Table 70.3). This toxicity is thought to be largely mediated by inhibition of COX-1, causing a decrease in protective gastric prostaglandins.[18] NSAID-related gastrointestinal adverse events have been estimated to cause approximately 200,000 to 400,000 hospitalizations per year.[19]

Studies have had varied results in attempts to compare risk of various NSAIDs for causing gastrointestinal complications, and there is no single unifying rank-order list that can be developed. Piroxicam, ketorolac, and indomethacin seem to frequently be listed as those at highest risk, with naproxen, ketoprofen, and diclofenac often listed as being in a more intermediate zone. Ibuprofen, shown to be less toxic to the gastrointestinal tract in many studies, approaches the risk of other agents when used at very high doses.[1,6,20,21] Gastrointestinal toxicity clearly correlates with increasing NSAID dose.[6] Indomethacin significantly increases risk at approximately 7 to 14 days; other NSAIDs increase risk in weeks to months.[1] NSAID-induced injury distal to the duodenum is much less common than gastric/duodenal injury but does occur as well.[21]

While much less prevalent than ulcer-related complications, NSAIDs may cause other gastrointestinal complications as well (patients with quiescent inflammatory bowel disease have been found to suffer lower bowel damage after long-term use),[6] and some studies have suggested that

---

Table 70.3 Risk Factors for Nonsteroidal Anti-inflammatory Drug–induced Gastrointestinal Complications

- Prior history of gastrointestinal event
- Age >60 years
- Concurrent use of corticosteroids
- Concurrent use of anticoagulants
- Dosage >2 times normal
- Duration of use

NSAIDS place patients with pre-existing diverticulosis at higher risk for complications of diverticulosis and perforation.[21] NSAIDs have also been rarely associated with hepatic toxicity, and some authorities recommend checking LFTs 8 to 12 weeks after initiation of any long-term NSAID therapy.[4] Hepatic toxicity, which at times may even progress to overt liver failure, has been seen.[4,6]

All NSAIDs, particularly indomethacin, have the potential to interfere with pharmacologic control of hypertension and heart failure due to involvement of prostaglandins in the modulation of vascular tone, tubular reabsorption of electrolytes, and other prostaglandin-dependent actions of diuretics.[5] Given lower interaction with prostaglandins, nonacetylated salicylates may be better options for patients on antihypertensive or cardiac regimens.[6]

NSAIDs carry the risk of renal complications. Interference with prostaglandin synthesis can interfere with fluid/electrolyte homeostasis and is more likely to occur in settings of intrinsic renal disease, hypoalbuminemia, and hypovolemia. Sulindac and nonacetylated salicylates have less effect on prostaglandins but may still affect renal function.[6] Inhibition of prostaglandin synthesis may affect renin levels, leading to hyperkalemia, which may be exacerbated in patients on a potassium-sparing diuretic. Interference with prostaglandins may also lead to salt retention, causing peripheral edema at rates of up to 2% to 3% in patients. Effects on antidiuretic hormone may lead to reduced excretion of free water and hyponatremia, which may be exacerbated in patients on thiazide diuretics. All NSAIDs have been associated with increased blood pressure, although this response is very difficult to predict on a patient-by-patient basis.[4]

NSAID-induced interstitial nephritis is extremely rare and thought to be immune mediated.[6] It may manifest as pyuria, hematuria, proteinuria, anasarca, or any combination of these. Eosinophilia, eosinophiluria, and fever, which are usually thought to accompany drug-induced allergic nephritis, often do not occur. Interstitial nephritis has been reported most commonly with fenoprofen but has been seen with other NSAIDs such as naproxen, tolmetin, and indomethacin. Acute renal failure, which is thought to be prostaglandin mediated, may also occur; patients on triamterene-containing diuretics may be at higher risk. NSAIDs should NOT be used in patients with a CrCl <30.[4]

NSAIDS that are highly lipid soluble will have increased central nervous system penetration and may cause changes in mentation, perception, and mood. Indomethacin has been associated with these effects, particularly in the elderly. Tinnitus may occur with higher doses of both salicylates and nonsalicylate NSAIDs; this is reversible with discontinuation.[4] Aseptic meningitis has been reported in the past; NSAIDs involved in those reports included ibuprofen, sulindac, and tolmetin.[5]

Patients with allergic rhinitis, nasal polyposis, or a history of asthma are thought to be at somewhat increased risk for NSAID-related anaphylaxis (rare). The mechanism is thought to be related to a decrease in synthesis of prostaglandin E (bronchodilators) or a shunting of arachidonic acid down the leukotriene pathway when COX is inhibited.[4] Although rare, there have also been several reports of pulmonary infiltrates with

SECTION 13 General Medical Problems

eosinophilia in association with NSAID exposure. These patients presented with a pneumonialike syndrome, including shortness of breath and at times high fever in association with a peripheral eosinophilia. Corticosteroids and discontinuance of drug led to a reversal of the process.[4,22]

If possible, avoidance of NSAIDs during pregnancy is recommended; if used, they should be discontinued 6 to 8 weeks before delivery. Their use has been associated with increased risk of miscarriage, and use during the third trimester may cause premature closure of the ductus arteriosus and persistent pulmonary hypertension in the neonate.[3]

Prevention of Nonsteroidal Anti-inflammatory Drug–induced Ulcers

Given the high burden of ulcerative complications related to NSAID use, there has been a large amount of interest through the years in preventing this side effect. One of the earliest attempts was the development of enteric-coated and buffered forms of aspirin. Enteric-coated aspirin is coated with a combination of inactive ingredients resistant to disintegration in an acidic environment, which delays the breakdown of aspirin until it reaches the duodenum. Endoscopic studies have demonstrated less gastric erosion and microbleeding in association with enteric-coated aspirin but no difference with buffered aspirin. While some observational studies have found differences, a 1996 study found no substantial difference in risk of major upper gastrointestinal bleeding according to type of aspirin preparation.[18]

Multiple studies have examined the possibility of pharmacologic prophylaxis of NSAID-induced ulcers. A 2002 Cochrane review on the subject found that proton pump inhibitors (such as omeprazole) and misoprostol (prostaglandin analog) were both effective in preventing endoscopic ulcers. H2 receptor antagonists (such as ranitidine) prevented endoscopic ulcers only when given in very high doses (300 mg twice daily). While PPIs were associated with significantly less dropout due to side effects, misoprostol was the only agent to prevent ulcer complications such as perforation, hemorrhage, and obstruction. Misoprostol only achieved this at a dose of 800 μg/day; lower doses were less effective but were still associated with significant diarrhea.[23] PPIs, misoprostol, COX-2–selective and COX-2–specific NSAIDs (but not H2 blockers, possibly due to low event reporting) were all found to protect against symptomatic ulcers, and all except COX-2 selective protected against endoscopic ulcers.[24] Misoprostol was shown to protect against serious gastrointestinal complications but again was associated with increased dropout rates. It should be noted that sucralfate and antacids have not been shown to be effective in preventing NSAID-induced ulcers.[21]

Thus, based on current data, misoprostol is probably the most effective prophylactic agent. However, due to issues of adherence secondary to side effects, PPIs are usually chosen as first-line agents for prophylaxis. While H2 receptor antagonists may relieve symptoms of dyspepsia, they may not protect against and may even increase the risk of serious gastrointestinal complications when given at standard doses.[23] Prophylaxis with pharmacotherapy is recommended only for patients at medium to

KEY POINTS

- Proton pump inhibitors (PPIs) are usually chosen as first-line agents for prophylaxis.

- If patients develop an NSAID-induced ulcer, it is preferable to stop NSAID therapy, as healing rates are better when the offending agent is stopped.

- Treatment for *Helicobacter pylori* is recommended for patients who develop NSAID-related ulcers and are found to be infected.

high risk of complication, as treating all patients receiving NSAIDs with prostaglandins or PPIs would be unnecessary and cost prohibitive. Anti-inflammatory doses of many NSAIDs have been given for up to 7 days to young, healthy volunteers without any reports of significant gastrointestinal bleeding or other serious events.

If patients develop an NSAID-induced ulcer, it is preferable to stop NSAID therapy, as healing rates are better when the offending agent is stopped. In those in whom the agent is continued, healing rates are significantly better in those treated with a PPI. Treatment for *H. pylori* is recommended for patients who develop NSAID-related ulcers and are found to be infected.[21]

Cyclooxygenase-2–specific Nonsteroidal Anti-inflammatory Drugs

COX-2–specific NSAIDs have been the subject of much recent debate. They were originally designed based on the presumption that preferential inhibition of COX-2 would provide decreased inflammation without associated involvement of pathways involving platelet aggregation, gastrointestinal mucosal protection, and renal perfusion.[25,26] There are five agents that have undergone study prior to date of this publication, the least COX-2 selective being celecoxib and the most being lumiracoxib.

COX-2–specific NSAIDS have been found in multiple studies to have equivalent, but not superior, efficacy in several disorders, including RA and OA.[9,14,27,28] Rofecoxib has been shown to reduce gastrointestinal complications when compared with other NSAIDs;[28] however, studies in rofecoxib, lumiracoxib, and celecoxib all suggest that the decrease in gastrointestinal side effects with COX-2–specific NSAIDS may be limited to patients who are not taking concomitant aspirin.[26,29–31]

Significant concerns have been raised in recent years regarding cardiovascular risks associated with the use of these medications, which have severely limited their use.[25,26,30] There are potential physiologic explanations, including unbalanced effects on mediators affecting platelets and vasculature, that could support such an effect.[25,26] In fact, at this time, only celecoxib remains available in the U.S. market, and some debate looms about its cardiac safety profile as well. While many organizations have previously recommended the use of COX-2 agents in patients with risk for gastrointestinal bleeding, the use of a PPI with a nonselective NSAID such as ibuprofen is a safer choice. COX-2–specific NSAIDs should be reserved for those who may have a contraindication for PPIs or misoprostol and a pressing need for NSAID therapy or for those at very low risk for cardiac complications based on age and risk factors. Their use in populations taking aspirin for cardioprotection is not appropriate.

Summary

NSAIDs are a key component to management strategies for pain and functional limitation in both acute and chronic musculoskeletal issues that present to primary care physicians. There are a variety of NSAIDs with varying pharmacologic properties that allow varied dosing. There are many drug–drug interactions involving NSAIDS that providers should be aware of given the frequency with which NSAIDs are prescribed. Many patients will respond to an NSAID from one class but not another. There is a very limited role for COX-2–specific NSAIDs in current management given concerns regarding cardiovascular risk. For patients at risk of gastrointestinal toxicity, treatment with a PPI can help to decrease this toxicity.

References

1. Richy F, Bruyere O, Ethgen O, et al. Time dependent risk of gastrointestinal complications induced by non-steroidal anti-inflammatory drug use: a consensus statement using a meta-analytic approach. *Ann Rheum Dis* 2004;63:759–766.
2. Smalley W, Griffin M. NSAIDs, Eicosanoids, and the gastroenteric tract. *Gastroenterol Clin North Am* 1996;25(2):373–396.
3. Drugs for rheumatoid arthritis. *Treatment Guidelines from The Medical Letter* 2005;3(40):83–90.
4. Simon L. Nonsteroidal anti-inflammatory drugs. In: Klippel JH, ed. *Primer on the Rheumatic Diseases.* Atlanta: Arthritis Foundation; 2001:582–592.
5. Brooks P, O'Day R. Nonsteroidal antiinflammatory drugs—differences and similarities. *N Engl J Med* 1991;324(24):1716–1723.
6. Furst D. Are there differences among nonsteroidal antiinflammatory drugs? *Arthritis Rheum* 1994;37(1):1–9.
7. Sachs C. Oral analgesics for acute nonspecific pain. *Am Fam Physician* 2005;71(5):913–918.
8. Mehallo C, Drezner J, Bytomski J. Practical management: nonsteroidal antiinflammatory drug (NSAID) use in athletic injuries. *Clin J Sports Med* 2006;16(2):170–174.
9. Garner S, Fidan DD, Frankish RR, et al. Rofecoxib for osteoarthritis. *Cochrane Database Syst Rev* 2005;(1): CD005115.
10. Towheed TE, Hochberg MC, Shea BJ, et al. Analgesia and non-aspirin, non-steroidal anti-inflammatory drugs for osteoarthritis of the hip. *Cochrane Database Syst Rev* 2006;(1):CD000517.
11. Watson M, Brookes ST, Faulkner A, et al. Non-aspirin, non-steroidal anti-inflammatory drugs for treating osteoarthritis of the knee. *Cochrane Database Syst Rev* 2006;(1):CD000142.
12. Felson D. Osteoarthritis of the knee. *N Engl J Med* 2006;354(8):841–848.
13. Garner S, Fidan DD, Frankish RR, et al. Celecoxib for rheumatoid arthritis. *Cochrane Database Syst Rev* 2002;(4):CD003831.
14. Garner S, Fidan DD, Frankish RR, et al. Rofecoxib for rheumatoid arthritis. *Cochrane Database Syst Rev* 2002;(2):CD003685.
15. Catella-Lawson F, Reilly MP, Kapoor SC, et al. Cyclooxygenase inhibitors and the antiplatelet effects of aspirin. *N Engl J Med* 2001;345(25):1809–1817.
16. Steinhubl S. The use of anti-inflammatory analgesics in the patient with cardiovascular disease: what a pain (editorial comment). *J Am Coll Cardiol* 2005;45(8):1302–1303.
17. Gabriel SL, Jaakkimainen L, Bombardier C. Risk for serious gastrointestinal complications related to use of nonsteroidal anti-inflammatory drugs: a meta-analysis. *Ann Intern Med* 1991;115:787–796.
18. Kelly JP, Kaufman DW, Jurgelon JM, et al. Risk of aspirin-associated major upper-gastrointestinal bleeding with enteric-coated or buffered product. *Lancet* 1996;348:1413–1416.
19. Lanza F. Gastrointestinal toxicity of newer NSAIDs. *Am J Gastroenterol* 1993;88(9):1318–1321.
20. Griffin MR, Piper JM, Daugherty JR, et al. Nonsteroidal anti-inflammatory drug use and increased risk for peptic ulcer in elderly persons. *Ann Intern Med* 1991;114(4):257–263.
21. Lanza F. A guideline for the treatment and prevention of NSAID-induced ulcers. *Am J Gastroenterol* 1998;93(11):2037–2046.
22. Goodwin S, Glenny R. Nonsteroidal anti-inflammatory drug-associated pulmonary infiltrates with eosinophilia. *Arch Intern Med* 1992;152(7):1521–1524.
23. Rostom A, Dube C, Wells G, et al. Prevention of NSAID-induced gastroduodenal ulcers (review). *Cochrane Database Syst Rev* 2000;(3):CD002296.
24. Hooper L, Brown TJ, Elliott R, et al. The effectiveness of five strategies for the prevention of gastrointestinal toxicity induced by non-steroidal anti-inflammatory drugs: systematic review. *BMJ* 2006;329(7472):948.
25. Furberg C, Psaty B, FitzGerald G. Parecoxib, valdecoxib, and cardiovascular risk. *Circulation* 2005;111:249.
26. Pratico D, Dogne J. Selective cyclooxygenase-2 inhibitors development in cardiovascular medicine. *Circulation* 2005;112:1073–1079.
27. Simon LS, Weaver AL, Graham DY, et al. Anti-inflammatory and upper gastrointestinal effects of celecoxib in rheumatoid arthritis. *JAMA* 1999;282(20):1921–1928.
28. Bombardier C, Laine L, Reicin A, et al. Comparison of upper gastrointestinal toxicity of rofecoxib and naproxen in patients with rheumatoid arthritis. *N Engl J Med* 2000;343:1520–1528.
29. Silverstein FE, Faich G, Goldstein JL, et al. Gastrointestinal toxicity with celecoxib vs nonsteroidal anti-inflammatory drugs for osteoarthritis and rheumatoid arthritis: the CLASS study: a randomized controlled trial. *JAMA* 2000;284(10):1247–1255.
30. Lo V, Meadows S. When should COX-2 selective NSAIDs be used for osteoarthritis and rheumatoid arthritis? *J Fam Pract* 2006;55(3):260–262.
31. Laine L. Ulcer formation with low-dose enteric-coated aspirin and the effect of COX-2 selective inhibition: a double-blind trial. *Gastroenterology* 2004127(2):395–402.

CHAPTER

71 The Use of Corticosteroid Preparations: Intra-articular and Soft Tissue Injections

Jennifer Kwan-Morley and Joan M. Von Feldt

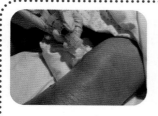 *A 69-year-old man who has a history of hypertension, diabetes, and hyperlipidemia presents with a 7-year history of bilateral knee pain. He notes that his pain is worse after physical activity and prolonged standing. He denies morning stiffness. He describes minimally warm knees with significant fluid. He has had only minimal relief with a physical therapy regimen, NSAIDs, and knee braces. He needs further management because the pain is starting to impair his activities of daily living.*

Intra-articular corticosteroid injections are the mainstay of many orthopaedic and rheumatology clinics and have been extensively used to treat various musculoskeletal conditions since the 1950s. The discovery of corticosteroids in 1949, for which Hench and Kendall won the Nobel prize in 1950, opened the door for treatment of inflammatory diseases and states. In 1951, Hollander[1] described the use of intra-articular corticosteroids for arthritic joints, and since then, their continued popularity is in part due to efficacy in pain relief, promptness of action, safety, and relative lack of systemic side effects. Since its discovery, the use of long-acting depot corticosteroids has found several niches.[2,3] Table 71.1 lists the many diseases that have been shown to benefit from steroid injections.

Corticosteroid Preparations in the United States

One of the biggest challenges facing practitioners is determining the ideal preparation of corticosteroid for use, the dosage and volume of corticosteroid needed, and whether or not to add lidocaine to the steroid mixture. A study of members of the American College of Rheumatology (ACR) showed that the type of intra-articular steroids used and whether or not the physician added lidocaine to the steroid was in part due to geographic location (type of steroid) and time of training (younger physicians tend to use lidocaine). In general, fluorinated compounds are less soluble and therefore

SECTION 13 General Medical Problems

381

Table 71.1 Diseases That Benefit from Steroid Injection

LOCATION	DISEASE
Intra-articular	Rheumatoid arthritis Systemic lupus erythematosus Crystal deposition Osteoarthritis Spondyloarthropathies
Bursa	Bursitis
Tendon	Overuse syndromes Tendinitis Epicondylitis Trigger finger *Never* inject the Achilles tendon
Soft tissue	Myofascial/Trigger points Tietze syndrome
Entrapment neuropathies	Carpal tunnel syndrome Cubital tunnel syndrome Tarsal tunnel syndrome

tend to be longer acting, which is preferable for intra-articular injections. However, given those characteristics, fluorinated compounds are less desirable for soft tissue injections, as their use can lead to more adverse reactions.[4] Table 71.2 lists commonly used preparations available in the United States.

Table 71.2 Commonly Used Preparations in the United States

PREPARATION	TRADE NAME	FLUORINATED	CONCENTRATION (mg/mL)	PREDNISONE EQUIVALENT
Soluble				
Hydrocortisone acetate	Hydrocortone	No	25, 50	5, 10
Dexamethasone sodium phosphate	Decadron Phosphate	Yes	4	40
Slightly Soluble				
Methylprednisolone acetate	Depo-Medrol	No	20, 40, 80	25, 50, 100
Triamcinolone diacetate	Aristocort Forte Hydeltra TBA or	Yes	40	50
Prednisolone tebutate	Predalone TBA	No	20	20
Relatively Insoluble				
Triamcinolone hexacetonide	Aristospan	Yes	20	25
Triamcinolone acetonide	Kenalog	Yes	40	50
Combination (soluble + insoluble)				
Betamethasone sodium phosphate + betamethasone acetate	Celestone Soluspan	Yes	6	50

Table 71.3 Volume of Steroid and Lidocaine into Joints

SIZE OF JOINT	EXAMPLES	VOLUME
Small	Interphalangeal, metacarpalphalangeal	0.1–0.5 cc
Medium	Elbow, wrist, ankle	1.0–1.5 cc
Large	Shoulder, knee	2.0–5.0 cc

INTRA-ARTICULAR INJECTIONS

The most important aspect of intra-articular injections is choosing the optimal dose of corticosteroids. This is in part determined by the size of the joint involved, the degree of inflammation, and the concentration of steroid used.[5] In general, joints are subdivided into small, medium, and large categories. The maximum volume that can be injected into the joints without overdistension of the surrounding capsule is listed in Table 71.3. Note that the values listed are for total volume into the joint. The ACR recommends maximal drainage of the joint prior to corticosteroid injection for maximal effect and to avoid overdistension of the joint capsule.

In addition to consideration of the total volume to be injected, the total dose of corticosteroid to be injected into a joint needs to be determined. This is based on the degree of inflammation and the prednisone equivalent of the preparation used.[6] Table 71.4 provides general guidelines for appropriate doses of corticosteroids.

Most physicians commonly use a mixture of depot corticosteroid with lidocaine for intra-articular injections. The reasons are twofold: immediate anesthesia confirms proper location, and it is beneficial for rapid patient relief. A common technique in injecting corticosteroids is a mix of lidocaine and steroid in a ratio of 2:1. For example, in a large joint such as a knee, a reasonable mixture would be 2 cc of 1% lidocaine with 1 cc of depot corticosteroid. It should be noted that occasionally the preservatives in lidocaine can cause flocculation of the corticosteroids; therefore, the mixture should be appropriately mixed prior to injection.

The last step in preparation for the injection is determining the needle size appropriate for the joint. Table 71.5 gives a general guideline for needle gauges.

Table 71.4 Doses of Depot Corticosteroids to Be Injected

LOCATION	EXAMPLES	PREDNISONE EQUIVALENT DOSE
Bursa	Subacromial	10–40
Tendon sheath	De Quervain	10–20
Small joints	Metacarpophalangeal	5–10
Medium joints	Wrist	15–20
Large joints	Knee	20–50

SECTION 13 General Medical Problems

Table 71.5 General Guideline for Needle Gauges

SIZE OF JOINT	NEEDLE SIZE (gauge)
Small (interphalangeal, metacarpophalangeal)	25–28
Medium (ankle)	19–22
Medium (wrist)	20–23
Large (knee)	18–21
Large (shoulder)	19–22

Intra-articular injections have been successful in patients with various rheumatic conditions for days to months. As a general rule of thumb, intra-articular corticosteroid injections of the same joint are reserved for use four times a year, or approximately every 3 months. This is in part due to the fact that steroids can cause tendon rupturing, and there have been reports that it can also accelerate osteoarthritis.

SOFT TISSUE INJECTIONS

Soft tissue injections are usually reserved for overuse syndromes. For example, common uses include periarticular injections, injections into the tendon sheath (but not the tendon itself, which can cause rupture), bursal injections, and certain fascial injections. A controversial area is the injection of local myofascial trigger points. As stated previously, the most important factor in choosing an injectable corticosteroid is to choose a nonfluorinated compound for soft tissues to avoid side effects such as atrophy or skin depigmentation. Table 71.6 lists examples of common soft tissue disorders.

Precautions

Although the use of injectable corticosteroids is very well tolerated and very safe (the estimated rate of infection for an intra-articular injection is

Table 71.6 Common Soft Tissue Disorders

DISORDER	NEEDLE SIZE (gauge)	TOTAL VOLUME (cc)
Subacromial bursa	20	3.0
Lateral epicondylitis	25	1.0
Olecranon bursa	20	2.0–3.0
De Quervain	25	1.0
Trigger finger	27	0.5
Trochanteric bursa	20	3.0–5.0
Anserine bursa	22	1.0
Plantar fasciitis	23–25	0.5–1.0

Table 71.7 Possible Side Effects

stemic absorption

ndon weakening

n hypopigmentation

bcutaneous atrophy

aphylaxis

eroid arthropathy

ection

teonecrosis

shing

stinjection flare

Table 71.8 Contraindications to Use of Intra-articular Corticosteroids

Absolute Contraindications

Surrounding infection
Sepsis
Skin breakdown
Known allergy to injection
Fracture
Severe joint deformity

Relative Contraindications

Inaccessible joint
Prior failed attempts
Joint instability
Blood clotting disorder

POSTINJECTION RECOMMENDATIONS

- Rest and decreased weight bearing of the joint[5]

- Ice to injection site[5]

- NSAIDs, if not a contraindication, or analgesics as needed[5]

- Follow-up for postinfection flares, which usually arise and resolve within 48 hours[5]

estimated at as low as 4 in 10,000 injections), there are known possible adverse side effects, as noted in Table 71.7. The absolute contraindications to the use of intra-articular corticosteroids are listed in Table 71.8.

References

1. Hollander JL, Brown EM, Jessar RA, et al. Hydrocortisone and cortisone injected into arthritic joints. Comparative effect of and use of hydrocortisone as a local antiarthritic agent. JAMA 1951;147:1629–1635.
2. Klippel, JH, Crofford LJ, Stone JH, et al. *Primer on the Rheumatic Diseases.* Atlanta: Arthritis Foundation; 2001.
3. Hunter JA, Blyth TH. A risk-benefit assessment of intra-articular corticosteroids in rheumatic disorders. *Drug Saf* 1999;21:353–365.
4. Cole BJ, Schumacher HR. *J Am Acad Ortho Surg* 2005;13(1):37–46.
5. Schumacher HR, Chen LX. Injectable corticosteroids in treatment of arthritis of the knee. *Am J Med* 2005;118:1208–1121.
6. West S. *Rheumatology Secrets.* Denver: Hanley and Belfus; 2002.

SECTION 13 General Medical Problems

Technical Injections and Casts/Splints

72 Injection Techniques for Joints and Bursa

Paul A. Lotke

Aspirations and/or injections of the joints and bursa are valuable tools for the treatment and diagnosis of problems related to bone and joint inflammation. The ability to remove synovial fluid, inspect it, and send the specimen to the laboratory analysis or culture helps the primary care physician to understand the underlying problem regarding the joint. The visual inspection of the fluid itself is a valuable tool. Bloody fluid indicates significant trauma or coagulopathy, cloudy fluid creates suspicion of infection or inflammatory arthritis, and clear yellow viscous fluid is usually associated with some transitory inflammation of a joint or bursa.

Intra-articular/intrabursal injections of cortisone preparation have been used for decades and can be very effective in giving prompt relief to inflamed joints, bursa, ligaments, or tendons. The agents are absorbed slowly, in general do not effect systemic cortisone levels, and have an excellent safety record. This section will review how to inject various parts of the body. Although the author describes his technique for injection, there are other approaches that are equally effective.

Sterile technique must be carefully observed. The tip of the needle and the skin insertion site must remain sterile. The skin is sterilized with an alcohol sponge, rubbing and cleansing the skin. Tincture of iodine or iodophor solution is applied as the final preparation. Gloves are not used unless protection is a concern. A physician may unknowingly contaminate sterile gloves and think that they are still sterile. Without gloves, instinct tells us to stay away from the critical areas, and they remain well prepped and sterile.

In the joints to be aspirated, remove most of the fluid first and then leave the needle in place, change the syringe to one with a cortisone preparation, and inject it into the space. It is not attempted to remove all of the fluid completely from a bursa or joint space, as it collapses and the needle may displace into the soft tissues. Failures of injections are frequently related to failure to enter or remain in the appropriate space. Avoid superficial injections, as they may go into the subcutaneous space and cause skin atrophy. When injecting the cortisone preparation, there should be no resistance in the flow from the syringe. If there is, the tip of the needle may be embedded into tendon or cartilage and should be redrawn slightly or redirected.

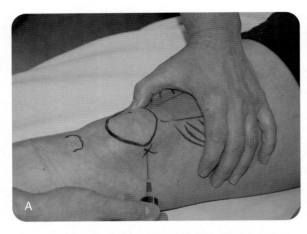

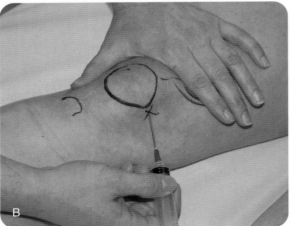

Figure 72.1 Knee joint. **A.** Tilted. **B.** Compressed.

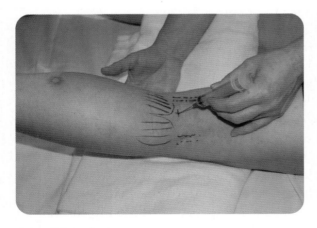

Figure 72.2 Popliteal cyst.

The size of the syringe and needle depends on the site to be aspirated. If injecting a tendon sheath in the hand, a 0.2 cc of cortisone in a 1-cc syringe with a 25-gauge needle should be used. On the other hand, if aspirating a swollen knee, an 18-gauge needle on a 60-cc syringe with 1 cc of cortisone preparation could be used.

Lower Extremity

KNEE

The knee is one of the most frequently aspirated joints. It is easy to inject, especially if there is fluid within the joint. Generally, the clinician can enter from the medial side with the knee fully extended. The author chooses a mid-patellar location, 1 to 2 cm medial to the inner border of the patella. The needle should be aimed to slide beneath the patella into the joint. The position of the needle can be confirmed by rocking it slightly under the patella without pain. Advantages of a medial approach are the lack of fat and a thin synovium in this area. The angle of medial patella facet facilitates entry. With minimal fluid in the joint, the patella is tilted to allow easier entry (Fig. 72.1A). If there is fluid in the joint, the supra-patella pouch can be compressed, which raises the patella and makes entry into the knee easier (Fig. 72.1B).

PREPATELLAR BURSITIS (HOUSEMAID'S KNEE)

Prepatellar bursitis presents as swellings over the anterior aspect of the patella or tibial tubercle. The swellings can be easily aspirated by directing a needle through healthy skin on the edge of the bursa.

POPLITEAL CYSTS

Popliteal cysts can be aspirated or injected relatively safely since they can be readily palpitated, especially with the patient lying prone with the knee extended. Direct entry is usually possible (Fig. 72.2).

ANKLE

It is easiest to enter the ankle joint from the anteromedial site. Choose a soft depressed spot about 1 cm above and lateral to the medial malleolus. The author directs the needle posteriorly and slightly lateral (Fig. 72.3).

POSTERIOR TIBIAL TENDINITIS

The tendon in the area immediately behind the medial malleolus can usually be palpated. Direct the needle distally into the tendon and sheath (Fig. 72.4).

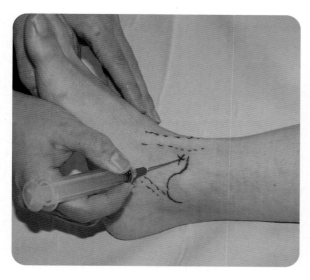

Figure 72.3 Ankle joint.

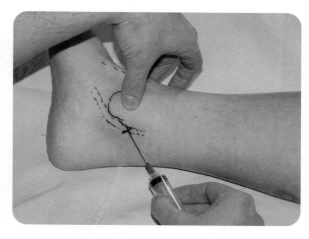

Figure 72.4 Posterior tibia.

GREAT TOE BURSA (BUNION)

The great toe bursa is easy to see and inject. Choose a location where there is some normal skin available, and aim into the bursa.

HIP

The hip joint is one of the more difficult joints to aspirate or inject because of the mass of the overlying soft tissues. This is best done under radiographic guidance. With the hip extended, use a 2.5-inch needle, palpate the artery, and insert the needle vertically 1.5 cm laterally to the artery and 1.5 cm distal to the inguinal ligament. A small amount of local anesthetic is a benefit and may be injected into the capsule as the joint is approached. If aspirating for possible infection, avoid local anesthetics, as they may contaminate the joint with a preservative (Fig. 72.5).

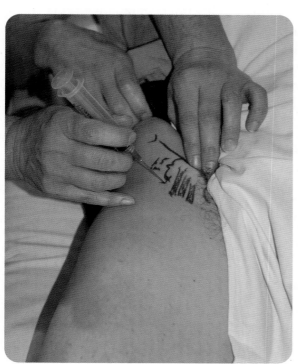

Figure 72.5 Hip joint.

TROCHANTERIC BURSA

This bursa is found next to the posterolateral aspect of the greater tuberosity of the femur. This bursa can be injected by aiming for the point of maximum tenderness. With the patient lying on the opposite side, palpate the area of tenderness, mark it with a pen, prep the puncture site, and direct the needle into the tender zone. Because this is a relatively large area, add 5 to 10 cc of a local anesthetic with the cortisone preparation, insert the needle directly onto the bone, and lift the needle slightly from the bone in order for it to be in the bursa. Broadly disperse the injection around the

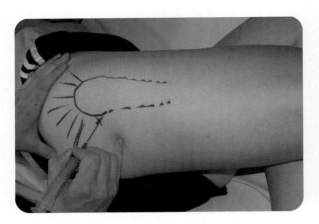

Figure 72.6 Trochanteric bursa.

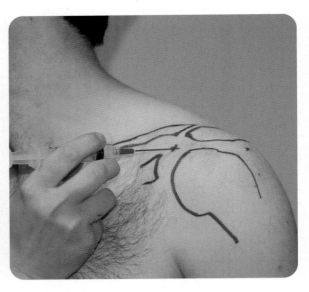

Figure 72.7 Shoulder joint.

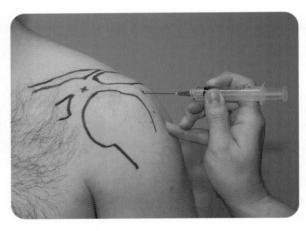

Figure 72.8 Subacromial bursa.

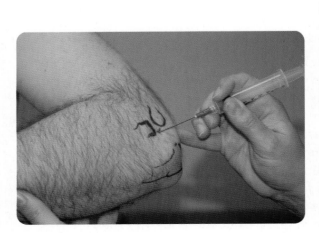

Figure 72.9 Elbow joint.

bursa. In general, if the needle is in the bursa, the patient should find relief of pain relatively soon after the injection (Fig. 72.6).

Upper Extremity

SHOULDER JOINT

The shoulder joint is easily injected and aspirated Using the anterior puncture site, which is 1.5 cm below the clavicle and 1.5 cm lateral to the coracoid prominence, direct the needle horizontally. It should be possible to palpate the humeral head and define the anatomy in thinner patients (Fig. 72.7).

SUBACROMIAL BURSA

The subacromial bursa may be entered anteriorly or laterally. The needle may be inserted from the lateral aspect into the midacromial, below the anterior bony edge, and directed into the soft tissue depression below the acromium (Fig. 72.8).

ELBOW JOINT

The elbow joint is best entered laterally. With the elbow held at 90 degrees of flexion, find the space just anterior and distal to the capitellum and into the triangular depression between the radial head, capitellum, and ulna (Fig. 72.9).

OLECRANON BURSA

The olecranon bursa is easy to aspirate. Choose a puncture site where there is good-quality skin, and direct the needle into the bursa.

TENNIS ELBOW (LATERAL EPICONDYLITIS)

Inject a small amount of cortisone directly into and around the point of maximal tenderness. The tip of the needle can be felt when it enters the tendon. If it is too deep, there will be resistance to the flow from the needle. If retracted slightly, the needle comes into the tendon sheath, and the injection can be made without resistance.

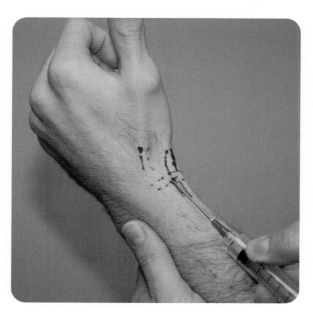

Figure 72.10 De Quervain tenosynovitis.

WRIST (DE QUERVAIN TENOSYNOVITIS)

The inflamed tendon sheath, at the base of the thumb, responds well to injection. The sheath is easy to palpate and inject, offering excellent relief. Extend the thumb a few times, and palpate the tendon. Choose a site that is just proximal to the wrist and proximal to a slight swelling of the tendon sheath and direct the needle distally into the tendon. Relax the needle and syringe, and move the thumb gently; the needle will move, and the clinician can be sure that the tendon space has been entered. Inject fluid without resistance; otherwise, slightly retract the needle tip until the bevel is in the tendon sheath, and reinject without resistance (Fig. 72.10).

CARPAL TUNNEL

For acute swollen, painful carpal tunnel syndrome, inject a small amount of cortisone into the carpal canal. On the palmar side, insert the needle approximately 2 cm proximal to the transverse carpal ligament at the level of the skin wrist crease. Direct the needle obliquely and distally, beneath the transverse carpal ligament. When in the sheath, test to be sure that there is no resistance. If there is resistance, retract the tip of the needle until the bevel is in the tendon sheath, and reinject without resistance (Fig. 72.11).

TRIGGER FINGERS

Trigger fingers are easy to inject and frequently resolve the triggering sensation caused by a nodule in the tendon. When moving the finger from flexion to extension, this nodule can be felt on the tendon. At the level of the palmar crease, direct the needle obliquely and distally into the tendon sheath. Move the finger slightly, and the needle/syringe will move slightly, indicating

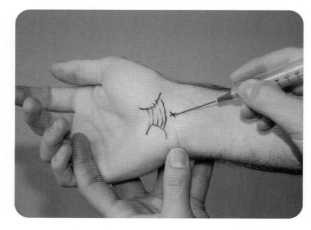

Figure 72.11 Carpal tunnel.

SECTION 14　Technical Injections & Casts/Splints

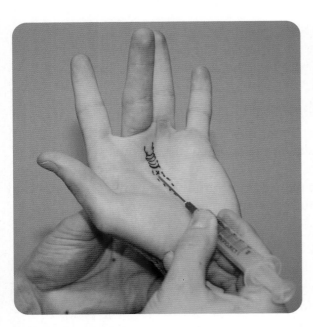

Figure 72.12 Trigger finger.

placement in the tendon. Inject without resistance. If there is resistance, retract the tip of the needle until the bevel is in the tendon sheath. This directs the fluid into the sheath. Occasionally, it is possible to feel the fluid extend distal into the finger (Fig. 72.12).

73 Splints and Braces

Paul A. Lotke

Shoulder

SIMPLE SHOULDER SLING

Treatment: Painful shoulders including bursitis, tendinitis, nondisplaced fractures, contusions in arm, and painful elbow

Comment: This is a classic, inexpensive, readily available device that can be made from almost any cloth fabric. It is inexpensive, versatile, and effective. Care should be taken not to keep patients in slings too long in order to avoid stiffness.

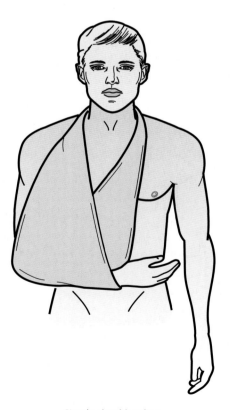

Simple shoulder sling.

SECTION 14 Technical Injections & Casts/Splints

ABDUCTION PILLOW SHOULDER IMMOBILIZER

Treatment: Fractures of the humerus, status post shoulder dislocation

Comment: This is a more constrained device that prevents abduction and external rotation of the arm. Therefore, it protects dislocations and allows fractures to heal. It is reasonably comfortable. Care should be taken to permit good underarm hygiene. Avoid using it for prolonged periods of time to prevent stiff shoulders. The harness can be released for short periods in order to begin pendulum exercises.

SLING AND SWATHE BANDAGE

Treatment: Post reduction shoulder dislocation, fractures of the humerus, postsurgical treatment of the humerus

Comment: A very effective immobilization of the shoulder and humerus. It keeps the humerus supported to the chest wall and prevents external rotation. Reasonably comfortable. Care for underarm hygiene.

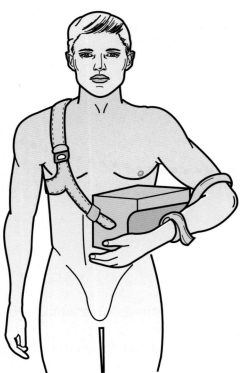

Abduction pillow shoulder immobilizer.

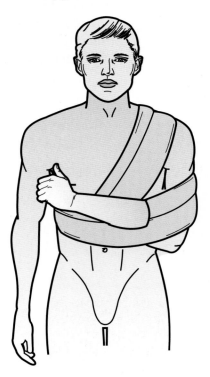

Sling and swathe bandage.

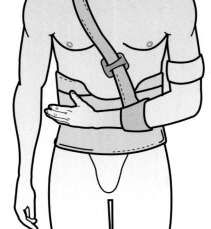

Shoulder immobilizer.

SHOULDER IMMOBILIZER

Treatment: Rotator cuff tear, status post repair rotator cuff tear

Comment: This is very bulky and somewhat cumbersome splint that is effective in maintaining abduction of the shoulder. It can be used for acute support of the rotator cuff.

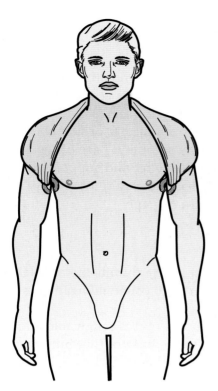

Figure-of-eight strap.

FIGURE-OF-8 STRAP

Treatment: Moderately displaced clavicle fractures, acromioclavicular joint separation

Comment: Readily available splinting that can be made of a variety of materials, including off-the-shelf foam padding or a padded stockinette. Available and reasonably effective in relieving symptoms.

Elbow

TENNIS ELBOW BAND

Treatment: Tennis elbow, medial and lateral epicondylitis

Comment: This is a band that can be placed over the forearm for symptomatic relief of epicondylitis/tennis elbow. It should only be used during activity and offers relief of symptoms during activity. It should not be worn for prolonged periods of time.

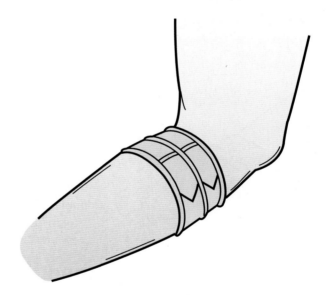

Tennis elbow band.

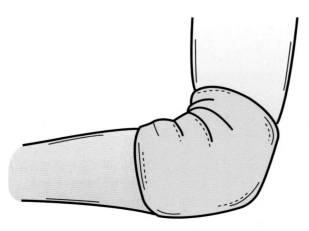

Neoprene pull-on elbow sleeve.

NEOPRENE PULL-ON ELBOW SLEEVE

Treatment: Minor sprains of the elbow or persistent swelling

Comment: Used for diffuse swelling about the elbow and strains or sprains of the elbow where patients need support to the elbow. Usable for rehabilitating a prior injury to the elbow.

Wrist

WRIST SPLINT

Treatment: Carpal tunnel syndrome, synovitis, wrist sprain, active inflammatory arthritis of the wrist

Comment: This is a very simple splint that is readily available. It can be made from plaster or fiberglass casting. It can stabilize the wrist and base of the thumb to give symptomatic relief and support of injury or inflammation. Patients can remove the splint periodically for skin hygiene.

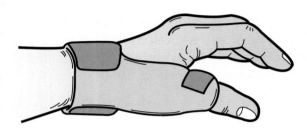
Wrist splint.

THUMB SPICA

Treatment: Injuries to the base of the thumb, metacarpal phalangeal arthritis, injuries to collateral ligaments of the thumb, synovitis

Comment: Simple, effective brace that is removable and gives excellent support to the base of the thumb. Useful for a variety of injuries and inflammation to the base of the thumb.

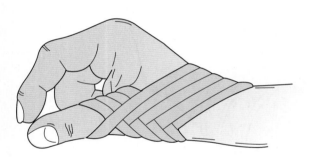
Thumb spica.

TAPING OF THE THUMB

Treatment: Strains and sprains about the thumb, prevention of injuries to the thumb; used for athletes with a history of recent thumb injury or thumb instability

Comment: Very simple taping can be used for short-term protection of the base of the thumb.

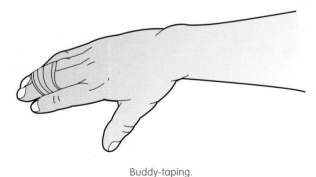
Taping of the thumb.

Hand

BUDDY TAPING OF THE FINGERS

Treatment: Finger sprains, status post dislocations

Comment: Two fingers can be taped against each other to offer support after severe sprains or dislocations of the fingers. The taping should be applied with the fingers flexed 30 to 45 degrees to prevent stiffness.

Buddy-taping.

STACK SPLINT

Treatment: Mallet finger

Comment: A premolded plastic orthotic can be placed over the end of the finger in order to reduce the deformity related to a mallet finger. Such orthotics are reasonably well tolerated and reasonably effective.

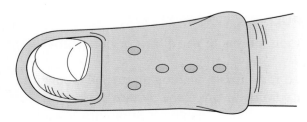
Stack splints.

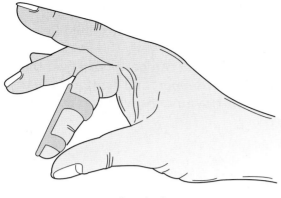

Dorsal splint.

DORSAL SPLINT

Treatment: Mallet finger

Comment: Can be used to help reduce the deformity related to mallet fingers. Careful padding prevents skin problems.

METAL FINGER SPLINT

Treatment: Severe sprains, status post dislocations of the proximal interphalangeal joint of the fingers

Comment: Relatively simple aluminum splint can be taped or fitted to any finger in order to give temporary protection. Avoid prolonged use in order to avoid stiffness.

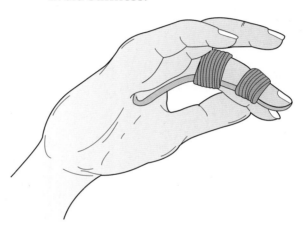

Metal finger splint.

Knee

ACE WRAP

Treatment: Swelling, pain, sprain about knee

Comment: This is a common, readily available wrap that can be used for minor aches and pains about the knee. Care should be taken not to wrap too tightly in order to prevent distal edema.

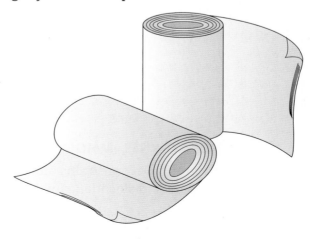

Ace wrap.

SECTION 14 Technical Injections & Casts/Splints

NEOPRENE PULL-ON KNEE SLEEVE

Treatment: Swollen knees, sprained knees, mild arthritis, mild ligament instability

Comment: There are a variety of sleeves that can be applied over the knee. These offer modest structural support and comfort for early arthritis or for active patients with symptoms who want to continue in recreational sports.

VELCRO KNEE CAGE

Treatment: Minor sprains about the knee

Comment: Available knee support that gives some symptomatic relief to patients with a sprain or swelling in the knee. Care should be taken not to pull the straps too tight.

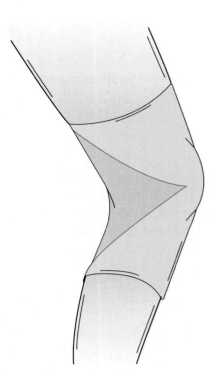

Neoprene pull-on knee sleeve.

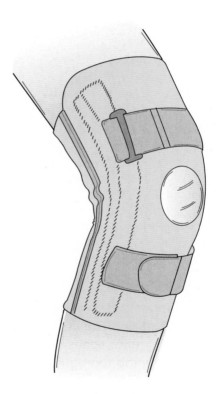

Velcro knee cage.

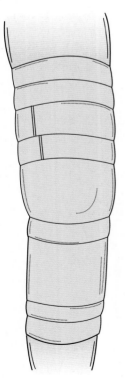

Velcro knee immobilizer.

VELCRO KNEE IMMOBILIZER

Treatment: Severe strains and sprains of the knee, quadriceps injuries, post patella dislocation, any injury that requires avoidance of flexion of the knee

Comment: Readily available splint that can be used to prevent flexion of the knee. It can be removed for skin hygiene.

HINGE KNEE SUPPORT

Treatment: Structural injuries to ligaments and tendons about the knee

Comment: A variety of hinge braces are available to either protect from ligament instability or to relieve symptoms related to unicompartmental arthritis. They can be used to protect from symptomatic deficiencies in the anterior cruciate ligament or early arthritis. They range in price from relatively inexpensive, simple hinges to derotational type braces. They are modestly effective, depending on the patient's age and structural deformities.

Ankle

NEOPRENE PULL-ON ANKLE SLEEVE

Treatment: Minor sprains of the ankle

Comment: An elastic sleeve can be placed over the ankle in order to give some sense of support after a sprain and also to help reduce swelling after a cast is removed or after prolonged activity.

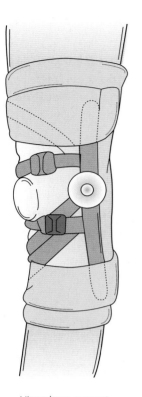

Hinge knee support.

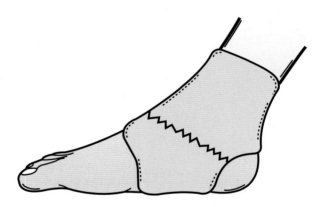

Neoprene pull-on ankle sleeve.

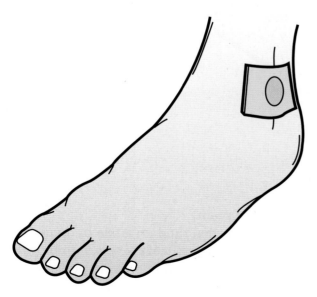

New skin/moleskin.

NEW SKIN/MOLESKIN

Treatment: Bony prominences, soft calluses, hammer toes, dorsal bunions

Comment: Padded moleskin can be applied to the feet in a variety of locations in order to prevent bony contact to soft tissue. It offers excellent relief and protects from painful contact from soft corns. Care should be taken to prevent skin irritation.

VELCRO ANKLE SPLINT

Treatment: Minor strains and sprains of the ankle

Comment: This is a simple, removable splint that can be used for minor sprains of the ankle. It is very supportive and well tolerated. It can be used during rehabilitation of the ankle as patients begin to engage in activity.

ROCKER-BOTTOM PLASTIC ANKLE IMMOBILIZER

Treatment: Severe sprains and nondisplaced fractures of the ankle

Comment: This is a very supportive splint that can be used as a brace in severe sprained ankles. The rocker bottom allows the patients to walk securely and reasonably comfortably. Depending on the injury, it can be removed for skin hygiene.

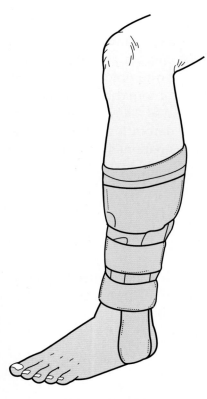

Velcro ankle splint.

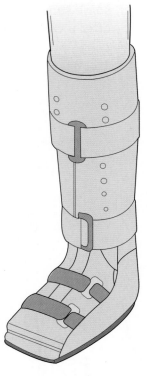

Rocker-bottom plastic ankle immobilizer.

UNNA BOOT

Treatment: Skin ulcers, severe ankle sprain

Comment: An Unna boot can be wrapped around an ankle to reduce swelling, allow venous ulcers to heal, and treat severe sprains. It can also be applied after casts are removed in order to prevent swelling. Care should be taken to apply the boot in a neutral position for the ankle.

Unna boot.

DROP FOOT BRACE

Treatment: Drop foot for transient peroneal palsy or chronic neurologic defect

Comment: A variety of drop foot braces are available. They can be made of plastic or wire springs that can be placed in or out of the shoe and around the calf in order to protect the foot from dropping. They are very effective and can be used for long periods of time if necessary.

Foot

HEEL CUSHION

Treatment: Achilles tendinitis, plantar fascitis, heel bone bruise

Comment: The soft insert can be placed into the sole of the shoe at the level of the heel in order to cushion against repeated injury. Can be used for short- or long-term painful heel problems.

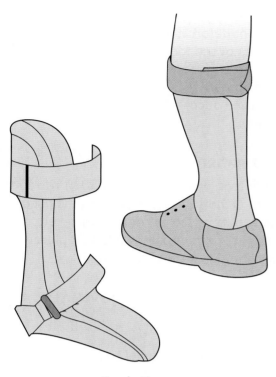

Drop foot brace.

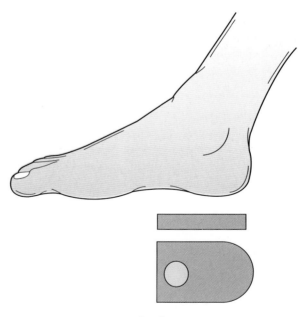

Heel cushions.

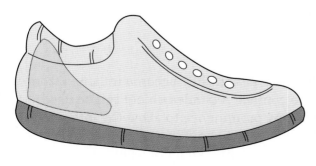

Heel cups.

HEEL CUP

Treatment: Plantar fasciitis, calcaneal spurs

Comment: Heel cups are relatively inexpensive and are placed in the shoe in order to provide protection to the heel. They offer transient benefit for patients who have plantar fasciitis and are variably effective.

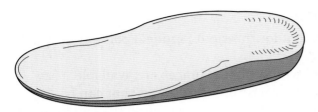

Padded insoles.

PADDED INSOLE

Treatment: Severe foot deformities from rheumatoid arthritis, arthritis of the foot, Charcot foot deformities

Comment: A custom-molded shoe insert is available that can be utilized successfully for patients with severe deformity.

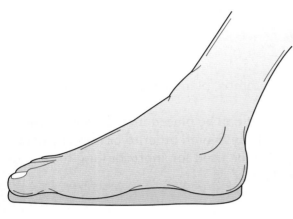

Padded arch supports.

PADDED ARCH SUPPORT

Treatment: Pronated feet, posterior tibial tendon rupture

Comment: A custom orthotic arch support can be used for long periods of time for patients with severe pronation. Supports can be removable and placed in shoes. They should be custom molded.

PLASTIC ORTHOTIC ARCH SUPPORT (OVER THE COUNTER OR CUSTOM MADE)

Treatment: Symptomatic flatfeet

Comment: Arch supports can give relief to patients who have symptoms related to the pronation of the foot. This can occur in the elderly with posterior tibial tendon loss or in young people with marked pronation and symptoms related to nerve stretching.

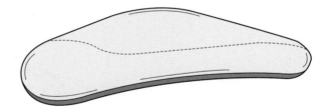

Plastic orthotic arch supports.

BUNION SHIELD

Treatment: Painful bunion

Comment: Bunions periodically become inflamed from tight shoe contact. A padded shield can be used over the bony prominence to allow the inflammation to resolve. Care should be taken to prevent repeated or constant contact of a shoe against the bunion prominence.

Bunion shields.

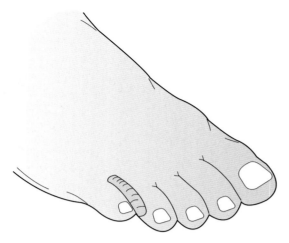

Toe spacers.

TOE SPACER

Treatment: Painful soft corns

Comment: A soft corn can be extremely painful and out of proportion to what can be palpated or visualized. Excellent relief can be found with soft padding between the toes.

BUDDY TAPING OF THE TOES

Treatment: Sprain, Fracture or dislocation of toes

Comment: Simple taping of minimal or nondisplaced fractures or dislocations of the toes. Useful for short-term support. Care on skin hygiene.

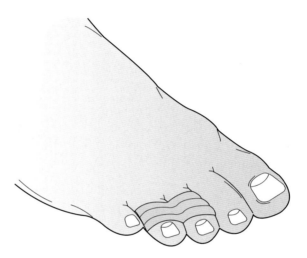

Buddy-taping of the toes.

METATARSAL PAD

Treatment: Metatarsalgia, painful plantar calluses on the metatarsal head

Comment: A soft pad can be placed just proximal to the metatarsal heads. This relieves the pressure on the metatarsal head as well as distributes the weight more evenly across the metatarsal heads. This is a very effective brace.

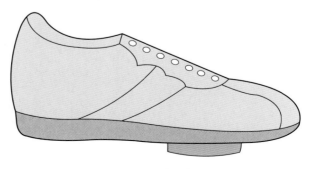

Metatarsal pad.

SECTION 14 Technical Injections & Casts/Splints

Rehabilitation and Home Physical Therapy

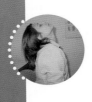

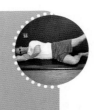

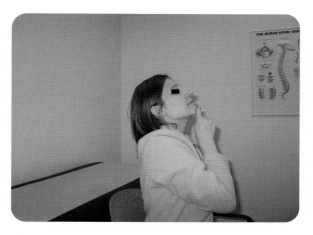

Figure 74.3 Cervical extension exercise, side view.

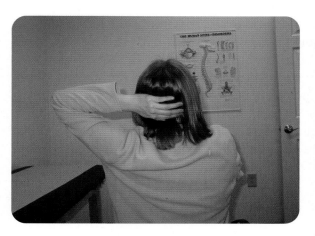

Figure 74.4 Cervical extension exercise, posterior view.

CERVICAL EXTENSION

The cervical extension exercise follows the retraction exercise when it causes a reduction or abolishment of the distal symptom. The same seated or standing position is used. The cervical spine is first fully retracted, with pressure maintained over the chin with the hand (Fig. 74.3). The patient's other hand is placed behind the occiput to control the angle and weight of the head. The exercise is progressed in intervals of 25%, 50%, 75%, or 100% of available range. The hand supporting the head stays in place (Fig. 74.4), and the position is maintained for a period of 30 to 60 seconds. This is repeated three times. Once the patient can fully extend the cervical spine and experience a reduction in distal symptoms, the support hand can be removed (Fig. 74.5).

Posture Maintenance

When the patient completes either the supine or seated retraction exercise, it is imperative that the cervical spine is maintained in a more retracted position in an effort to decrease intradiscal pressure, improve lordosis of the cervical spine, and minimize distal symptoms (Fig. 74.6). Most patients intuitively understand that improving their posture can help their symptoms. However, maintaining good posture is extremely difficult, physically demanding, and requires reinforcement from the physician and physical therapist.

General Range-of-motion Exercises

ROM exercises are utilized when a patient lacks adequate cervical mobility to perform activities of daily living. There are six cervical ROM

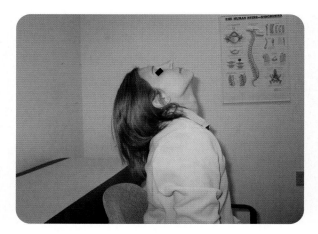

Figure 74.5 Full end-range cervical extension.

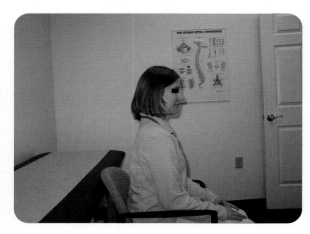

Figure 74.6 Improved sitting posture (cervical spine more retracted).

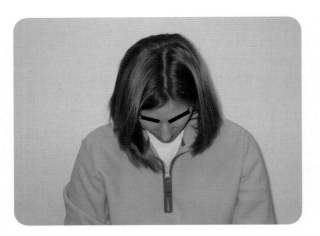

Figure 74.7 Cervical flexion.

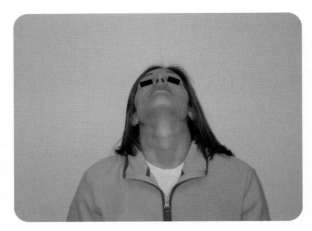

Figure 74.8 Cervical extension.

exercises: flexion, extension, left and right rotation, and left and right side bending. The exercises should be performed in the available painfree ROM. The goal of the exercises is to restore or improve on cervical ROM. They should be performed in one set of ten repetitions, three times daily. The end-range position is held for 10 seconds. Concentration should be placed only on the motions that are restricted (Figs. 74.7–74.12). Patients with cervical stenosis may benefit from cervical flexion ROM exercises where the narrowed spinal canals are in a more open position.

General Advice

Patients who complain of cervical pain should be advised to refrain from sleeping prone. The prone position places the patient's cervical spine in an end-range rotation and usually a degree of extension. This position will tend to exacerbate cervical problems.[5]

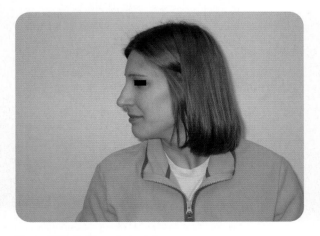

Figure 74.9 Right cervical rotation.

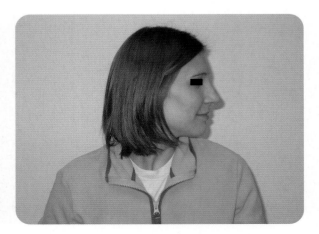

Figure 74.10 Left cervical rotation.

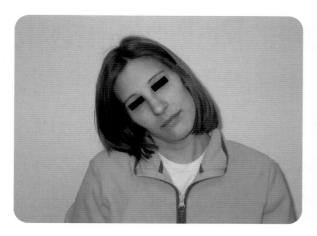

Figure 74.11 Right cervical side bending.

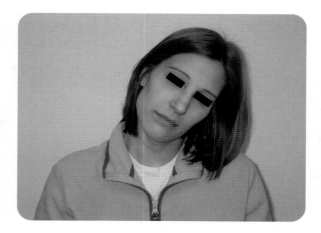

Figure 74.12 Left cervical side bending.

References

1. Schenk R, Kelley J, Kruchowsky T, et al. An evidence-based algorithm for examination of the cervical spine. *Orthop Practice* 2002;14:4.
2. Harms-Ringdahl K, Ekholm J. Intensity and character of pain and muscular activity levels elicited by maintained extreme flexion position of the lower-cervical–upper-thoracic spine. *Scand J Rehabil Med* 1986;18(3):117–126.
3. Kisner C, Colby LA. *Therapeutic Exercise: Foundations and Techniques*. Philadelphia: FA Davis; 1985.
4. Sprague R. Mobilization of the cervical and upper thoracic spine. In: Donatelli RA, Wooden MJ, eds. *Orthopedic Physical Therapy*. New York: Churchill Livingstone; 1989:109–114.
5. DiMaggio A. Strategic Orthopaedics: Cervical and Thoracic Pain. Strategic Orthopaedics II, course notes. October 13–14, 2001.

SECTION 15 Rehabilitation

CHAPTER 75 Shoulder Rehabilitation

Brian G. Leggin

Shoulder disorders affect 7% to 27% of the general population and account for 1.0% to 2.5% of patients presenting to general medical practitioners annually.[1,2] It is the third most common cause of musculoskeletal consultation in primary care.[3] Up to 53% of these patients are then referred to physical therapy.[2] A study to determine the course of shoulder disorders in general practice and the prognostic indicators of outcome revealed that 23% of all patients showed complete recovery after 1 month.[4] After 1 year, 59% of patients showed complete recovery.[4] A more rapid recovery seemed to be related to preceding overuse or slight trauma and early presentation. A high risk of persistent or recurrent complaints was found for patients with concomitant neck pain and severe pain during the day of presentation.[4]

This chapter will discuss a rehabilitation approach for the most common shoulder disorders. Early intervention is a critical component to recovery of shoulder pathology. However, the quantity of rehabilitation does not always equate to quality. Each patient requires a different level of intervention. Supervised therapy three times per week is not necessary for all patients. Many patients only need instruction in a home program and periodic evaluation and progression of the rehabilitation program. Therefore, it is incumbent on therapists, physicians, and the patient to administer the appropriate amount of rehabilitation following the onset of a shoulder injury.

The importance of patient education cannot be emphasized enough. The patient needs to learn about the healing process and the importance of rest from positions or activities that may contribute to the inflammatory process. They should also be instructed in proper positioning of the arm for comfort. Many patients report that while at rest or sleeping, the most comfortable position is with the arm supported in the plane of the scapula. From a biomechanical standpoint, this also appears to be a more advantageous position. Patients should be instructed to perform activities such as working with a computer or driving with their affected arm supported at the elbow.

Range of motion (ROM) and stretching exercises are designed to prevent adhesions and/or fibrosis, reduce pain, allow collagen healing, and increase tissue length. When restoring normal ROM of the shoulder, the clinician

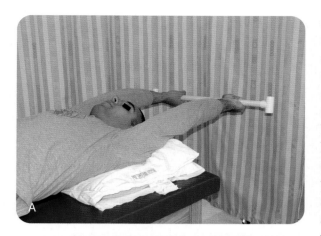

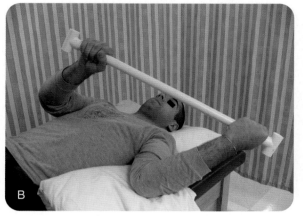

Figure 75.1 Phase I ROM exercises. **A:** Supine forward elevation. **B:** Supine external rotation at 45 degrees.

should consider which structure might limit the motion. Studies have shown that external rotation with the arm at the side is most limited by the subscapularis and the coracohumeral ligament.[5–7] External rotation with the arm at 45 degrees appears to be limited by the subscapularis and middle fibers of the anterior glenohumeral ligament.[7] The inferior glenohumeral ligament limits external rotation when the arm is abducted to 90 degrees.[7] Gerber and colleagues[5] simulated capsular contractures in cadavers and measured changes in elevation and rotation ROM. They found that restriction of the anterior capsule restricted external rotation ROM and that posterior contractures restricted internal rotation ROM. Contracture of the superior capsular structures limited rotation motions with the arm adducted.[5] Contracture of the inferior structures yielded restriction in abduction and rotation in the more elevated positions.[5]

The author's ROM exercises have been divided into phase I and phase II. Phase I exercises include supine passive or active assisted forward elevation and external rotation (Fig. 75.1). Phase II ROM exercises include extension, internal rotation, and cross body adduction (Fig. 75.2). The patient is asked to take the extremity to a position of tolerable stretch and hold the position for 10 to 20 seconds. Each exercise is repeated ten times, two to three times per day at home.

There are several methods that therapists can use for improving strength and neuromuscular control. These include manual resistance, elastic resistance, free weights, and machines. Regardless of the method, the underlying principle guiding the therapist is that exercises should begin in nonprovocative or supported positions with a gradual progression toward potentially provocative or functional positions.

The author's strengthening exercise program is also categorized by phases and utilizes elastic resistance. Elastic resistance is more portable for the patient to use and has yielded good results in those with shoulder pain.[8] Phase I exercises include external and internal rotation with the arm at the side and extension with elastic resistance (Fig. 75.3). Patients are typically asked to perform ten repetitions with the lightest resistance. They are able to add a second set of ten when the first set is performed without difficulty. A third set is added when there is no difficulty with the first two. When all three sets become easy, the patient may progress to the next level of resistance. Phase II of the strengthening exercise program is added when the patient can perform all three of the phase I exercises with the third level of resistance. These exercises emphasize strengthening of the deltoid and rotator cuff in more functional positions and include abduction to 45 degrees, forward elevation below the shoulder level, and external rotation with the arm supported at 45 degrees (Fig. 75.4). Most patients will realize an improvement in symptoms and function with

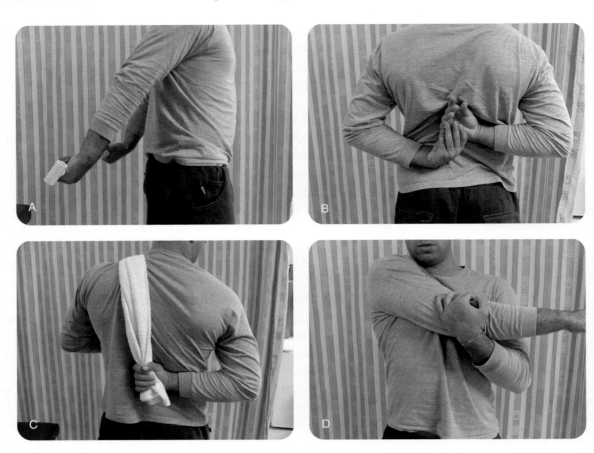

Figure 75.2 Phase II ROM exercises. **A:** Extension. **B:** Internal rotation with opposite hand or towel (**C**). **D:** Cross body adduction.

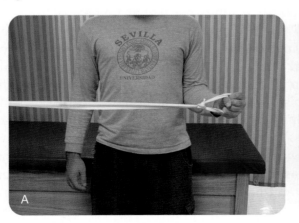

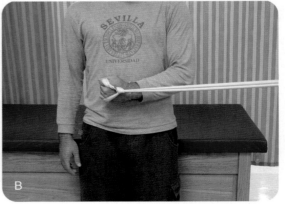

Figure 75.3 Phase I strengthening exercises. **A:** External rotation. **B:** Internal rotation. **C:** Extension.

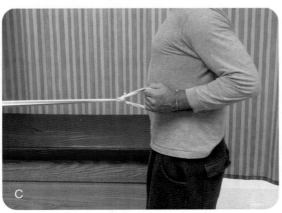

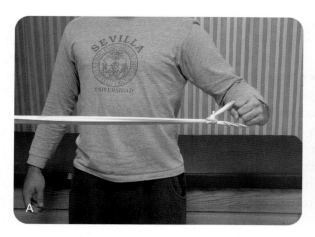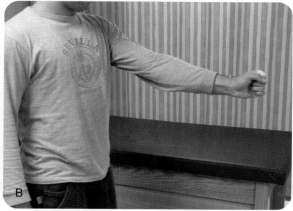

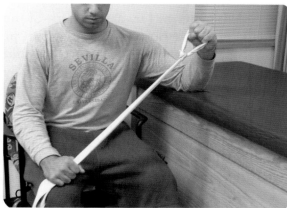

Figure 75.4 Phase II strengthening exercises. **A:** Abduction. **B:** Forward elevation. **C:** External rotation at 45 degrees.

phase I strengthening exercises. Therefore, there is no need to progress to the phase II exercises.

Rotator cuff disease ranks as one of the most common shoulder disorders encountered by medical practitioners. The presence of rotator cuff disease is highly correlated with age.[9] It has been documented that the average age of patients with rotator cuff disease but no rotator cuff tear is 48.7 years, 58.7 years for those with a unilateral rotator cuff tear, and 67.8 years for those with a bilateral tear.[9] Patients with rotator cuff disease but no tear typically present with pain, particularly at night; limited ROM reaching behind and up the back; and weakness of external rotation. These patients can be instructed in phase II ROM exercises and phase I strengthening exercises.[8]

The clinical presentation of patients with a rotator cuff tear will vary depending on the size of the tear. Typically, the patient will complain of pain at night and with activities when the arm is away from the body, similar to patients without a rotator cuff tear. However, patients with a rotator cuff tear may have difficulty reaching above shoulder level, and external rotation weakness will be more pronounced. These patients may need to regain passive forward elevation as well as the ability to reach up the back and across the body. Therefore, patients with a rotator cuff tear should be instructed in phase I and II ROM exercises and phase I strengthening exercises.

Primary frozen shoulder, also known as *adhesive capsulitis*, most frequently affects people between 40 and 65 years old.[11,12] Women appear to be affected by this process more than men.[12,13] Patients with primary frozen shoulder commonly report an insidious onset and then a progressive increase in pain and gradual loss of motion. A minor traumatic event may coincide with the patient's first recognition of symptoms. Pain, specifically sleep-disturbing night pain, frequently motivates patients to seek medical advice. They are usually comfortable with the arm at the side or with midrange activities. The normal course of a frozen shoulder has been described to have three stages: stage 1, the "freezing" stage, which is characterized by progressive increase in unrelenting pain and loss of motion; stage 2, the "frozen" stage, which is characterized by a slow improvement in pain, but there is continued stiffness; and stage 3, the "thawing" stage, which is characterized by slow return of motion.

Patients with frozen shoulder should be instructed in phase I and II ROM exercises. They should also be cautioned to stay within their limits of pain. Patients in the first stage, or "freezing" stage, may not realize much improvement in ROM. The goal for exercise at this stage is to limit the loss of motion and keep the patient as comfortable as possible. In many cases, an injection of corticosteroid into the glenohumeral joint may help to ease the pain and allow progression of the exercises.[14]

Multidirectional glenohumeral instability may be manifested in a variety of ways.[15] The patient is often athletic, and gymnasts, swimmers, and weight trainers may be predisposed to this condition.[15] An instability episode may have occurred without significant injury and spontaneously reduced or was self-reduced.[15] Hypermobile shoulder can become symptomatic without unusual trauma and possibly even from activities of daily living.[15] A strengthening exercise program has been shown to provide enough glenohumeral stability to allow 87% of patients to return to normal activities without instability.[16] Therefore, patients with multidirectional instability should be instructed in phase I strengthening exercises and progressed to phase II when appropriate.

This chapter has provided recommendations for effective exercises in the treatment of shoulder disorders. It should not be assumed that the patient will leave the office and be able to perform these exercises adequately to allow return to normal function. Therefore, it may be prudent to schedule a follow-up visit to evaluate the performance of the exercises. It may also be helpful to refer the patient to physical therapy for instruction in the exercises and supervised progression.

References

1. Luime J, Hendriksen I, Verhagen A, et al. Prevalence and incidence of shoulder pain in the general population: a systematic review. *Scand J Rheumatol* 2004;33:73–81.
2. Van der Windt D, Koes B, de Jong B, et al. Shoulder disorders in general practice: incidence, patient characteristics, and management. *Ann Rheum Dis* 1995;54(12):959–964.
3. Mitchell C, Adebajo A, Hay E, et al. Shoulder pain: diagnosis and management in primary care. *BMJ* 2005;331:1124–1128.
4. Van der Windt D, Koes B, Boeke A, et al. Shoulder disorders in general practice: prognostic indicators of outcome. *Br J Gen Pract* 1996;46(410):519–523.
5. Gerber C, Werner C, Macy J, et al. Effect of selective capsulorrhaphy on the passive range of motion of the glenohumeral joint. *J Bone Joint Surg Am* 2003;85(1):48–55.

6. Harryman DTD, Sidles JA, Harris SL, et al. The role of the rotator interval capsule in passive motion and stability of the shoulder. *J Bone Joint Surg Am* 1992;74(1):53–66.

7. Turkel SJ, Panio MW, Marshall JL, et al. Stabilizing mechanisms preventing anterior dislocation of the glenohumeral joint. *J Bone Joint Surg Am* 1981;63(8):1208–1217.

8. McClure P, Bialker J, Neff N, et al. Shoulder function and 3-dimensional kinematics in people with shoulder impingement syndrome before and after a 6-week exercise program. *Phys Ther* 2004;84: 832–848.

9. Yamaguchi K, Ditsios K, Middleton W, et al. The demographic and morphological features of rotator cuff disease. A comparison of asymptomatic and symptomatic shoulders. *J Bone Joint Surg Am* 2006;88:1699–1704.

10. Neviaser RJ. Painful conditions affecting the shoulder. *Clin Orthop* 1983(173):63–69.

11. Neviaser RJ, Neviaser TJ. The frozen shoulder. Diagnosis and management. *Clin Orthop* 1987;(223):59–64.

12. Binder A, Bulgen D, Hazleman B. Frozen shoulder: an arthrographic and radionuclear scan assessment. *Ann Rheum Dis* 1984;43:365.

13. Lundberg BJ. The frozen shoulder: clinical and radiographic observation: the effect of manipulation under general anesthesia: structure and glycosaminoglycan content in the joint capsule. *Acta Orthop Scand* 1969;119:1–59.

14. Carette S, Moffet H, Tardif J, et al. Intraarticular corticosteroids, supervised physiotherapy, or a combination of the two in the treatment of adhesive capsulitis of the shoulder. A placebo-controlled trial. *Arthritis Rheum* 2003;48(3):829–838.

15. Cordasco F. Understanding multidirectional instability of the shoulder. *J Athl Train* 2000;35(3):278–285.

16. Burkhead W, Rockwood C. Treatment of instability of the shoulder with an exercise program. *J Bone Joint Surg* 1992;74:890–896.

SECTION 15 Rehabilitation

76 Elbow Rehabilitation

Laura Walsh and Gayle K. Severance

Lateral Epicondylitis

Lateral epicondylitis, often called *tennis elbow*, affects 1% to 3% of the population, with <5% to 10% being tennis players. It affects women (40%–50%) more often than men. The greatest incidence is between 35 and 55 years of age.[1-3]

Lateral epicondylitis typically presents with pain at the lateral epicondyle of the humerus and may radiate proximal or distal. The wrist and digit extensors are involved, most notably the extensor carpi radialis brevis. The pain typically lasts from 6 months to 2 years.[2,3]

Current literature suggests that the histopathology is a degenerative condition rather than inflammatory. Therefore, lateral epicondylitis is more of a tendinosis, indicating degenerative changes, than a tendinitis, indicating inflammatory changes. Studies have found a prevalence of fibroblasts cells and atypical vascular formation, termed *angiofibroblastic tendinosis*, at the lateral epicondyle rather than inflammatory cells.[2,3]

Onset can be an acute event or a gradual process. Physical findings include tenderness 1 to 2 cm distal to the lateral humeral epicondyle, which may radiate proximally or distally. The pain usually increases with repetitive and resistive gripping activity, wrist extension, wrist radial deviation, and/or forearm supination. Patients experience a decrease in function and strength due to pain rather than actual weakness. Strength typically returns when the pain has resolved. Early intervention is optimal for recovery and return of function.[2,3]

Conservative treatment consists of two splinting options. A wrist splint with the wrist in slight extension puts the extensors on rest (Fig. 76.1). A forearm cuff (tennis elbow strap) is used to deflect the pull of the extensor tendon and decrease pain with use (Fig. 76.2). A wrist splint is preferred to allow for rest and healing of the degenerative tissue, but if a patient cannot wear the wrist splint due to job demands, the forearm cuff may be used for work. The affected arm should be allowed to rest until the pain has significantly resolved.[4]

In addition to the wrist splint and forearm cuff, stretches are recommended to decrease pain and tightness in the affected muscles, tendons, and surrounding tissue. The stretches are to be done slowly, with no

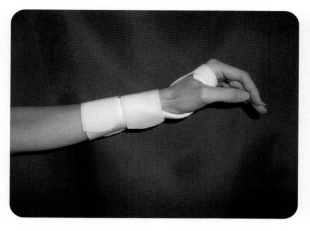

Figure 76.1 Wrist splint. Place on the volar surface of the wrist. Wear with use to rest the painful area.

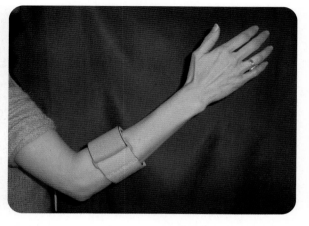

Figure 76.2 Forearm cuff. Place approximately 2 to 3 inches below the elbow crease with the extra pad over the muscle bulk. Wear with activity.

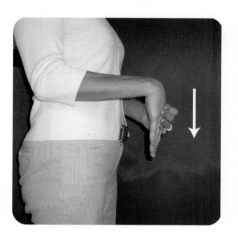

Figure 76.3 Step 1: Bend the elbow. Let the wrist drop down. Use the opposite hand to gently push until a gentle stretch is felt.

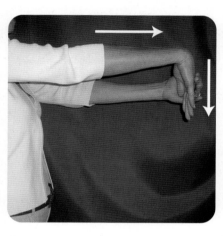

Figure 76.4 Step 2: Hold the arm out straight. Use the opposite hand to gently push the wrist down until a gentle stretch is felt.

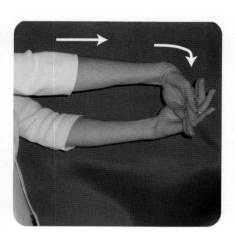

Figure 76.5 Step 3: Keeping the arm straight and the wrist bent, turn the fingers outward until a gentle stretch is felt.

increase in pain. If the stretches are painful, the patient should proceed more gently or discontinue. Stretches are performed in five to ten repetitions, holding the position for 5 seconds and repeating five times daily. The stretches vary in intensity and should be progressed as tolerated[5,6] (Figs. 76.3–76.5).

Radial Neck Fracture

A radial neck fracture is commonly caused by a fall on an extended and supinated outstretched hand. This type of fracture will impact the mobility of the elbow and the forearm due to the articular connection between the radius, ulna, and humerus. Range-of-motion (ROM) exercises should begin as soon as the fracture is stable. Stability is determined by the referring physician.

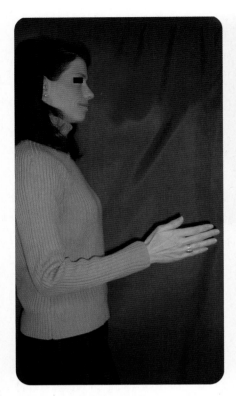

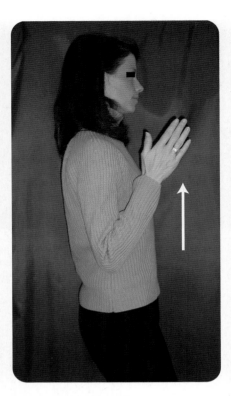

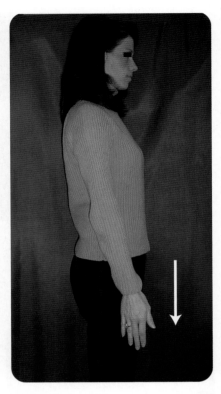

Figure 76.6 Starting position. Begin with the elbow tucked into the side, with the thumb pointing at the ceiling.

Figure 76.7 Elbow flexion. Bend the elbow up as if trying to touch the thumb to the shoulder.

Figure 76.8 Elbow extension. Straighten the elbow as if the fingers are pointing to the floor.

The radius articulates with the capitellum of the humerus at the elbow; therefore, elbow flexion and extension are diminished with a fracture of the radial neck. Gentle active motion of the elbow into flexion and extension will be necessary to regain full functional motion[7] (Figs. 76.6–76.8).

Proximally, in the forearm, the radius articulates with the ulna at the proximal radioulnar joint. Distally, the ulna and the radius again articulate in the forearm, forming the distal radioulnar joint. This is a pivot joint formed between the head of the ulna and the ulnar notch at the distal end of the radius. In addition to these two bony articulations in the forearm, a very thick, tight ligament called the *interosseous membrane* lies between the two bones. When performing forearm rotation, the radius rotates around the ulna, pulling on all of the previously mentioned structures. It is easy to understand why it is difficult for the radius to rotate around the ulna after a radial neck fracture. Forearm supination and pronation exercises are essential to regaining full motion after a radial neck fracture[7,8] (Figs. 76.9–76.11).

Exercises can gradually be advanced by using the uninjured hand to help guide the upper extremity toward the desired position if ROM

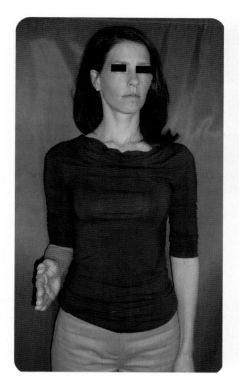

Figure 76.9 Starting position. Begin with the arm tucked at the side, elbow bent at 90 degrees with the thumb on top.

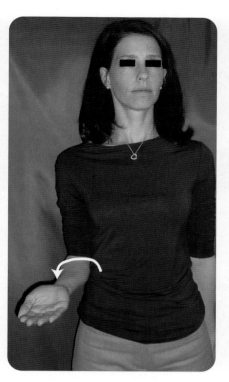

Figure 76.10 Supination. Turn the palm up to face the ceiling.

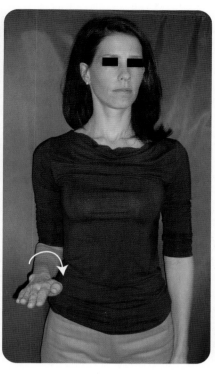

Figure 76.11 Pronation. Turn palm down to face the ground.

deficits persist. Force should be applied in a gentle and comfortable manner. Uncomfortable stretching may cause cocontraction and guarding of the surrounding muscles, which is counterproductive.

The exercise program should be performed in five to ten repetitions each. The desired end position should be held for a minimum of 5 to 10 seconds. The exercise program should be performed five times a day.

In addition to the exercises, light use of the affected upper extremity for activities of daily living such as folding laundry, turning door handles, and reaching to place objects into closets or cupboards is encouraged.

In the event that motion is not improving with the ROM exercises, a splinting regimen may be introduced. The purpose of a splint is to give a steady, comfortable pull into the direction of the desired motion.[9,10] A flexion splint and/or an extension splint should be considered (Figs. 76.12, 76.13). Literature supports the concept that the longer the wear time of the splint, the better the results.[9] A balanced schedule of splint-wearing time, ROM exercises, and functional activity should be established to provide guidelines for the patient.[9,10]

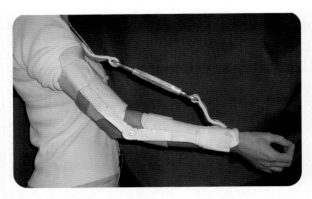

Figure 76.12 Static progressive elbow extension turnbuckle splint.

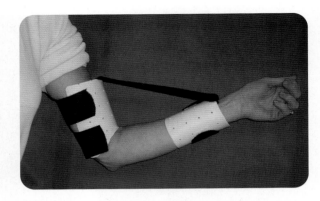

Figure 76.13 Static progressive elbow flexion splint.

References

1. Fedorczyk J. Therapist's management of elbow tendinitis. In: Mackin EJ, Callahan AD, Skirven TM, et al., eds. *Rehabilitation of the Hand and Upper Extremity*, 5th ed. St Louis: Mosby; 2002.
2. Struijs PAA, Smidt N, Arola H, et al. Orthotic devices for the treatment of tennis elbow. *Cochrane Database Syst Rev* 2001;(2):CD001821.
3. Boyer M, Hastings H. Lateral tennis elbow: "is there any science out there?" *J Shoulder Elbow Surg* 1999;8(5):481–491.
4. Smidt N, Windt D, Assendelft W, et al. Corticosteroid injections, physiotherapy, or wait and see policy for lateral epicondylitis: a randomized controlled trial. *Lancet* 2002;359(9307):657–662.
5. Cyr LM, Ross RG. How controlled stress affects healing tissues. *J Hand Ther* 1998;11:125–130.
6. Davila SA, Johnson-Jones K. Managing the stiff elbow: operative, nonoperative, and postoperative techniques. *J Hand Ther* 2006;19(2):268–281.
7. Michlovitz S, Harris BA, Watkins MP. Therapy interventions for improving joint range of motion: a systematic review. *J Hand Ther* 2004;17(2):118–131.
8. Vardakas DG, Varitimidis SE, Goebel F, et al. Evaluating and treating the stiff elbow. *Hand Clin* 2002;18(1):77–85.
9. Griffith. Therapist management of the stiff elbow. In: Hunter JM, Mackin EJ, Callahan AD, et al., eds. *Rehabilitation of the Hand and Upper Extremity*, 5th ed. St. Louis: Mosby; 2002:1245–1262.
10. Page C, Backus SI, Lenhoff MW. Electromyographic activity in stiff and normal elbows during elbow flexion and extension. *J Hand Ther* 2003;16(1):5–11.

CHAPTER 77 Hand and Wrist Rehabilitation

Gayle K. Severance and Laura Walsh

Ganglia of the Wrist

Ganglia of the wrist is a synovial cyst that arises from the synovial lining of the tendon sheath or the joint space. The cause of a wrist ganglion is not determined. It can be located on the dorsal surface (dorsal wrist ganglion) or the volar surface (volar wrist ganglion) of the wrist. The cyst contains a thick, clear, mucuslike fluid that is similar to the fluid found in the joint.[1]

Usually, the more active the wrist, the larger the cyst becomes. With rest, the lump generally decreases in size. Conservative treatment focuses on resting the wrist with a volar wrist splint and activity modification. A splint holds the wrist in the functional position (approximately 15–30 degrees of extension), and the digits are free. A patient may be sent to hand therapy for a custom-made splint (Fig. 77.1), or a prefabricated model can be purchased over the counter (Fig. 77.2). A custom-made splint is preferred to ensure proper positioning.[2] Activity modification includes limiting or avoiding repetitive and resistive wrist and digit use.

If the condition does not resolve with conservative therapy, surgery to remove the cyst may be necessary. Wrist motion may be limited after surgery. The patient will benefit from postoperative hand therapy to regain full functional motion, and address postoperative edema and adherant or sensitive scarring. Wrist flexion will be more limited with a dorsal ganglion cyst removal, and wrist extension is more difficult with volar wrist ganglion removal. Ulnar and radial deviation may also be limited. The patient should be instructed in range of motion in all planes of the wrist (Fig. 77.3–77.6).

Carpal Tunnel Syndrome

Carpal tunnel syndrome (CTS) is compression of the median nerve as it passes through the carpal canal located in the volar wrist. Symptoms include numbness and tingling in the thumb, index, middle, and radial half of the ring fingers. Pain in the volar wrist area is often reported. CTS can cause atrophy of the thenar muscles in the more severe stages. Typically, symptoms begin at night while sleeping and then may advance to the daytime hours.[3]

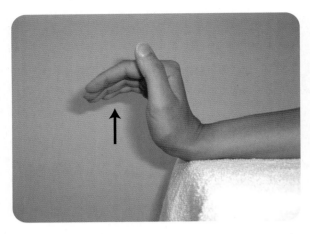

Figure 77.1 Extension. Gently bend the wrist up, keeping the fingers in a loose fist for wrist extension.

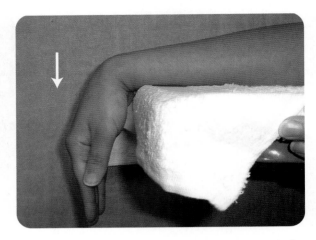

Figure 77.2 Flexion. Gently bend the wrist down, allowing the fingers to relax open for wrist flexion.

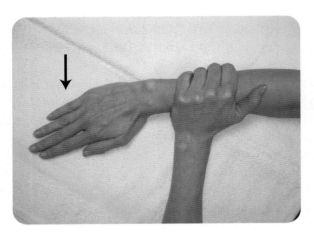

Figure 77.3 Ulnar deviation. Move the hand toward the small finger for ulnar deviation.

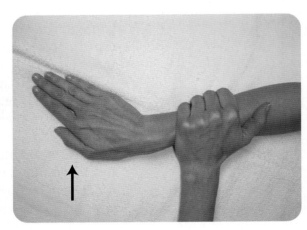

Figure 77.4 Radial deviation. Move the hand toward the thumb for radial deviation.

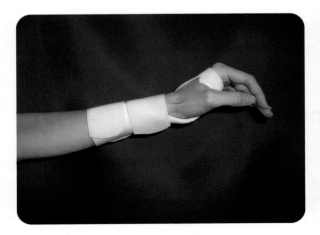

Figure 77.5 Custom-made volar wrist splint with wrist in slight extension.

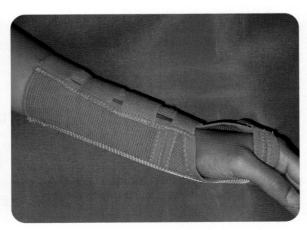

Figure 77.6 Prefabricated volar wrist splint.

CTS can be treated conservatively if the symptoms are mild to moderate. Once an individual reaches the stage of muscle wasting, symptoms are at the severe stage and conservative treatment will not be successful.[4]

Conservative treatment for CTS includes splinting, activity modification, nerve glides, and tendon glides.[5] Splinting the wrist in neutral is suggested. Any degree of wrist flexion or extension will increase pressure on the median nerve in the carpal canal, compromising the median nerve function. Splints can be purchased over the counter (Fig. 77.6), although a custom-made splint (Fig. 77.5) provided by a hand therapist is preferred to ensure proper positioning. Patients are advised to wear the splint while sleeping and during aggravating activities. For those individuals with more advanced symptoms, increased time in the splint may be appropriate. However, prolonged splint wear may lead to wrist stiffness, so a splint weaning schedule should be established.[3]

Activity modification is an important adjunct to splinting in the conservative treatment of CTS. The patient is instructed to modify activity by decreasing or avoiding repetitive gripping, prolonged wrist flexion or extension, and use of vibratory tools.[3]

A home exercise program including median nerve and tendon glides is recommended. The median nerve glide is a series of movements that maximizes the excursion of the median nerve through the carpal canal (Figs. 77.7–77.12). The goal of the median nerve glide is to prevent or reduce fibrotic adhesion formation on the median nerve. These adhesions can form on the nerve due to the body's inflammatory response to compression and irritation of the nerve.[5]

Tendon glides are equally important. Nine tendons course through the carpal canal along with the median nerve. These tendons can be affected by fibrosis as well. Tendon gliding exercises can help to prevent or reduce adhesions and promote tendon excursion.[5]

If conservative treatment does not decrease the symptoms after 2 to 3 months, surgical intervention may be necessary. Individuals who have a carpal tunnel release will need postoperative hand therapy. A hand therapy program will address wound care, edema, pain, sensory issues, range of motion, and strengthening and functional activities.[4]

MEDIAN NERVE GLIDE

Perform the nerve glide five times, hold the end position for 5 seconds, and repeat five times daily (Figs. 77.7–77.12).

TENDON GLIDE

Perform each position five times, hold each position for 5 seconds, and repeat five times daily (Figs. 77.13–77.17).

SECTION 15 Rehabilitation

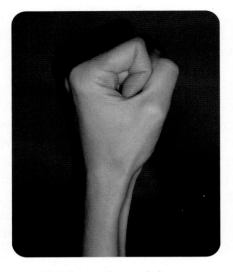

Figure 77.7 Begin with a gentle fist.

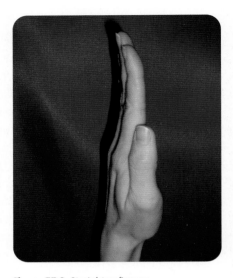

Figure 77.8 Straighten fingers.

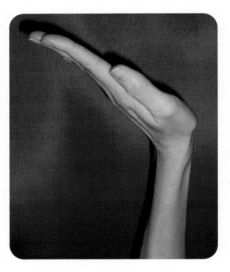

Figure 77.9 Move the wrist back while keeping the fingers straight.

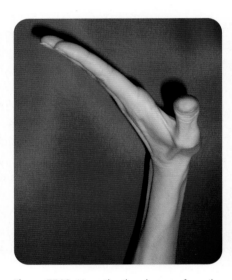

Figure 77.10 Move the thumb away from the hand.

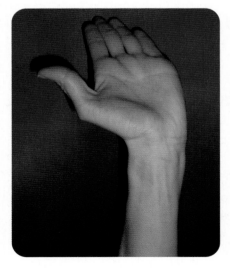

Figure 77.11 Turn the palm to face the clinician.

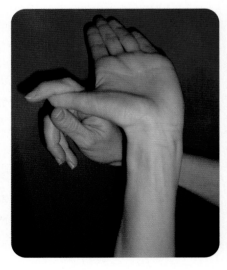

Figure 77.12 Gently push out on the thumb.

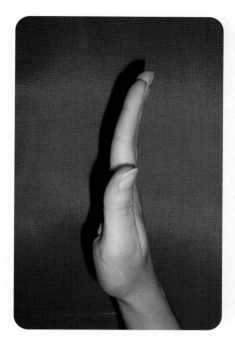

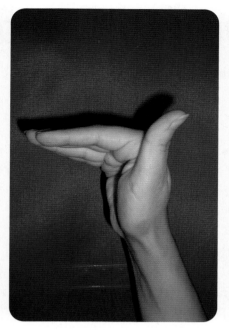

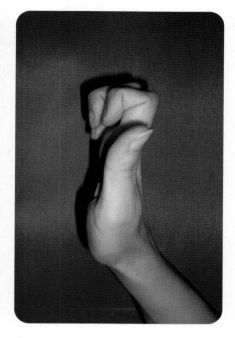

Figure 77.13 Start and finish each fisted position with fingers straight.

Figure 77.14 Table top

Figure 77.15 Hook fist.

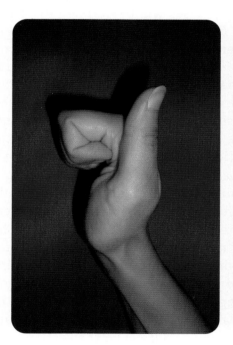

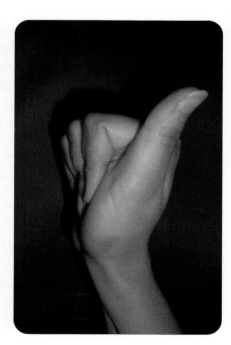

Figure 77.16 Full fist.

Figure 77.17 Straight fist.

SECTION 15 Rehabilitation

References

1. Bush D. Soft tissue tumors of the forearm and hand. In: Hunter JM, Mackin EJ, Callahan AD, eds. *Rehabilitation of the Hand and Upper Extremity*, 5th ed. St. Louis: Mosby; 2002:954–970.
2. Burke FD, Melikyan EY, Bradley MJ, et al. Primary care referral protocol for wrist ganglia. *Postgrad Med J* 2003;79:329–331.
3. Omer G. Diagnosis and management of cubital tunnel syndrome. In: Hunter JM, Mackin EJ, Callahan AD, eds. *Rehabilitation of the Hand and Upper Extremity*, 5th ed. St. Louis: Mosby; 2002:672–678.
4. Eversmann W. Proximal median nerve compression. *Hand Clin* 1992;8:307–315.
5. Chin DH, Jones NF. Repetitive motion hand disorders. *J Calif Dent Assoc* 2002;30(2):149–160.

78 Lumbar Rehabilitation

Timothy J. Bayruns and Won Sung

It is well documented that 80% of Americans will eventually have low back pain.[1] Lumbar pain is the number one reason why patients visit an orthopaedic or neurosurgeon and the number two reason why patients see a primary care physician.[2] The vast majority of low back pain complaints will resolve in approximately 6 weeks.[3] Exercises that are applicable to a specific patient need may not only help to decrease pain and symptoms but also may improve function.[4] In this chapter, a variety of home exercises will be outlined to assist patients in returning to a more active life.

Werneke and colleagues[5] described the concept of centralization. This occurs when a lumbar injury produces radiating and expanding pain that becomes worse with certain movements or positions and "centralizes" or reduces in intensity and size with other movements or positions. Typically, sitting, bending, and lifting will increase and spread or peripheralize the complaints, while prone lying, extension in lying, or standing trunk extension can centralize the complaints[6,7] (refer to the section on Extension-based Exercises).

Spinal stenosis is an example of a flexion-based degenerative condition brought on by one or more processes, causing a decrease in the available free space in the lumbar spine.[8] These include foraminal or central canal narrowing and decreased elasticity in ligamentous or capsular structures. Pressure exerted on the spinal cord, nerve root, or both can lead to pain, decreased activities of daily living, muscle weakness, or other limiting symptoms.[9] Standing, walking, or lying flat typically bring on the complaints, while sitting, bending, or any trunk flexion postures reduce the symptoms[10] (refer to the section on Flexion-based Exercises).

A large portion of "lumbago" patients will have no clear-cut pathology.[11,12] Recent research has shown that an exercise program of "stabilization" can help to decrease pain and limitation.[13,14] Other patients also respond to movement into a pattern that has helped to "centralize" their pain.[5] The importance of treating patients with back pain can therefore be based more on how people respond to treatment versus a diagnosis-specific exercise routine (refer to the section on Stabilization Exercises).

The preceding exercises are a very general, and certainly, a non-exhaustive collection designed to get a patient mobile. A true intervention and treatment plan should only be implemented once a through examination has been performed. There are many other mechanical, anatomical, and physiologic factors that need to be considered prior to initiation of a guided intervention. This is especially true with the complicated patient, that would require personal and specific guidance.

Extension-based Exercises

LYING PRONE

The patient with back pain with or without referred pain lies on the stomach, and the clinician looks for the back pain to decrease or, for distal symptoms, to begin centralizing to the lumbar spine (Fig. 78.1).

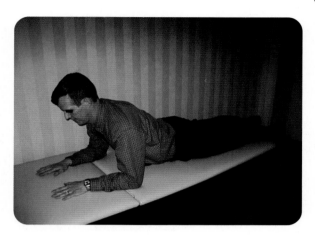

Figure 78.1

EXTENSION IN LYING

If the patient does not feel worse lying prone, the patient with back and/or leg symptoms goes into extension, fully extending the arms and letting the stomach sag. Reduction in back and/or leg symptoms are sought here, and if successful, this should be performed on a regular basis (10–20 repetitions every 1–2 hours) (Fig. 78.2).

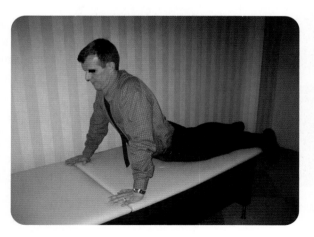

Figure 78.2

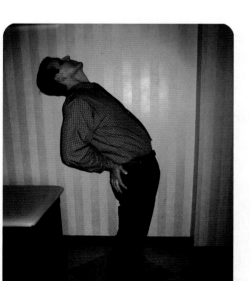

Figure 78.3

EXTENSION IN STANDING

If the patient responds well to extension in lying, extension in standing is another exercise that can be performed to reduce and maintain symptom reduction. In some instances, due to confounding factors, the patient who responds to extension in lying may have an increase in symptoms with extension in standing. If that is the case, the patient is urged to continue with extension in lying on a regular basis (Fig. 78.3).

Flexion-based Exercises

SINGLE KNEE TO CHEST/DOUBLE KNEE TO CHEST

Flexion-based exercises are typically used with patients who are stenotic. Again, the patient is asked to perform a motion, and the clinician is looking for a reduction in pain or centralization. These exercises can also help to stretch the extensor muscles of the trunk that may be in spasm (Figs. 78.4, 78.5).

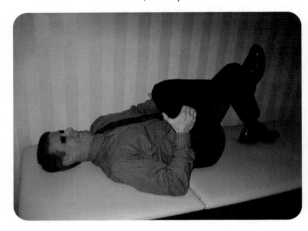

Figure 78.4

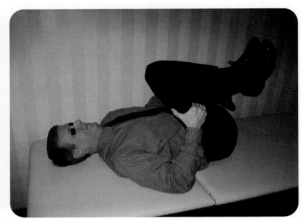

Figure 78.5

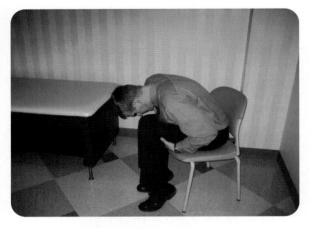

Figure 78.6

SEATED TRUNK FLEXION

This is a variation of the knee-to-chest exercises that can be performed seated. Some patients who report classic symptoms of stenosis, such as increased pain with walking, often find this to be a helpful exercise to perform as they sit (Fig. 78.6).

LOW TRUNK ROTATION/HIP DROPS

Although the lumbar spine does not rotate, a rotational exercise helps to stretch trunk muscles with oblique orientations (Fig. 78.7).

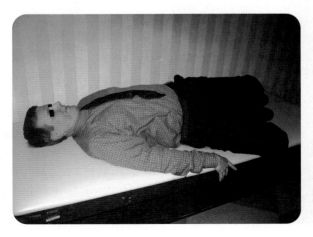

Figure 78.7

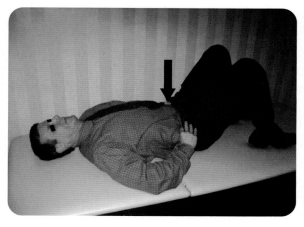

Figure 78.8

Stabilization Exercises

ABDOMINAL DRAWING IN

In the supine position, the patient is asked to pull the navel toward the spine, which leads to recruitment of the abdominal musculature. This drawing-in exercise causes recruitment of all abdominal musculature but minimizes rectus abdominus firing while possibly getting more recruitment of the transversus abdominus. This can also be performed in quadruped, and the patient is asked to pull the navel toward the spine (Fig. 78.8).

BRIDGING

The patient lies supine, performs the drawing-in maneuver, and raises the buttocks off the mat, eliciting a contraction of the gluteals and trunk extensors. As this becomes easy, the patient can perform a bridge and then extend the leg to go into a single limb support, requiring the gluteals and trunk stabilizers to work harder (Figs. 78.9, 78.10).

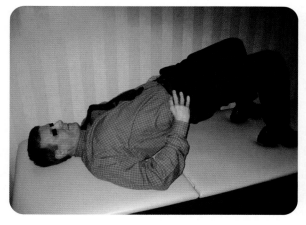

Figure 78.9

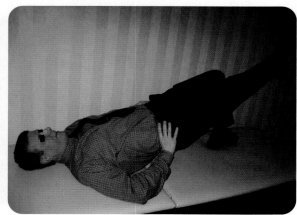

Figure 78.10

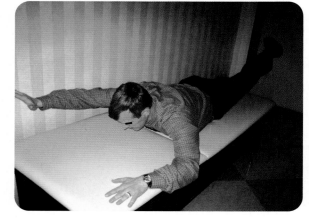

Figure 78.11

PRONE LEG EXTENSIONS/ALTERNATING ARM AND LEG EXTENSIONS

The patient lies prone and alternately extends the arm and legs, facilitating firing of the trunk stabilizers, specifically the lumbar extensors (Fig. 78.11).

SECTION 15 Rehabilitation

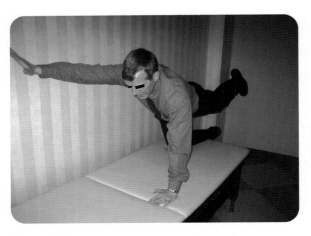

Figure 78.12

QUADRUPED ALTERNATING LEG EXTENSIONS/ALTERNATING ARM AND LEG EXTENSIONS

The patient starts in the quadruped position and is asked to perform the drawing-in exercise. As the abdominal contraction is held, the patient lifts one leg off the surface and is asked to maintain a stable trunk. By raising the opposite arm and leg off the mat, the patient is required to increase the firing of trunk stabilizers (Fig. 78.12).

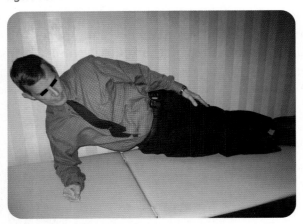

Figure 78.13

SIDE BRIDGING

In this particular exercise, the patient is asked to lie on the side with the elbow under the shoulder. The patient is then asked to lift the trunk off of the mat. This exercise has been shown to recruit the quadratus lumborum, which is an important trunk stabilizer, as well as the oblique abdominal muscles (Fig. 78.13).

References

1. Lewis JS, Hewitt JS, Billington L, et al. A randomized clinical trial comparing two physiotherapy interventions for chronic low back pain. *Spine* 2005;30(7):711–721.
2. National Institute of Neurological Disorders and Stroke. Available at *www.nlm.nih.gov/medlineplus/ency/article/003108.htm,* accessed 3/3/08.
3. Waddell G. A new clinical model for treatment of low back pain. *Spine* 1987;12:632–644.
4. Long A, Donelson R, Fung T. Does it matter which exercise? A randomized control trial of exercise for low back pain. *Spine* 2004;29(23):2593–2602.
5. Werneke M, Hart DL. Centralization phenomenon as a prognostic factor for chronic low back pain and disability. *Spine* 2001;26(7):758–764.
6. Cole AJ, Herring SA. *The Low Back Pain Handbook: a Guide for the Practicing Clinician.* Philadelphia: Henry and Belfus; 1997:151–168.
7. McKenzie R. *The Lumbar Spine: Mechanical Diagnosis and Therapy.* Waikanae, New Zealand: Spinal Publications; 1981:68–90.
8. National Institute of Arthritis and Musculoskeletal and Skin Diseases. Available at *www.niams.nih.gov/health_info/spinal_stenosis/default.asp,* accessed 3/3/08.
9. Alvarez JA, Hardy RH. Lumbar spine stenosis: a common cause of back and leg pain. *Am Fam Physician* 1998;57:1825–1834.
10. Snyder DL, Doggett D, Turkelson C. Treatment of degenerative lumbar spinal stenosis. *Am Fam Physician* 2004;70(3):517–520.
11. Venes D. *Taber's Cyclopedic Medical Dictionary,* 20th ed. (Thumb-indexed). Philadelphia: FA Davis; 2005:1207.
12. Flores L, Gatchel RJ, Polatin PB. Objectification of functional improvement after non-operative care. *Spine* 1997;22(14):1622–1633.
13. Golby LJ, Moore AP, Doust J, et al. A randomized control trial investigating the efficiency of musculoskeletal physiotherapy on chronic low back disorder. *Spine* 2006;31(20):1083–1093.
14. Slade SC, JL Keating. Trunk strengthening exercises for chronic low back pain: a systematic review. *J Manipulative Physiol Ther* 2006;29(2):163–173.

79 Hip Rehabilitation

Brian J. Eckenrode and Christopher J. Kauffman

Rehabilitation of a patient with hip pathology depends on a number of factors, including age, type of pathology, and activity level. The focus of physical therapy should address the patient's impairments and functional limitations to improve quality of life. Due to the contribution of the trunk and entire lower extremity to mobility, many of the exercises described in Chapters 78 and 80 may be appropriate for the individual with hip pathology as well.

Hip osteoarthritis has been identified as a major cause of disability among the older population.[1] Management should be directed at maintaining functional mobility, decreasing pain, prevention of deformity, and joint protection techniques. Patients often exhibit pain with weight bearing, loss of motion, and strength deficits to the hip, which impacts their functional mobility, such as rising from a chair, bathing, dressing, and the use of stairs.[2] Adaptive equipment such as canes and walkers and home modifications may benefit the patient through improving their independence at home and in the community.

The use of an assistive device can reduce the amount of joint stress/reaction force when placed in the contralateral extremity (Fig. 79.1). This requires less activity of the hip abductors, and loads placed on the hip are reduced with the use of a cane. Weight loss is also important for this population, as for every pound of body weight reduced, there is a 3-pound decrease in load through the hip. This population may want to consider activities that minimize stress on the hip joint (i.e., swimming, pool exercises, biking).

Exercise has been shown to reduce pain and disability in patients with osteoarthritis and should focus on improving the patient's hip range of motion (ROM) while avoiding pain and symptoms.[3,4] The heel slide description in Chapter 80 shows an example of a gentle hip and knee ROM exercise. Hip flexor stretching is also important, as tight hip flexors will impair the kinematics between the lumbar spine, pelvis, and hips.

Strengthening of the hip joint should emphasize the gluteus medius, hip adductors, and hip extensors as well as the remainder of the lower extremity and core musculature.[1] The gluteus medius acts as the primary stabilizer of the hip and pelvis in single-limb stance and is important for gait. Side-lying hip abduction is performed by having the patient lie on

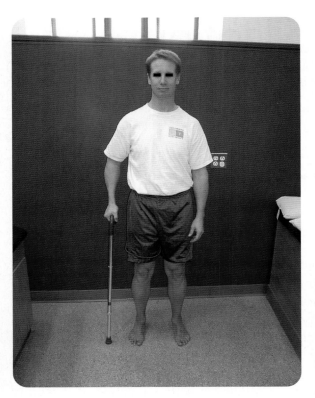

Figure 79.1 An assistive device such as a cane should be placed in the contralateral upper extremity in order to effectively decrease loads placed on the involved hip and/or leg.

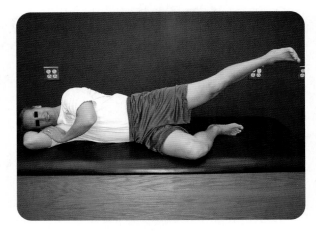

Figure 79.2 Side-lying hip abduction strengthening exercise.

their side with the top leg straight and then raising the top leg up toward the ceiling (Fig. 79.2). The leg should be raised to approximately 25 to 40 degrees and held for 2 to 3 seconds, repeating ten repetitions in one to three sets. It is important to keep the leg neutral (in line) with the trunk and not to deviate into flexion. The "clamshell exercise" is another exercise to strengthen the hip abductors and external rotators. The patient is again in a side-lying position with both legs bent and the heels together. The top knee is raised by rotating the hip, keeping the heels together while preventing the pelvis from rolling (Fig. 79.3). Have the patient hold this position for 2 to 3 seconds, repeating ten repetitions in one to three sets. Hip extensor strengthening can be performed with the patient supine with the knees bent (Fig. 79.4A). The patient then raises the hips upward while keeping the feet on the bed, creating a "bridge" (Fig. 79.4B). The bridge position is held for 2 to 3 seconds, then the patient lowers the pelvis and hips down. With all of these strengthening exercises, it is suggested that ten repetitions are performed, progressing sets and resistance as able one to two times per day.

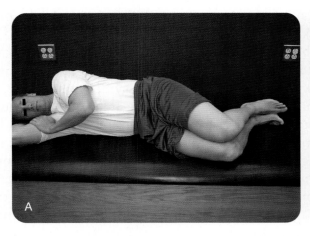
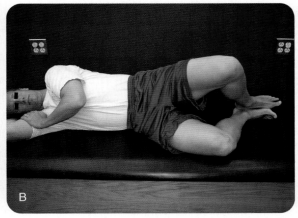

Figure 79.3 Side-lying "clamshell" exercise to address the abductors and external rotators of the hip.

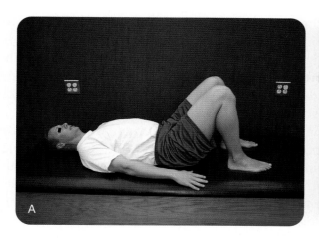
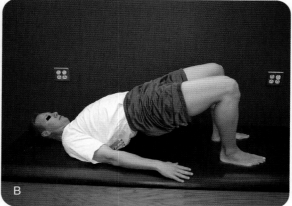

Figure 79.4 A: Start position for the bridge exercise. **B:** End position for the bridge exercise.

A referral to physical therapy may consist of patient education, gait assessment and training, modalities to assist with pain, joint mobilization techniques and stretching to improve hip ROM, and strengthening exercises to address areas of weakness. Specific manual physical therapy techniques have been shown to decrease pain, improve ROM, and increase functional activity in patients with hip osteoarthritis.[5,6]

For individuals with hip trochanteric bursitis or snapping hip syndrome, activity modification is one of the more substantial changes that a clinician can make. Modifying a patient's particular sport or exercise can remove a potential irritant and reduce repetitive trauma. Examples of modifications would be advising on a rest period from activity, managing the amount of time an activity is performed, managing the way the activity is performed, or modifying the training environment.

In conjunction with activity modification, cryotherapy can also be helpful to reduce pain and inflammation present with conditions such as snapping hip and trochanteric bursitis.[7] Specific to trochanteric bursitis, a referral to physical therapy for the performance of iontophoresis and/or ultrasound may also be helpful to reduce inflammation, decrease pain, and promote return to previous activity levels.[8,9]

Consideration should also be given to managing any biomechanical abnormalities pending the etiology of the conditions of snapping hip or trochanteric bursitis as well as the deficits noted during physical examination.[10] Rehabilitation should give special consideration to normalizing flexibility. Repeated low-load, long-duration stretches performed at a painfree intensity may be helpful to improve soft tissue flexibility and reduce symptom irritation. Commonly affected musculature for snapping hip are the iliotibial band, gluteus maximus, and iliopsoas; for trochanteric bursitis, the iliotibial band is most affected.[11] Any identified lumbar mobility deficits should also be addressed, as the hip joint may be compensating for lumbar spine deficits.

Further normalization of biomechanical abnormalities through addressing identified strength deficits surrounding the hip may be helpful. Performance of lumbopelvic stabilization exercises in conjunction

SECTION 15 Rehabilitation

with hip-strengthening activities may be of benefit since improved pelvic positioning provides the hip musculature with a stable base from which to function[12] (Figs. 79.2–79.4). Improvement of core strength also may reduce the abnormal stress on the hip joint region by reducing the need for the surrounding hip joint to accommodate for any deficits leading from poor core strength.

Regarding snapping hip due to intra-articular pathology, conservative rehabilitation options such as those found with labral pathology appear to be limited, since most labral tears do not appear to heal conservatively.[10] Considering the prevalence of chondral damage adjacent to labral tears due to the friction imposed on the adjacent articular cartilage, it is reasonable to avoid excessive loading of the hip joint to avoid any potential wear and tear.[13,14] Activity modification and addressing ROM, joint mobility, flexibility, and strength deficits may also be helpful and are of importance for patients who may be preoperative in nature.[15,16] A referral to a physical therapist may be beneficial for pain management and to address musculoskeletal deficits that limit functioning.

References

1. Arokoski JP. Physical therapy and rehabilitation programs in the management of hip osteoarthritis. *Eura Medicophys* 2005;41(2):155–161.
2. Lin YC, Davey RC, Cochrane T. Tests for physical function of the elderly with knee and hip osteoarthritis. *Scand J Med Sci Sports* 2001;11(5):280–286.
3. Roddy E, Zhang W, Doherty M, et al. Evidence-based recommendations for the role of exercise in the management of osteoarthritis of the hip or knee—the MOVE consensus. *Rheumatology (Oxford)* 2005;44(1):67–73.
4. Van Baar ME, Dekker J, Oostendorp RA, et al. The effectiveness of exercise therapy in patients with osteoarthritis of the hip or knee: a randomized clinical trial. *J Rheumatol* 1998;25(12):2432–2439.
5. Hoeksma HL, Dekker J, Ronday HK, et al. Comparison of manual therapy and exercise therapy in osteoarthritis of the hip: a randomized clinical trial. *Arthritis Rheum* 2004;51(5):722–729.
6. MacDonald CW, Whitman JM, Cleland JA, et al. Clinical outcomes following manual physical therapy and exercise for hip osteoarthritis: a case series. *J Orthop Sports Phys Ther* 2006;36(8):588–599.
7. Nadler SF, Weingand K, Kruse RJ. The physiologic basis and clinical applications of cryotherapy and thermotherapy for the pain practitioner. *Pain Physician* 2004;7(3):395–399.
8. Costello CT, Jeske AH. Iontophoresis: applications in transdermal medication delivery. *Phys Ther* 1995;75(6):554–563.
9. Li LC, Scudds RA. Iontophoresis: an overview of the mechanisms and clinical application. *Arthritis Care Res* 1995;8(1):51–61.
10. Paluska SA. An overview of hip injuries in running. *Sports Med* 2005;35(11):991–1014.
11. Winston P, Awan R, Cassidy JD, et al. Clinical examination and ultrasound of self-reported snapping hip syndrome in elite ballet dancers. *Am J Sports Med* 2007;35(1):118–126.
12. Mascal CL, Landel R, Powers C. Management of patellofemoral pain targeting hip, pelvis, and trunk muscle function: 2 case reports. *J Orthop Sports Phys Ther* 2003;33(11):647–660.
13. McCarthy J, Noble P, Aluisio FV, et al. Anatomy, pathologic features, and treatment of acetabular labral tears. *Clin Orthop Relat Res* 2003;(406):38–47.
14. McCarthy JC, Noble PC, Schuck MR, et al. The Otto E. Aufranc Award: the role of labral lesions to development of early degenerative hip disease. *Clin Orthop Relat Res* 2001;(393):25–37.
15. Enseki KR, Martin RL, Draovitch P, et al. The hip joint: arthroscopic procedures and postoperative rehabilitation. *J Orthop Sports Phys Ther* 2006;36(7):516–525.
16. Lewis CL, Sahrmann SA. Acetabular labral tears. *Phys Ther* 2006;86(1):110–121.

80 Knee Rehabilitation

David S. Logerstedt and Christopher J. Kauffman

The knee can be described as the central link between the hip and the ankle joints. Because the knee has mobility and stability responsibilities, it is the primary functional link involved in gait, stair climbing, and standing and sitting activities. A patient typically presents to the primary care physician with complaints of pain and/or swelling, which can have a significant effect on the function of the knee.[1–4] In addition, dysfunction to the knee can be the result of range of motion (ROM) loss, strength deficits, instability, decreased flexibility in the surrounding musculature, and dysfunctions in the adjacent joints. One goal is to restore functional motor patterns that patients will encounter in activities of daily living and occupational, recreational or athletic endeavors by reduced microtrauma and recurrent injury on joint structures. A home exercise program can be provided to a patient to address physical impairments and functional limitations.

In addressing ROM loss related to knee swelling, degenerative joint changes, overuse injuries, or acute knee injuries, restoration of knee extension and flexion are paramount for normal function. The restoration of full passive knee extension is paramount, as limitations in knee extension contribute to gait dysfunctions and patellofemoral symptoms.[5] Loss of knee extension can be addressed with low-load, long-duration stretch by utilizing the heel prop technique (Fig. 80.1). Place a rolled-up towel under the heel while the patient is lying supine. This position should be maintained for 10 to 12 minutes two to three times daily until full extension is restored. Knee flexion can be restored by employing the heel slide (Fig. 80.2). Place a towel or strap around the ankle, and grasp either end of the towel or strap while seated in the long-sitting position. Actively slide the heel toward the buttocks, assisting by pulling on the ends of the towel until mild resistance is felt. Hold this position for 10 seconds for ten repetitions two to three times daily.

Flexibility exercises can assist in restoring normal joint motion.[6] Although decreased flexibility may not be a risk factor for the development of knee disorders or injuries, increased flexibility and ROM provides for cartilage nutrition and health, protection of joint structures from damaging impact loads, and function and comfort in daily activities.[7,8] Quadriceps stretching is performed in the prone position with a strap attached to the ipsilateral ankle and grasping the other end of the strap over the

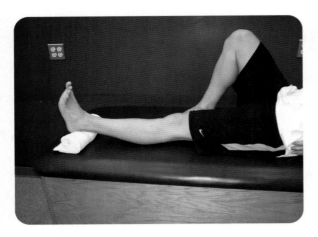

Figure 80.1 Heel prop.

ipsilateral shoulder (Fig. 80.3). The knee is flexed while being given active assistance with the strap and provides mild overpressure as a stretch is felt in the anterior thigh. Hamstring stretching is performed in the supine position, and the knee is bent toward the chest while grasping behind the knee with both hands (Fig. 80.4). Actively extend the knee until feeling a stretch sensation in the posterior thigh. Both stretching exercises should be held for 30 to 45 seconds and repeated twice. Stretching can be performed daily.

Muscle weakness has been associated with painful knee osteoarthritis and joint effusion. Quadriceps weakness may increase the risk of the development of knee osteoarthritis. Patients who present to the clinic may not be able to tolerate weight-bearing exercises; therefore, nonweight-bearing exercises within safe ROM can facilitate appropriate muscle activation without compromising joint integrity. Isometric quadriceps setting is an effective method of facilitating initial quadriceps activation. The quadriceps muscle is contracted by pressing the back of the knee into the floor or bed (Fig. 80.5). Instruction should be given to watch for the superior glide of

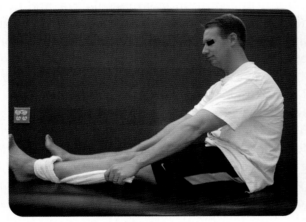

Figure 80.2 Heel slide.

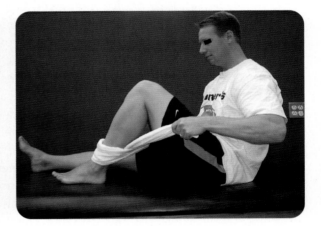

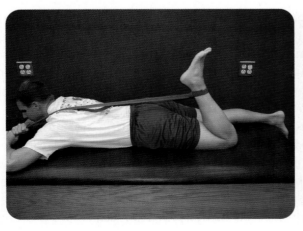

Figure 80.3 Quad stretch.

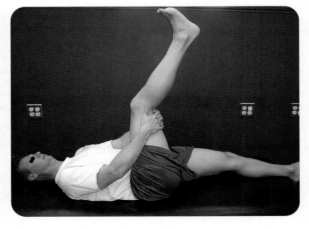

Figure 80.4 Hamstring stretch.

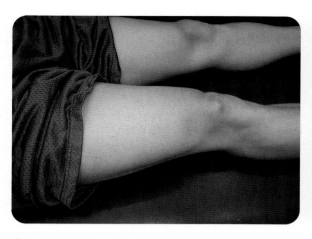
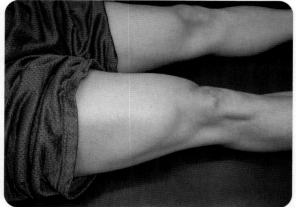

Figure 80.5 Quad set.

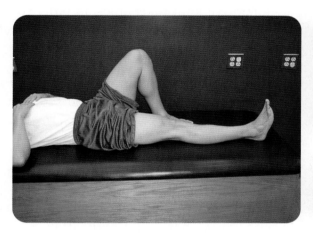
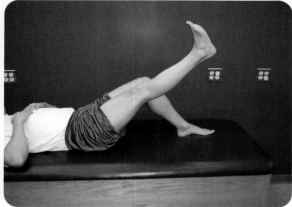

Figure 80.6 Straight-leg raise.

the patella when the exercise is performed correctly. Care should be taken that the hip extensor muscles are not activated, resulting in an incorrect extension moment on the knee. The straight-leg-raise flexion can promote quadriceps activation without irritating the tibiofemoral or patellofemoral joint.[9] The nonexercising knee is flexed to 90 degrees. The exercising leg is maintained in an extended position while lifting from the hip. The exercising extremity is lifted to the level of the opposite knee and held for 3 seconds (Fig. 80.6). The extremity is lowered slowly until the heel slightly touches. This is initially performed for ten repetitions in two sets, progressing as the activity becomes easier.

If the patient presents with mild to moderate symptoms and demonstrates a straight-leg-raise flexion without an extensor lag, the patient can progress to weight-bearing exercises. One the most effective is the squat (Fig. 80.7). Squatting encourages equal weight-bearing between the legs, reduces shear forces across the tibiofemoral joint, minimizes patellofemoral compressive forces, and enhances cocontraction of the quadriceps and hamstrings.[10–12] The squat should be performed to 45 degrees of knee flexion.

Patellofemoral pain syndrome is one of the more common knee conditions presenting to a practitioner's office. In order to achieve and maintain

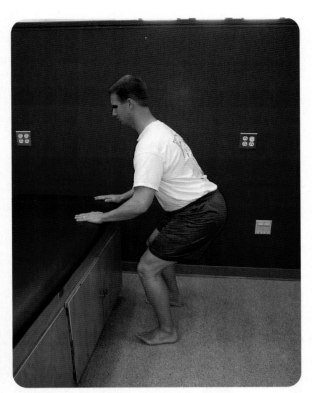

Figure 80.7 Squat.

good functional results, a core component to conservative management is quadriceps strengthening.[13–17] Examples of general quadriceps strengthening exercises, best performed without increasing symptoms, are straight-leg raises (Fig. 80.6) or mini-squats (Fig. 80.7). Referral for physical therapy evaluation can be beneficial to further educate patients on safe performance of higher-level quadriceps-strengthening exercises.

A current concept gaining attention is that of segmental interaction.[18] With segmental interaction, abnormal motion of the tibia and femur in the transverse and frontal planes results in a change in the dynamic Q angle at the knee, therefore altering normal patellofemoral joint mechanics. In order to restore normal mechanics and limit abnormal patellofemoral stress, it is important to consider proximal and distal stability of the lower extremity.

To promote improved proximal stability at the hip, a variety of exercises can be utilized, with focus of those exercises being to improve the strength and recruitment of the hip external rotators to normalize femoral positioning during dynamic activities. Such exercises that can be performed easily at home are clamshell exercises and bridges while having the hips in a position of abduction and external rotation (refer to Figs. 79.3 and 79.4). Performance of such exercises with lumbopelvic stabilization is important, as this allows the musculature to function off of a stable base and at an optimal position.

Distal stability is provided by controlling foot alignment.[19–21] Studies have found that controlling foot positioning, primarily foot pronation, may be of benefit to individuals with patellofemoral pain, but this is likely only in a subpopulation.[21] A trial of over-the-counter orthotics may be beneficial, with custom orthotics considered if symptom reduction is noted. Addressing flexibility and strength deficits of the surrounding foot and ankle musculature as well as gait deficits may also promote improved dynamic stability.

Lower extremity positioning and normal patellofemoral joint mechanics can also be influenced by tight musculature.[22,23] Musculature that is identified to have an influence includes the quadriceps, hamstrings, iliopsoas, iliotibial band, gastrocnemius, and soleus. Stretches targeting the particular musculature, if tight, may be beneficial (Figs. 80.3, 80.4).

Lastly, for almost all knee disorders, the role of cryotherapy cannot be overemphasized. Cryotherapy appears to be effective in the treatment of acute and chronic joint swelling, tendon and ligament inflammation, and muscle injury.[24] A cold pack can be applied for 15 to 20 minutes three to four times daily as a palliative modality. However, care should be taken with patients who have cold sensitivities, neuropathies, or fragile skin, as a cold reaction may occur.

References

1. Manal TJ, Snyder-Mackler L. Failure of voluntary activation of the quadriceps femoris muscle after patellar contusion. *J Orthop Sports Phys Ther* 2000;30(11):655–660; discussion 661–653.
2. O'Reilly SC, Jones A, Muir KR, et al. Quadriceps weakness in knee osteoarthritis: the effect on pain and disability. *Ann Rheum Dis* 1998;57(10):588–594.
3. Palmieri RM, Tom JA, Edwards JE, et al. Arthrogenic muscle response induced by an experimental knee joint effusion is mediated by pre- and post-synaptic spinal mechanisms. *J Electromyogr Kinesiol* 2004; 14(6):631–640.
4. Spencer JD, Hayes KC, Alexander IJ. Knee joint effusion and quadriceps reflex inhibition in man. *Arch Phys Med Rehabil* 1984;65(4):171–177.
5. Noyes FR, Dunworth LA, Andriacchi TP, et al. Knee hyperextension gait abnormalities in unstable knees. Recognition and preoperative gait retraining. *Am J Sports Med* 1996;24(1):35–45.
6. Geffen SJ. Rehabilitation principles for treating chronic musculoskeletal injuries. *Med J Aust* 2003; 178(5):238–242.
7. Murphy DF, Connolly DA, Beynnon BD. Risk factors for lower extremity injury: a review of the literature. *Br J Sports Med* 2003;37(1):13–29.
8. Felson DT, Lawrence RC, Hochberg MC, et al. Osteoarthritis: new insights. Part 2: treatment approaches. *Ann Intern Med* 2000;133(9):726–737.
9. Soderberg GL, Cook TM. An electromyographic analysis of quadriceps femoris muscle setting and straight leg raising. *Phys Ther* 1983;63(9):1434–1438.
10. Borsa PA, Lephart SM, Irrgang JJ, et al. The effects of joint position and direction of joint motion on proprioceptive sensibility in anterior cruciate ligament-deficient athletes. *Am J Sports Med* 1997;25(3): 336–340.
11. Palmitier RA, An KN, Scott SG, et al. Kinetic chain exercise in knee rehabilitation. *Sports Med* 1991; 11(6):402–413.
12. Wilk KE, Escamilla RF, Fleisig GS, et al. A comparison of tibiofemoral joint forces and electromyographic activity during open and closed kinetic chain exercises. *Am J Sports Med* 1996;24(4):518–527.
13. Fulkerson JP. Diagnosis and treatment of patients with patellofemoral pain. *Am J Sports Med* 2002; 30(3):447–456.
14. Kannus P, Natri A, Paakkala T, et al. An outcome study of chronic patellofemoral pain syndrome. Seven-year follow-up of patients in a randomized, controlled trial. *J Bone Joint Surg Am* 1999;81(3):355–363.
15. Natri A, Kannus P, Jarvinen M. Which factors predict the long-term outcome in chronic patellofemoral pain syndrome? A 7-year prospective follow-up study. *Med Sci Sports Exerc* 1998;30(11):1572–1577.
16. Powers CM. Rehabilitation of patellofemoral joint disorders: a critical review. *J Orthop Sports Phys Ther* 1998;28(5):345–354.
17. Witvrouw E, Danneels L, Van Tiggelen D, et al. Open versus closed kinetic chain exercises in patellofemoral pain: a 5-year prospective randomized study. *Am J Sports Med* 2004;32(5):1122–1130.
18. Powers CM. The influence of altered lower-extremity kinematics on patellofemoral joint dysfunction: a theoretical perspective. *J Orthop Sports Phys Ther* 2003;33(11):639–646.
19. Messier SP, Davis SE, Curl WW, et al. Etiologic factors associated with patellofemoral pain in runners. *Med Sci Sports Exerc* 1991;23(9):1008–1015.
20. Powers CM, Chen PY, Reischl SF, et al. Comparison of foot pronation and lower extremity rotation in persons with and without patellofemoral pain. *Foot Ankle Int* 2002;23(7):634–640.
21. Sutlive TG, Mitchell SD, Maxfield SN, et al. Identification of individuals with patellofemoral pain whose symptoms improved after a combined program of foot orthosis use and modified activity: a preliminary investigation. *Phys Ther* 2004;84(1):49–61.
22. Fredericson M, Yoon K. Physical examination and patellofemoral pain syndrome. *Am J Phys Med Rehabil* 2006;85(3):234–243.
23. Tyler TF, Nicholas SJ, Mullaney MJ, et al. The role of hip muscle function in the treatment of patellofemoral pain syndrome. *Am J Sports Med* 2006;34(4):630–636.
24. Bleakley C, McDonough S, MacAuley D. The use of ice in the treatment of acute soft-tissue injury: a systematic review of randomized controlled trials. *Am J Sports Med* 2004;32(1):251–261.

SECTION 15 Rehabilitation

CHAPTER 81 Foot and Ankle Rehabilitation

Heather L. Smith

Rehabilitation of musculoskeletal injuries of the foot and ankle require multiple intervention techniques to address impairments that may include strength deficits, decreased balance, and gait abnormalities. Foot and ankle injuries often present with multiple impairments that need to be addressed in order to ensure full recovery from injury and prevent recurrence. Basic rehabilitation techniques can be employed by the patient, as instructed per the physician, to provide improved function following injury.

One of the most common injuries of the foot and ankle is the ankle sprain. According to the National Institute of Arthritis and Musculoskeletal and Skin Diseases, approximately 850,000 Americans sprain their ankles on an annual basis. The severity of ankle sprain is variable, with the more severe ankle sprains requiring longer periods of rest and immobilization.[1] Compression and elevation can be applied in the acute phase to decrease edema and ecchymosis. Gentle strengthening exercises such as ankle range of motion (ROM) in four directions (Figs. 81.1–81.4), and seated heel raises (Fig. 81.5) can be initiated in the first 1 to 2 weeks. Early movement has been advocated in the research to improve and restore motion and decrease joint edema.[2,3] Progressive weight-bearing exercises can be added beginning in weeks 2 to 4, depending on the severity of the sprain. As the patient's ROM improve and pain decreases, single-limb balance, and bilateral, progressing to unilateral, heel raises and lunges can be added (Fig. 81.6–81.9). In the case of severe sprains, which may present with residual strength and balance deficits and gait abnormalities, further assessment by a physical therapist may be required.[4]

The importance of rehabilitation and exercise to the ankle sprain patient has been well documented.[2] Ankle sprains can lead to persistent conditions such as chronic ankle instability if the joint is not returned to its premorbid status. Research demonstrates that decreased strength, not only at the ankle but at the hip as well, can occur after a sprain, directly impacting the patient's ability to balance.[5,6]

Another common foot and ankle issue is Achilles tendinopathy. Acute tendinitis of the Achilles can occur, but the chronic nature of tendinosis makes the condition more likely to be seen and require rehabilitation. Achilles tendinosis is not an inflammatory condition but

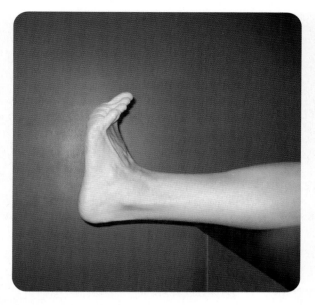

Figure 81.1 Active dorsiflexion.

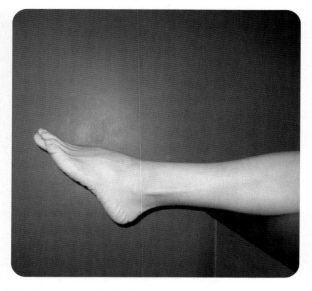

Figure 81.2 Active plantar flexion.

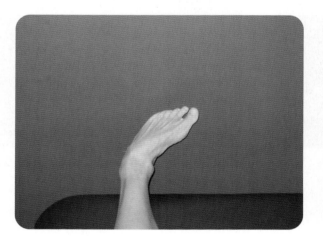

Figure 81.3 Active inversion.

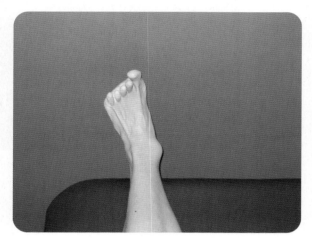

Figure 81.4 Active eversion.

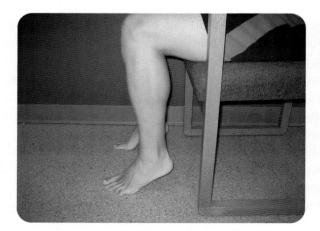

Figure 81.5 Seated heel raise.

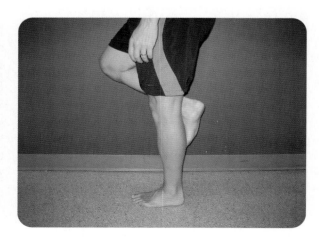

Figure 81.6 Single-limb stance for balance.

SECTION 15 Rehabilitation

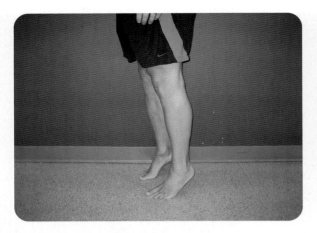

Figure 81.7 Standing bilateral heel raise.

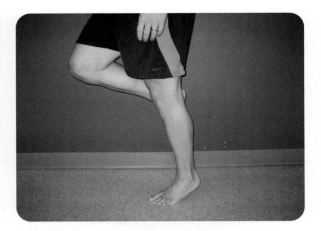

Figure 81.8 Standing single-limb heel raise.

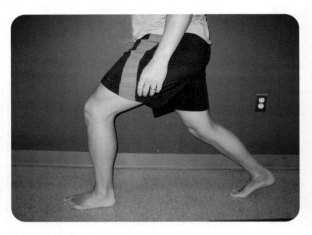

Figure 81.9 Standing lunge.

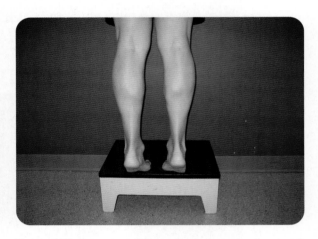

Figure 81.10 Eccentric Achilles strengthening exercise part 1: standing bilateral plantar flexion.

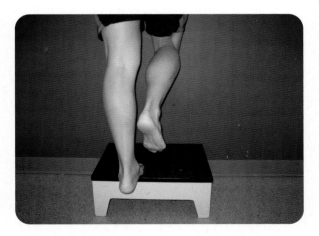

Figure 81.11 Eccentric Achilles strengthening exercise part 2: standing unilateral controlled lowering.

rather a degenerative condition of the tendon. Research in this area has been abundant in the last several years and demonstrates the efficacy of the use of eccentric strengthening with these patients.[7,8] Evidence of restoration of the tendon to more normal presentation on MRI has been demonstrated following a strict eccentric training program.[9,10] The program is performed as a modified version of the heel raise. The patient is instructed to perform this exercise on the edge of the stair, rising up on both feet (Fig. 81.10), holding at the top, and slowly lowering to the bottom by using only the involved leg (Fig. 81.11). The exercise should be performed daily and should be done for ten repetitions (starting with one set working up to three sets), with both a straight-leg and a bent-knee position. These exercises should be performed for no less than 8 to 12 weeks. In addition, stretching of the calf musculature can be employed as needed (Figs. 81.12, 81.13).

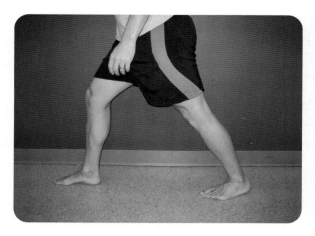

Figure 81.12 Standing gastrocnemius stretch.

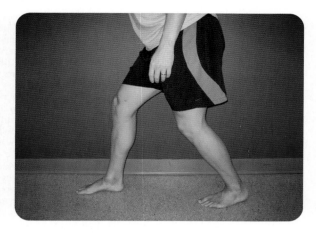

Figure 81.13 Standing soleus stretch.

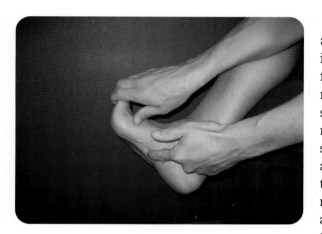

Figure 81.14 Seated dorsiflexion stretch of the great toe.

Lastly, overuse injuries of the foot and ankle, such as plantar fasciitis should be reviewed. Plantar fasciitis is fairly common and typically occurs more in the flat-footed individual. The treatment for plantar fasciitis is multifaceted and should include patient education for shoe-wear modification, stretching, and the use of a night splint.[11] Patients should wear shoes with a slightly elevated heel to place the fascia in a shortened and less stressed position with weight-bearing activities. As well, the use of a heel cup to add heel height may be useful. Stretching of the fascia is also important and should be performed consistently. In addition to the calf stretches discussed previously, stretching the great toe into dorsiflexion (Fig. 81.14) will provide a more specific stretch to the plantar fascia.[12] Use of a night splint provides a low-load, prolonged stretch that is often effective in relieving the "start-up" or morning pain often associated with this diagnosis.[13] Patients can obtain such a splint from a variety of online and durable medical equipment vendors.

Other foot and ankle injuries that have not been covered in this chapter may benefit from strengthening, ROM, and balance exercises. Foot and ankle injury patients should be instructed in edema and pain control techniques in the acute phase, followed by appropriate exercises to address their ROM, strength, and balance deficits. The exercises provided offer the primary care physician a range of useful tools in addressing some of the more common musculoskeletal injuries associated with this body region. Physical therapy intervention should be considered for those patients with significant functional deficits.

References

1. Beynnon BD, Renstrom PA, Haugh L, et al. A prospective, randomized clinical investigation of the treatment of first-time ankle sprains. *Am J Sports Med* 2006;34(9):1401–1412.
2. Mattacola CG, Dwyer MK. Rehabilitation of the ankle after acute sprain or chronic instability. *J Athl Train* 2002;37(4):413–429.

3. Zoch C, Fialka-Moser V, Quittan M. Rehabilitation of ligamentous ankle injuries: a review of recent studies. *Br J Sports Med* 2003;37(4):291–295.
4. Delahunt E, Monaghan K, Caulfield B. Altered neuromuscular control and ankle joint kinematics during walking in subjects with functional instability of the ankle joint. *Am J Sports Med* 2006;34:1970–1976.
5. Bernier JN, Perrin DH. Effect of coordination training on proprioception of the functionally unstable ankle. *J Orthop Sports Phys Ther* 1998;27(4):264–275.
6. Konradsen L, Olesen S, Hansen HM. Ankle sensorimotor control and eversion strength after acute ankle inversion injuries. *Am J Sports Med* 1998;26(1):72–77.
7. Alfredson H, Pietila T, Jonsson P, et al. Heavy-load eccentric calf muscle training for the treatment of chronic Achilles tendinosis. *Am J Sports Med* 1998;26(3):360–366.
8. Ohberg L, Lorentzon R, Alfredson H. Eccentric training in patients with chronic Achilles tendinosis: normalised tendon structure and decreased thickness at follow-up. *Br J Sports Med* 2004;38(1):8–11; discussion 11.
9. Shalabi A, Kristoffersen-Wiberg M, Aspelin P, et al. Immediate Achilles tendon response after strength training evaluated by MRI. *Med Sci Sports Exerc* 2004;36(11):1841–1846.
10. Shalabi A, Kristoffersen-Wilberg M, Svensson L, et al. Eccentric training of the gastrocnemius-soleus complex in chronic Achilles tendinopathy results in decreased tendon volume and intratendinous signal as evaluated by MRI. *Am J Sports Med* 2004;32(5):1286–1296.
11. Cole C, Seto C, Gazewood J. Plantar fasciitis: evidence-based review of diagnosis and therapy. *Am Fam Physician* 2005;72(11):2237–2242.
12. Digiovanni BF, Nawoczenski DA, Malay DP, et al. Plantar fascia-specific stretching exercise improves outcomes in patients with chronic plantar fasciitis. A prospective clinical trial with two-year follow-up. *J Bone Joint Surg Am* 2006;88(8):1775–1781.
13. Probe RA, Baca M, Adams R, et al. Night splint treatment for plantar fasciitis. A prospective randomized study. *Clin Orthop Relat Res* 1999;(368):190–195.

Patient Information Sheets

Monica Ferguson

Lumbar Disc Herniation

What is lumbar disc herniation?

The spine is made up of bones, called *vertebrae*, with a disc in between each vertebra that provides cushioning. The lumbar spine is the name for the group of five vertebrae that make up your lower back. In a disc herniation, the disc slips out of place and can push on a nerve in the spine. This is usually caused by a wearing down of the disc, or degeneration, as we age.

What are the symptoms?

- Pain in the lower back
- Pain may travel down the buttocks and into one or both legs
- Numbness or tingling going down the leg
- Leg weakness

How is it treated?

- A couple of days of rest may be helpful for severe pain, but prolonged rest is not recommended.
- Anti-inflammatory medication, like ibuprofen or naproxen. Talk to your doctor before using this type of medication.
- Pain medication such as acetaminophen (Tylenol)
- Stronger pain medications, such as narcotics, are sometimes used for a short period of time.
- Steroid injection. This is done under x-ray guidance to direct the medication to the right place.
- Physical therapy
- Surgery to remove the disc

When can I expect to feel better?

- You should start feeling better after a few weeks of treatment.

Warning signs to contact your doctor immediately:

- Loss of bowel or bladder control
- Numbness in the groin or genital area

Cervical Degenerative Joint Disease

What is cervical degenerative joint disease?

Cervical degenerative joint disease is another name for osteoarthritis affecting the neck. Osteoarthritis is a "wear and tear" form of arthritis that results from our bones deteriorating, or wearing down, as we age.

What are the symptoms?

- Neck pain
- Neck stiffness
- Headache, especially in the back of the head
- Numbness or weakness in the arms, hands, and even the legs
- Symptoms may be worse when upright from supporting the head

How is it treated?

- Rest. Wearing a soft cervical collar may help, but it should not be worn all the time.
- Pain medication such as acetaminophen (Tylenol).
- Anti-inflammatory medication, like ibuprofen or naproxen. Talk to your doctor before using this type of medication.
- Physical therapy, which may include hot or cold treatments, massage, and exercises

When can I expect to feel better?

- Symptoms should improve after a few weeks of treatment but may flare again without warning.

Cervical Muscle Strain

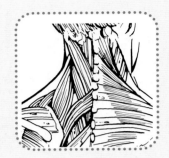

What is cervical muscle strain?

Cervical muscle strain is a sprain in the muscles of the neck. It is usually caused by a sudden, unexpected movement that causes the neck to extend and flex, often to an extreme position. It may also be caused by holding the neck in the same position for a long time. It may be accompanied by a sprain of the ligaments in the neck. Ligaments are slightly elastic bands of tissue that connect bones to other bones, holding them in place.

What are the symptoms?

- Pain in the back of the neck
- Pain is often worse a day or two after the injury
- Neck stiffness
- Headache, especially in the back of the head
- Numbness in the arm or hand

How is it treated?

- Ice may help for the first few days. Apply for 20 minutes three or four times a day.
- Anti-inflammatory medication, like ibuprofen or naproxen. Talk to your doctor before using this type of medication.
- Muscle relaxants
- A soft cervical collar can be used initially to support the head, allowing the neck muscles to rest. However, prolonged use should be avoided, as it can lead to neck stiffness.
- Stretching exercises
- Physical therapy

When can I expect to feel better?

- You should improve after 4 to 6 weeks of treatment.
- It may take months to recover following a more severe injury.

Warning signs to contact your doctor:

- Persistent numbness or weakness in the arm or hand
- Worsening symptoms after the first few days
- Lack of improvement

Hip Degenerative Joint Disease

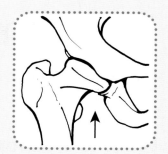

What is hip degenerative joint disease?

Hip degenerative joint disease is another name for osteoarthritis affecting the hip. Osteoarthritis is a "wear and tear" form of arthritis that results from our bones deteriorating, or wearing down, as we age.

What are the symptoms?

- Pain in the buttock, groin, or thigh
- Pain is usually worse with activities and improves with rest
- Stiffness of the hip
- Walking with a limp

How is it treated?

- Weight loss
- Changing your activities. You may need to avoid certain activities that make your pain worse.
- Physical therapy. Aquatic exercises can be particularly helpful.
- Pain medication such as acetaminophen (Tylenol)
- Anti-inflammatory medication, like ibuprofen or naproxen. Talk to your doctor before using this type of medication.
- Surgery to replace the hip

When can I expect to feel better?

- Symptoms should improve after a few weeks of treatment but may flare again without warning.

Trochanteric Bursitis

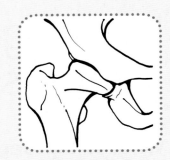

What is trochanteric bursitis?

Trochanteric bursitis is an inflammation of the bursa in the hip. A bursa is a fluid-filled sac that cushions a joint.

What are the symptoms?

- Pain affecting the side of the hip
- The pain is often worse with lying on the hip or with prolonged activities such as walking or running.

How is it treated?

- Rest. Avoid activities that make the pain worse.
- Anti-inflammatory medications, like ibuprofen or naproxen. Talk to your doctor before using this type of medication.
- Icing the area, if the bursitis was caused by an injury
- A steroid injection into the bursa
- Some patients find physical therapy to be helpful.
- Surgery is very rarely necessary.

When can I expect to feel better?

- You should start feeling better with treatment after a few days, but it can take up to 6 weeks to fully recover.
- Following an injection, the pain may be immediately relieved and then return after several hours, once the local anesthetic wears off. The steroid should start relieving the pain after a couple of days.

Low Back Pain

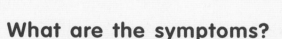

What is low back pain?

Low back pain refers to pain affecting the lumbar spine, which is a group of five bones in the lower back. It is usually caused by a strain of the muscles or a sprain of the ligaments and tendons that surround the lumbar spine. It may also be related to the discs between the bones and the nerves that come out of the spine.

What are the symptoms?

- Sharp or dull pain in the lower back
- Pain may be worse with movement, especially bending or lifting.
- Stiffness is often present.
- Numbness going down one or both legs

How is it treated?

- A couple of days of rest may be helpful for severe pain, but prolonged rest is not recommended.
- Pain medication such as acetaminophen (Tylenol)
- Anti-inflammatory medication, like ibuprofen or naproxen. Talk to your doctor before using this type of medication.
- Stronger pain medications, such as narcotics, are sometimes used for the first few days.
- Heat or ice
- Muscle relaxants
- Stretching and strengthening exercises
- Physical therapy

When can I expect to feel better?

- An acute episode of back pain will usually improve significantly after a few days but will often take 4 to 6 weeks to improve completely.
- Low back pain may become chronic and last for years.

Warning signs to contact your doctor:

- Worsening pain despite treatment
- Leg weakness
- Loss of bowel or bladder control

Chondromalacia

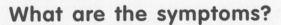

What is chondromalacia?

Chondromalacia is damage to the cartilage under the kneecap, which is called the *patella*. This condition is also called *chondromalacia patella*. It often affects young people, especially athletes, and is usually caused by overuse or an injury such as a fall. In older people, it may be caused by arthritis in the knee.

What are the symptoms?

- Pain under or around the kneecap
- The pain is often worse when walking up or down stairs, kneeling, squatting, or getting out of a chair.
- Grinding or grating when extending the knee

How is it treated?

- Rest. Avoid activities that aggravate the pain.
- Anti-inflammatory medication, like ibuprofen or naproxen. Talk to your doctor before using this type of medication.
- Physical therapy consisting of exercises that strengthen and stretch the muscles in the thigh.
- Rarely, surgery may be required.

When can I expect to feel better?

- Most people will feel better after a few weeks of some combination of rest, medications, or physical therapy and can safety start to resume their prior activities.

Prepatellar Bursitis

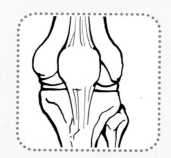

What is prepatellar bursitis?

Prepatellar bursitis is inflammation of a bursa in the knee. A bursa is a fluid-filled sac that cushions a joint. The patella is another name for the kneecap. Prepatellar bursitis is often caused by kneeling for long periods of time.

What are the symptoms?

- Pain with activity but not usually at rest
- Swelling over the kneecap
- Stiffness in the knee

How is it treated?

- Rest. Avoid activities that aggravate the pain.
- Icing the knee. Apply for 20 minutes, three or four times a day.
- Anti-inflammatory medication, like ibuprofen or naproxen. Talk to your doctor before using this type of medication.
- Drainage of the bursa
- Surgical removal of the bursa

When can I expect to feel better?

- You should start to feel better after a few days and should be able to resume your usual activities after a few weeks.

Knee Degenerative Joint Disease

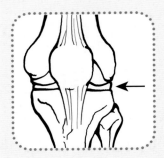

What is knee degenerative joint disease?

Knee degenerative joint disease is another name for osteoarthritis affecting the knee. Osteoarthritis is a "wear and tear" form of arthritis that results from our bones deteriorating, or wearing down, as we age.

What are the symptoms?

- Pain in the knee
- Swelling
- Stiffness, especially first thing in the morning, that improves with use
- Pain may become worse with activities such as walking and climbing stairs.

How is it treated?

- Weight loss
- Pain medication such as acetaminophen (Tylenol)
- Anti-inflammatory medication, like ibuprofen or naproxen. Talk to your doctor before using this type of medication.
- Knee exercises
- Physical therapy
- Supportive treatments such as using a cane or knee brace
- Injections into the joint (steroids to reduce inflammation and pain or a special fluid to help lubricate the joint)
  1. Steroids to reduce inflammation and pain
  2. A special fluid to help lubricate the joint
- Surgery to replace the knee

When can I expect to feel better?

- Symptoms should improve after a few weeks of treatment but may flare again without warning.

Ankle Sprain

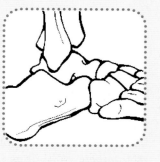

What is an ankle sprain?

An ankle sprain occurs when the ligaments of the ankle are stretched beyond their normal limits. Ligaments are slightly elastic bands of tissue that connect bones to other bones. In the ankle, they help to keep the ankle bones in place. In a severe sprain, some of these ligaments can actually tear. Most sprains are caused by the ankle twisting suddenly or unnaturally.

What are the symptoms?

- Pain in the ankle
- Tenderness to touch
- Swelling
- Inability to walk or stand on the ankle

How is it treated?

- RICE (Rest, Ice, Compression, Elevation)
  1. Rest the ankle by not walking or standing on it.
  2. Apply ice for 20 minutes, three or four times a day.
  3. Use an Ace wrap or compression bandage to help support the ankle and decrease swelling.
  4. Elevate your ankle ideally above the level of your heart.
- Anti-inflammatory medication, like ibuprofen or naproxen. Talk to your doctor before using this type of medication.
- More severe sprains may require a brace or soft cast to prevent the ankle from moving.
- Rarely, surgery may be necessary.
- Physical therapy will help to improve strength and movement in the ankle and help prevent future sprains.

When can I expect to feel better?

- Most sprains improve after 2 to 4 weeks of treatment, but more severe sprains can take up to 6 months to heal.

Metatarsalgia

What is metatarsalgia?

Metatarsalgia is the medical term for pain under the ball of the foot. The long bones of the foot are called *metatarsals*. Activities that put a lot of pressure on the front of the foot, such as running or jumping, can result in pain and inflammation in this part of the foot. Wearing high heels or shoes that are too tight can also cause this condition.

What are the symptoms?

- Pain in the ball of your foot
- Sharp or shooting pain in your toes
- Feeling like you are walking on pebbles

How is it treated?

- Rest. Avoid activities that aggravate the pain.
- Ice. Apply for 20 minutes, three or four times a day.
- Anti-inflammatory medication, like ibuprofen or naproxen. Talk to your doctor before using this type of medication.
- Wearing appropriate footwear. Avoid high heels, and look for shoes that have adequate space for your toes.
- Metatarsal pads
- Arch supports or orthotics

When can I expect to feel better?

- Symptoms should start to improve within a few days of treatment.

Plantar Fasciitis

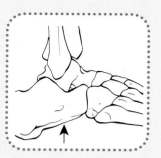

What is plantar fasciitis?

Plantar fasciitis is inflammation of the fibrous band of tissue connecting your heel to your toes, which is known as the *plantar fascia*. The term *plantar* refers to the sole of your foot.

What are the symptoms?

- Sharp pain in the bottom of the heel of your foot
- Pain is usually most severe on arising from prolonged rest, such as after getting up in the morning after sleeping or after sitting for a long time.
- Pain may occur after but not during exercise.

How is it treated?

- Rest. Avoid activities that provoke the pain such as prolonged standing, walking, or jogging.
- Icing, particularly after a flare-up of the pain. Apply for 20 minutes, three or four times a day.
- A splint worn at night
- Orthotics, or inserts, that fit into your shoe
- Physical therapy
- Anti-inflammatory medication, like ibuprofen or naproxen. Talk to your doctor before using this type of medication.
- Steroid injection
- Rarely, surgery

When can I expect to feel better?

- Most people feel better after a couple of months of treatment, and almost all feel better within a year.

Shoulder Tendinitis

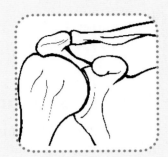

What is shoulder tendinitis?

Tendinitis is inflammation of a tendon, which is a band of tissue that connects a muscle to a bone. In shoulder tendinitis, the tendons of the shoulder muscles, known as the *rotator cuff*, become inflamed. This typically occurs because the tendons get pinched by surrounding structures in the shoulder joint, thus it is often referred to as an *impingement*. Finally, the bursa (a fluid-filled sac that cushions a joint) in the shoulder can also be affected, resulting in bursitis, or inflammation of the bursa.

What are the symptoms?

- Pain in the shoulder or upper arm, especially with reaching overhead
- Pain is often worse when sleeping on the affected shoulder at night.
- Stiffness in the shoulder

How is it treated?

- Rest. Avoid activities that aggravate the pain, such as throwing or overhead lifting.
- Ice. Use for 20 minutes at a time, three or four times a day.
- Anti-inflammatory medication, like ibuprofen or naproxen. Talk to your doctor before using this type of medication.
- Steroid injection
- Physical therapy
- Surgery

When can I expect to feel better?

- Pain may subside within a few days of treatment, but it usually takes several weeks to months for the symptoms to go away completely.

Frozen Shoulder

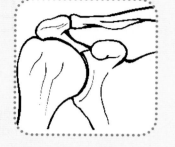

What is frozen shoulder?

Frozen shoulder is a condition in which the shoulder becomes painful and difficult to move. The tissue that envelops the shoulder joint is called a *capsule*. This capsule becomes inflamed and then scarred in frozen shoulder. For this reason, another name for this condition is *adhesive capsulitis*. The causes of frozen shoulder are not well understood.

What are the symptoms?

- Pain in the shoulder, which may be worse when sleeping on the affected shoulder
- Limited movement in the shoulder
- The symptoms of frozen shoulder can be divided into three stages:
  1. *Freezing stage*—the most painful stage
  2. *Frozen stage*—pain may subside but stiffness worsens
  3. *Thawing stage*—shoulder motion slowly returns to normal

How is it treated?

- Anti-inflammatory medication, like ibuprofen or naproxen. Talk to your doctor before using this type of medication
- Pain medication such as acetaminophen (Tylenol)
- Heat
- Physical therapy
- Steroid injection
- Manipulation of the shoulder under anesthesia
- Surgery, if there is no improvement with medication and physical therapy

When can I expect to feel better?

- Pain will usually subside within a few months, but it sometimes can take 2 years or more to recover from this condition. Many patients will have a slight limitation in movement in their shoulder for several years.

Tennis Elbow

What is tennis elbow?

Tennis elbow is an "overuse" injury affecting the elbow. Tendons are bands of tissue that connect muscles to bones. Tennis elbow occurs where the tendons of the muscles in your lower arm attach to the bony prominence on the outside of your elbow, called the *lateral epicondyle*. For this reason, tennis elbow is also known as *lateral epicondylitis*. The cause is thought to be inflammation in these tendons or tiny tears in them from a repetitive activity.

What are the symptoms?

- Pain on the outside of the elbow and tenderness to touch in that area
- Pain may go down your arm.
- Pain is often worse with grasping or lifting objects.

How is it treated?

- Rest. Avoid activities that make the pain worse.
- Icing the area. Use ice for 20 minutes at a time, three or four times a day.
- Pain medication such as acetaminophen (Tylenol)
- Anti-inflammatory medication, like ibuprofen or naproxen. Talk to your doctor before using this type of medication.
- Elbow and wrist braces
- Exercises or physical therapy
- Steroid injection
- Surgery to release the affected tendon. Surgery is only considered if the pain is still severe after at least 6 months of trying other treatments.

When can I expect to feel better?

- You should feel significantly better after 4 to 6 weeks of using medications and resting the elbow.

Carpal Tunnel Syndrome

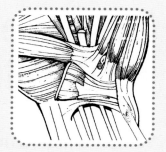

What is carpal tunnel syndrome?

In carpal tunnel syndrome, the main nerve that goes to the hand becomes pinched as it passes through a narrow area in the wrist known as the *carpal tunnel*. The symptoms are caused by pressure on this nerve, which is called the *median nerve*.

What are the symptoms?

- Numbness or tingling in the hand and fingers
- Pain in the hand and fingers
- Weakness in the hand and a tendency to drop objects
- Pain may extend up the arm to the shoulder.
- Pain may awaken you from sleep.
- You may find that shaking the hand relieves the symptoms.

How is it treated?

- Anti-inflammatory medication, like ibuprofen or naproxen. Talk to your doctor before using this type of medication.
- Wrist splint. This is worn at night and during activities that cause symptoms.
- Steroid injection into the carpal tunnel
- Surgery should be considered if your symptoms are severe or persistent despite the mentioned treatments.

When can I expect to feel better?

- You should start feeling better after a few weeks of treatment.

De Quervain Tendinitis

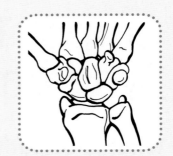

What is de Quervain tendinitis?

Tendinitis is inflammation of a tendon. A tendon is a band of tissue that connects a muscle to a bone. In de Quervain tendinitis, the tendons that go across the wrist to the thumb become inflamed. It is often caused by repetitive activities involving the wrist.

What are the symptoms?

- Wrist pain on the side of the thumb
- Pain may be worse with using the hand and thumb or with certain movements of the wrist.

How is it treated?

- Rest. Avoid activities that make the pain worse. Using a splint may help.
- Anti-inflammatory medication, like ibuprofen or naproxen. Talk to your doctor before using this type of medication.
- Steroid injection
- Surgery should be considered if symptoms are severe or do not improve.

When can I expect to feel better?

- You should feel better after 2 to 3 weeks of using medication and wearing a splint.
- A steroid injection should provide almost immediate relief that will last for months. In some cases, the relief may be permanent.

Trigger Finger

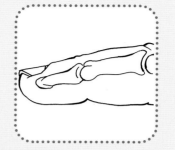

What is trigger finger?

Trigger finger is a condition in which one of your fingers gets caught in a bent position. With a trigger finger, as you try to straighten your finger, your muscle contracts but the tendon gets stuck in the narrow tunnel, called a *sheath*, that it must pass through in each finger. Tendons are bands of tissue that connect muscles to bone, causing movement when the muscles contract. The tendon may then snap or pop, like a trigger being released, as it is forced through this narrow tunnel.

What are the symptoms?

- Stiffness and catching in your fingers or thumb
- Symptoms are usually worse in the morning or after a period of inactivity.
- Pain in the palm of your hand at the base of the affected finger
- You may feel a lump at the base of the affected finger.
- In severe cases, the finger may become stuck in a bent position.

How is it treated?

- Rest. Wearing a splint may help.
- Pain medication such as acetaminophen (Tylenol)
- Anti-inflammatory medication, like ibuprofen or naproxen. Talk to your doctor before using this type of medication.
- Steroid injection into the sheath
- Trigger finger release to widen the sheath. This can be done with a needle in the doctor's office or surgically.

When can I expect to feel better?

- Symptoms should improve after resting and using medications for a couple of weeks.
- If you receive a steroid injection, you can expect to improve after a couple of days.

Index

Page numbers in *italics* indicate figure; those followed by t indicate table.